MATERIA MEDICA

Henderson's

MATERIA MEDICA

J. K. W. FERGUSON, M.B.E., M.A., M.D., F.R.S.C.
G. H. W. LUCAS, M.A., Ph.D., F.C.I.C.
Department of Pharmacology
University of Toronto

UNIVERSITY OF TORONTO PRESS
Toronto   1951

Preface

NO BOOK HAS YET BEEN PUBLISHED which describes all the drugs and medicinal preparations in use in the English speaking countries. To find details about even important ones, it may be necessary to consult the British Pharmacopoeia, the United States Pharmacopoeia, the British Pharmaceutical Codex, New and Non-Official Remedies, and possibly other compilations. It is hardly reasonable to expect a student or a practitioner to keep at hand all these volumes in addition to a text-book of pharmacology. Yet some source of detailed information is necessary if the prescribing of drugs is to be done accurately. It was this thought that prompted the late Professor V. E. Henderson to write his Materia Medica. The early editions of Professor Henderson's book were based entirely on the British Pharmacopoeia. In later editions he added new drugs which had not yet gained pharmacopoeial recognition. In planning the present volume the authors felt that to achieve, at this time, the original purpose of the book it was essential to include the preparations of the United States Pharmacopoeia.

The many differences in content, terminology and standards between the United States Pharmacopoeia and the British Pharmacopoeia made it necessary to evolve a method of presentation which we believe to be unusual. It was designed to facilitate rapid comparisons between British and American terminology and standards, and to do so in a concise manner. Another circumstance which made it necessary to rewrite the book almost entirely was a decision by the Faculty of Medicine of the University of Toronto in 1947 that henceforward medical students should be taught to write prescriptions in English instead of in Latin.

The appearance of the U.S.P. XIII in 1947 and the British Pharmacopoeia 1948 in September of this year, has introduced a large number of new names, standards, doses and procedures. Both of these volumes are of great importance in Canada. It is hoped that our Materia Medica will help students to grasp the scope and importance of these indispensable books, and help practitioners to learn more quickly of the changes which have received official approval.

We wish to express our thanks to the various members of the Department of Pharmacology who have critically examined the text in various stages of its preparation, particularly Miss D. Caldecott and Dr. H. W. Smith. We wish also gratefully to acknowledge many useful suggestions by Dean R. O. Hurst of the Ontario College of Pharmacy and to thank Mr. G. Bales, Phm.B., F.C.I.C., for his careful and helpful scrutiny of the typescript.

J.K.W.F.
G.H.W.L.

Toronto, 1948

Preface to the Second Edition

SINCE THE PUBLICATION of the previous edition of this book in 1948, the 14th revision of the United States Pharmacopoeia has become official on November 1, 1950, and the Addendum, 1951, to the British Pharmacopoeia on September 1, 1951. It has not been possible to include in this edition of *Materia Medica* any of the changes effected by the Addendum. However, most of the new drugs of the Addendum are described according to information from other sources.

It has been possible to add most of the 200 new items described in the U.S.P. XIV; however it has not been feasible (nor has it been considered necessary for the purposes of this book) to include many minor changes such as small alterations in molecular weights, melting points, solubilities, etc.

It should be noted that the Canadian Supplement to the British Pharmacopoeia, which was published during World War II, has been discontinued. Some 54 preparations are now specified in the Regulations under the Food and Drugs Act of Canada. These appear from time to time in the Canada Gazette. We have, therefore, introduced the abbreviation Can.Gaz. to indicate the source of certain information. The abbreviation Can.Supp. still appears where the information is really from the Canadian Supplement rather than the more recent Regulations.

The authors again wish to express their thanks to Mr. Gerald Bales, F.C.I.C., for his careful scrutiny of the typescript, and to Miss Dorothy Caldecott for her able assistance in the preparation of this edition.

J.K.W.F.
G.H.W.L.

Toronto, 1951

Acknowledgements

THE USE IN THIS VOLUME of certain portions of the text of the United States Pharmacopoeia, 14th revision, official Nov. 1, 1950, is by virtue of permission received from the Board of Trustees of the United States Pharmacopoeial Convention Inc. The said Board of Trustees is not responsiblr for any inaccuracy of quotations nor for any errors in the statements of quantities or percentage strengths.

The use of certain portions of the text of New and Non-Official Remedies in this volume is by virtue of permission received from the Council on Pharmacy and Chemistry of the American Medical Association. The Council on Pharmacy and Chemistry is not responsible for any inaccuracy of quotations nor for any errors in the statement of quantities or percentage of strengths.

"Permission to use for comment parts of the text of The National Formulary, Ninth Edition, in this volume has been granted by the Council of the American Pharmaceutical Association. The American Pharmaceutical Association is not responsible for any inaccuracy of quotation nor for any errors in the statement of quantities or percentage strengths."

Quotations from the British Pharmacopoeia are by the kind permission of the British Pharmacopoeia Commission.

Contents

One

Definitions, Weights & Measures

IN THE LEGAL SENSE a *drug* is any substance intended for administration to man or beast for the treatment, prevention or diagnosis of disease. Such substances are sometimes referred to collectively as the *Materia Medica*. Over a thousand, possibly two thousand, drugs are in more or less common use, and their various preparations, combinations and trade names number several thousand more. The possibilities for confusion and misunderstanding, not to mention misrepresentation and deceit, are very great. In the interests of honesty and to discourage unnecessary multiplication of drugs, representatives of the medical and pharmaceutical professions have combined to publish in their respective countries, books known as *pharmacopoeias*. In such books attempts are made to establish uniform nomenclature and to provide adequate descriptions and tests for drugs which are regarded as sufficiently important and useful to justify such attention. Many authorities, particularly in the U.S.A., feel that the name *pharmacopoeia* should be reserved for publications recognized by some national government as providing legal standards for drugs in that country. The British Pharmacopoeia (B.P.), a publication of the General Medical Council, is accorded such recognition in the United Kingdom and in most other parts of the British Commonwealth. The United States Pharmacopoeia (U.S.P.) and the Codex Medicamentarius occupy similar positions in the U.S.A. and in France respectively. It should be noted, however, that there is in preparation, under the auspices of the U.N.O., an International Pharmacopoeia, the legal status of which may be hard to define.

A drug may be described as *official* in any country if it appears in the national Pharmacopoeia or its Supplements. In the United States a drug is sometimes said to be "official in the National Formulary." The National Formulary (N.F.) is thus regarded as a subsidiary official publication. The term *officinal* is more inclusive and may be applied to any drug in common use.

In Canada the B.P. enjoys a senior but not exclusive legal status. Under the Food and Drugs Act of Canada, any drug offered for sale under a name recognized in the B.P. must conform to B.P. standards unless the label specifically states that it conforms to another acceptable standard, e.g. U.S.P.

From time to time it has been necessary for the Canadian Government to establish standards or names for drugs which differ from those in the B.P. These are published in the *Canada Gazette* and take precedence over the B.P. in Canada.

The preparation of a pharmacopoeial monograph consisting of description, tests and standards, often entails an enormous amount of work. For this reason and others, several years may elapse between the introduction of even an important drug and its publication in a Pharmacopoeia. A quicker means of providing authoritative guidance to the doctor and the pharmacist is supplied by an annual publication of the American Medical Association, called New and Non-Official Remedies (N.N.R.). Another book of great value to the doctor and the pharmacist is the British Pharmaceutical Codex (B.P.C.), a large volume published by the Pharmaceutical Society of Great Britain. It includes brief accounts of how drugs are used as well as formulae and lists of trade names.

Another reference book of great value is the United States Dispensatory (U.S.D.), which is even more voluminous and informative than the B.P.C. The Canadian Formulary (C.F.), a publication of the Canadian Pharmaceutical Association, provides formulae and specifications of interest in Canada and not readily available in other publications.

Pharmacology, in the narrow sense, is the science of the action of drugs on living organisms and thus used is synonymous with *Pharmacodynamics.* It is sometimes used in a broader sense to include pharmacy, pharmacognosy and posology as well as pharmacodynamics.

Pharmacy is the art and science of the preparation of substances for administration as medicines. This work has passed almost entirely out of the hands of the doctor, and to a large extent out of the hands of the retail pharmacist, into those of the pharmaceutical manufacturer.

Pharmacognosy is the science of the recognition and identification of drugs and their sources; it often includes a knowledge of the crude plant or animal material from which the drugs originate.

The doctor and the retail pharmacist nowadays rely on the integrity of manufacturers and the vigilance of government inspectors to guard the quality of the drugs they buy.

Posology is the science of dosage of drugs. The word is seldom used now but the subject it represents is constantly being enlarged and modified in current medical literature. Certain principles of the subject are discussed in Chapter v.

Therapeutics includes the art and science of applying all available knowledge and skill to the treatment of disease.

METROLOGY

Pharmacopoeias specify for their particular zones of influence the systems of weights and measures to be used in the prescribing and dispensing of medicines. The Metric System is given preference by both the B.P. and the U.S.P. and is steadily gaining general acceptance. New drugs are now issued by manufacturers in metric dosage units and current medical literature makes more use of metric terminology than of the older systems. To avoid confusion between grammes and grains, the B.P. has adopted the spelling of gramme rather than gram, which is accepted in chemistry and physics. For the same reason the abbreviation G. instead of g. is advised. The U.S.P. advises the use of Gm. as an abbreviation in prescribing.

Metric Weights   *Imperial Equivalent*

1 milligram (mg.) equals 0.001 gramme	0.015 gr.
1 gramme (Gm.) equals 0.001 kilogram (kg.)	15.432 gr.
1 kilogram (kg. or kilo.), equals 1,000 grammes	2.2046 lb.

Metric Volumes

1 millilitre (ml.) equals 0.001 litre	16.9 min.
1 litre (1.) is the volume of 1 kilogram of water at 4°C. . .	35.196 fl. oz.
1 millilitre equals 1.000027 cc.	

The term mil is an accepted abbreviation for millilitre in prescription writing, but cc. is much more commonly used on this continent.

The older systems of weights and measures used in pharmacy are a mixture of the Imperial System and the older Apothecary System. An added source of confusion in Canada is the fact that the U.S. Apothecary measures of volume differ from the Imperial volumes, although the units bear the same names. The U.S. Avoirdupois weights are, however, the same as the Imperial Avoirdupois weights.

Avoirdupois Weights   *Metric Equivalent*

1 grain (gr.)	64.7987 mg.
437.5 gr. make 1 ounce (oz.) Avoir.	28.349 Gm.
480 gr. make 1 ounce (℥) Apoth.	31.1035 Gm.
60 gr. make 1 drachm (Ʒ) Apoth.	3.888 Gm.
7,000 gr. make 16 oz. or 1 lb. Avoir.	453.59 Gm.

Imperial System Volumes

1 minim (min. or M.) is the volume of 0.9114 gr. of water at 62°F.	0.0592 ml.
60 min. make 1 fluid drachm (fl. dr. or Ʒ)	3.5515 ml.
8 fl. dr. make 1 fluid ounce (fl. oz. or ℥)	28.4123 ml.
20 fl.oz. make 1 pint (pt. or O.)	568.2454 ml.
8 pints make 1 gallon (gal. or C.)	4.5459 l.

In dispensing, the pharmacist may use two more weights, the half drachm, Ʒ s̄s̄ (30 grains) and the scruple, Ͻ (20 grains). The scruple is never written in a prescription.

The fl. oz. (℥) is the volume of 437.5 gr. of water at 62°F. In prescriptions the sign ℥ is read as fluid ounce if the substance is a liquid but as the Apothecary ounce (480 gr.) if the substance is a solid. Similarly, in a prescription, Ʒ means fluid drachm (60 min.) if the substance is a liquid, or one drachm (60 gr.) if the substance is a solid.

The student should memorize the following approximate equivalents for rapid mental conversions.

$$1 \text{ gr.} = 60 \text{ or } 65 \text{ mg.}$$
$$1 \text{ Ʒ} = 4 \text{ Gm. or cc.}$$
$$1 \text{ ℥} = 30 \text{ Gm. or cc.}$$
$$1 \text{ Gm. or cc.} = 15 \text{ gr. or min.}$$

Domestic measures. A teaspoon is a convenient but variable measure. It has long been the practice to consider it equivalent to one fluid drachm (3.6 cc.). Consequently medicine glasses show 8 teaspoons to a fluid ounce. Domestic science, however, has standardized the kitchen teaspoon at 5 cc. and decreed that 3 teaspoons make 1 tablespoon or 15 cc., and 6 teaspoons make a fluid ounce. *For purposes of dosage the teaspoonful may be considered roughly equivalent to 4 cc.*

The kitchen measuring cup holds 8 fluid ounces or roughly 240 mils, as does an ordinary tumbler. The ordinary teacup contains about six fluid ounces (180 cc.).

A minim is often considered roughly equivalent to one drop, but the size of a drop varies with the viscosity of the liquid and its surface tension and also with the size of the orifice at which it is formed. A given dropper may yield 17 drops of water from one cc., or 14 drops of glycerin, or 47 drops of alcohol. If a physician orders 10 minims of a medicine to be taken at a dose, a good pharmacist will determine the number of drops from the dropper provided, which equals 10 minims, and write the dose on the label as that number of drops.

The B.P. specifies that liquids are to be measured by volume and solids by weight. Unless otherwise specified, a 10% solution of a solid in a liquid would be made up with 10 Gm. of solid in a final volume of 100 cc. of solution. To make one fluid ounce of the same strength of solution, a pharmacist would weigh out 10% of 437.5, grains or 44 grains and add liquid to a final volume of 480 minims, which is the volume of 437.5 grains of water.

Measures in the United States. The U.S. fluidounce is the volume of 454.6 gr. of water at 25°C., while the U.S. minim is the volume of 0.947 gr. of water at 25°C. For this reason the U.S. pint containing 16 fluidounces is not 4/5 but approximately 5/6 of the Imperial pint and the U.S. gallon 5/6 of the Imperial gallon. The abbreviations for the fluidrachm, and fluidounce in the U.S.A. are f℥, and f℥ respectively.

Two

Materials & Methods of Pharmacy

MANY SUBSTANCES USED IN PHARMACY ARE NOT PURE CHEMICALS, nor can their composition be defined in terms of pure chemicals. Such substances are often called *galenicals* in memory of the Greek physician Galen, who prepared many medicines by simple processes of extraction. This term is used rather loosely and may be extended to include any preparations of a type in use before the development of modern chemistry. It does not include modern preparations such as vaccines or antitoxins, which are sometimes called *biologicals*.

When substances cannot be defined by their composition, they may be defined by certain properties, or by their origin and mode of preparation. A number of classes of material used in pharmacy are defined below.

Volatile or Essential Oils (e.g. Oil of Anise, Oil of Peppermint). At one time all such oils were obtained by distillation of plants. Many are now manufactured synthetically. They are soluble in ether and chloroform, fairly soluble in alcohol, but only slightly soluble in water.

Fixed Oils (e.g. Castor Oil, Olive Oil). These oils cannot be distilled by heating without decomposition. They are for the most part fluid esters of fatty acids and glycerol and are often obtained by expression from fruits or seeds. They are freely soluble in ether and chloroform but insoluble in water.

Fats (e.g. Lard)—are soft, but not liquid, esters of higher fatty acids and glycerol and have the same solubility characteristics as the fixed oils.

Waxes (e.g. Beeswax)—are solid esters of fatty acids and higher alcohols. They are slightly soluble in alcohol but insoluble in water.

Mineral Oils (e.g. Liquid Paraffin)—are liquid mixtures of hydrocarbons obtained from petroleum. They are unsaponifiable and hence do not become rancid. No generic term seems to have evolved yet for the soft paraffins. They might well be called mineral greases. A series of paraffin waxes is also used in pharmacy.

Resins (e.g. Scammony Resin)—are solid materials obtained by oxidation of certain oils. Some contain weak acids. They are soluble in alcohol, ether, and alkaline solutions but are insoluble in pure water.

Oleoresins (e.g. Oleoresin of Male Fern)—are resins mixed with essential oils.

Balsams or Aromatic Resins (e.g. Benzoin, Balsam of Tolu)— are resins or oleoresins which contain benzoic or cinnamic acid or both.

Gums (e.g. Acacia and Tragacanth)—are solid or semi-solid exudates of plants and are complex carbohydrates. They dissolve partly or completely in water, forming mucilages or adhesive jellies. They are insoluble in alcohol.

Gum-resins (e.g. Myrrh)—are mixtures of gums and resins.

Glycosides (or glucosides) (e.g. Strophanthin, Digitoxin, Salicin, Santonin)—are substances which on hydrolysis by alkalis or acids liberate a reducing sugar, such as glucose. The residual part of the split molecule is known as a *genin*; e.g. on hydrolysis digitoxin yields digitoxigenin + digitoxose.

Alkaloids (e.g. Morphine and Strychnine)—are nitrogenous organic bases usually of cyclic structure. They are usually only slightly soluble in water but their salts, particularly with strong acids, are usually soluble in water. The free alkaloids are soluble in alcohol and chloroform.

Tannins or Tannic Acids—are weak acids with an astringent taste. They occur commonly in barks and roots, are freely soluble in alcohol and water, and form precipitates with certain iron salts, with alkaloids and with proteins.

METHODS OF PREPARING DRUGS

Extraction—is the process of removing soluble constituents of a crude drug by means of a solvent (menstruum). Four types of extraction are used by the pharmacist:

i. **Infusion**—A finely divided drug is treated with hot or cold water for a certain time. The fluid is then filtered off and retained and the solid material rejected.

ii. **Decoction**—The drug is boiled in water for a short time and the resulting fluid separated and retained.

iii. **Maceration**—The solvent is poured upon the drug and kept in contact with it for a specified time, with occasional agitation. The fluid is filtered off. The solid portion or marc is pressed. The fluid thus obtained is added to the filtrate and the marc is rejected.

iv. **Percolation**—The drug is packed in a conical vessel (a percolator) with a small outlet at its lower end. The solvent is poured on the drug and allowed to run out slowly until a certain volume has been collected. The marc is usually pressed and the fluid obtained added to the percolate.

Expression—Pressure is applied to a drug in such a manner as to squeeze out the liquids which are required.

Desiccation—A drug is dried by currents of hot or cold air, or by exposure to reduced atmospheric pressure with arrangements to absorb the water vapour released.

Distillation—is a process for separating volatile substances from non-volatile or less volatile material by means of heat. The volatile substances are condensed on a cold surface and collected. Steam and vacuum distillation are modern variations of importance in pharmaceutical industry.

Pulverization—means reduction of a solid to a very finely divided state (powder). The degree of fineness is denoted by the finest sieve through which the powder can pass. Sieves are designated by the number of meshes to the linear inch, e.g. 20, 40, 60, 80 and 100. Pulverization is accomplished on a small scale by the use of the mortar and pestle, but pharmaceutical manufacturers use various kinds of mills.

Trituration—may mean the same as pulverization but more commonly means powdering and mixing intimately, two or more drugs.

Vehicle—is the liquid or mixture of liquids in which a drug is dissolved or suspended. In ointments the soft or greasy substance in which a more active drug is incorporated is usually called the *base*. In pills the material used to hold the drug is called the *excipient*.

Official Preparations

Titles followed by the letters U.S.P. or B.P. appear in the one publication but not in the other. Absence of initials means that the same title is used in both publications but sometimes with slightly different meaning.

Aromatic Waters—Aquae Aromaticae—(e.g. Peppermint Water) —are solutions of volatile substances in water. They are usually prescribed as flavours but some may be prescribed for an action, e.g. Peppermint Water may be used as a carminative. When used as flavours, little attention is paid to dosage. Enough is given to produce the flavour desired. Most of the Waters contain an aromatic oil which is only slightly soluble in water, into which it may be introduced by one of three methods. (1) By the old methods, the oil and the water were distilled together (Distilled Waters). Enough oil passed over with the water to saturate it. (2) A Concentrated Water is diluted 40 times with water. The Concentrated Water is a solution of the aromatic oil in diluted alcohol and is a convenient stock solution for the use of the pharmacist. (3) The aromatic oil is ground with an insoluble solid, such as talc. In this way the oil is made to present a large surface to hasten solution. Water is added and after sufficient agitation is separated by decanting or filtering. When prescribing an Aromatic Water, do not use the word Distilled. Let the pharmacist prepare it any way he chooses. Concentrated Waters are not prescribed.

Capsules—Capsulae. A number of preparations in the U.S.P. are specified as capsules, e.g. Pentobarbital Capsules. Capsule may also mean the container in which a powder or liquid may be swallowed. Capsules may be hard or soft. Hard capsules come in two parts which fit together. They can be filled by the retail pharmacist. Soft capsules are moulded and filled in the factory.

Some drugs are supplied by manufacturers in *enteric coated* capsules. These may be gelatin capsules hardened, sometimes with formaldehyde, sometimes with some varnish, for the purpose of delaying their disintegration until they are beyond the stomach and well into the small intestine.

Collodion—Collodium—(e.g. Flexible Collodion)—A solution of pyroxylin in ether and alcohol, alone or with other drugs. It is applied to the skin and when the ether and alcohol have evaporated a thin film is left on the surface.

Cream—Cremor (e.g. Penicillin Cream)—A thick liquid or thin ointment.

Elixir—Elixir—(e.g. Elixir of Cascara Sagrada)—A sweet, flavoured liquid often containing some alcohol—usually less than 20%—with or without other active drugs. Those containing active drugs may be given without modification. The others are employed as flavoured vehicles.

Emulsion Emulsio B.P., Emulsum U.S.P.—(e.g. Emulsion of Liquid Paraffin)—An emulsion consists of two liquid phases, one of which is finely divided and dispersed in the other, e.g. minute oil droplets in water. The system is made more or less stable by some emulsifying agent such as acacia, tragacanth or sodium lauryl sulphate.

Extract U.S.P. or **Dry Extract B.P.**—Extractum or Extractum Siccum—These are semisolid or dry powdered preparations made by extracting a drug and evaporating off the solvent. They are used principally for making pills and tablets.

Fluidextract U.S.P. or **Liquid Extract B.P.**—Fluidextractum or Extractum Liquidum—An extract prepared by maceration or percolation with a suitable solvent and usually adjusted to contain a specified concentration of active principle. The liquid extract is always more concentrated than a tincture of the same drug. If a tincture is available, it is usually preferable to use it in a prescription, unless there is a definite pharmaceutical reason to the contrary.

Gelatin—Gelatinum—(e.g. Gelatin of Zinc)—A solid preparation containing gelatin and glycerin.

Gel U.S.P.—Gelatum—(e.g. Aluminum Hydroxide Gel U.S.P.)— The official examples of this type of preparation are the colloidal gels of aluminum hydroxide and aluminum phosphate.

Glycerin B.P. or **Glycerite U.S.P.**—Glycerinum or Glyceritum— (e.g. Glycerin of Tragacanth)—A solution of a drug in glycerin. The glycerin has useful properties as a preservative and solvent, as well as being hygroscopic.

Infusion B.P.—Infusum—(e.g. Concentrated Infusion of Quassia) —An extract made by infusion.

Inhalation U.S.P.—Inhalatio—(e.g. Epinephrine Inhalation)— A preparation to be inhaled from a nebulizer as a mist or aerosol.

Injection—Injectio—(e.g. Injection of Insulin)—A liquid preparation intended for administration by hypodermic, intramuscular or intravenous injection.

Lamellae B.P.—Lamellae—(e.g. Lamellae of Cocaine)—Thin discs of gelatin and glycerin containing some drug. The disc is placed in the conjunctival sac and allowed to dissolve and in this way a local effect of the drug is secured.

Liniment—Linimentum—A liquid preparation for rubbing into the skin to produce a local effect.

Lotion B.P.—Lotio—A liquid preparation frequently containing suspended material, for application to the skin.

Lozenges B.P.—Trochisci — (e.g. Lozenge of Tannic Acid)—

Flat tablets made of sugar and acacia, incorporating one or more active drugs; to be dissolved slowly in the mouth.

Mixture—Mistura—A liquid preparation to be taken by mouth; a physician should use this term in a prescription only when the preparation is to be swallowed.   In the U.S.A. Mixture means any inhomogeneous liquid but in practice is applied only to preparations for oral use, e.g. Chalk Mixture.

Mucilage—Mucilago—(e.g. Mucilage of Acacia)—A viscous solution of gums or starch, used in making pills, lotions or suspensions.

Ointment—Unguentum—(e.g. Zinc Oxide Ointment)—A soft but non-liquid preparation for external application.   The common ointment bases often contain soft paraffin (Petrolatum U.S.P) or Wool Fat.   *Eye Ointments* (Oculenta) are recognized by the B.P. They are made with soft yellow paraffin as the base, since white paraffin may contain traces of irritant bleaching material.

Oxymel B.P.—Oxymel—(e.g. Oxymel of Squill)—A solution of a drug in honey.

Paste B.P.—Pasta—(e.g. Tannic Acid Paste)—A soft preparation for external application, usually stiffer or thicker than the ordinary ointments.

Pills—Pilulae—(e.g. Compound Rhubarb Pill)—Spheroidal pellets usually sugar coated, containing one or more drugs held together by some sticky substance known as the excipient.   They are no longer prepared to order by the pharmacist, and only types and sizes known to be available from manufacturers should be ordered.

Plaster U.S.P.—Emplastrum—(e.g. Mustard Plaster)—Plasters consist of suitably adhesive material (usually prepared rubber latex) spread on a fabric.   When pressed against the skin they stick.   Medicated plasters are less frequently used now than formerly.

Poultice B.P.—Cataplasma—(e.g. Kaolin Poultice)—A poultice is a soft mass employed to convey moist heat to an affected part. The only official poultice is that of kaolin.   Others of linseed, bran or mustard are often made up as required.

Powder B.P.—Pulvis—(e.g. Powder of Ipecac and Opium), or

Powders U.S.P.—Pulveres—(e.g. Compound Effervescent Powders)—One or more drugs finely powdered.   The pharmacopoeial powders are all for oral administration but the term may be applied to powders for other uses.

Solution—Liquor—Official solutions and some well-known non-official solutions are designated as Liquores. Solutions made up on prescription and some standard solutions are known as Solutiones.

Spirit—Spiritus—(e.g. Spirit of Chloroform)—Solutions of volatile substances containing 80-90% of alcohol. They are prepared either by simple solution or by distillation. An exception is Whiskey (not official), viz. Spiritus Frumenti, which is much weaker in alcoholic content. Whiskey, Spirit of Chloroform and Spirit of Nitrous Ether are miscible with water in all proportions. Others contain essential oils which may separate on dilution with water.

Suppository—Suppositorium—(e.g. Glycerin Suppository)—A solid object properly shaped for insertion into an orifice of the body where it melts, liberating a drug for local action or absorption. Suitable bases are Oil of Theobroma (a solid at room temperature), Glycerinated Gelatin or Sodium Stearate. Rectal suppositories weigh about 2 Gm.; vaginal suppositories (also called pessaries) weigh about 5 Gm.; urethral suppositories (bougies) are enlongated rods 7 or 14 cm. in length.

Syrup—Syrupus—(e.g. Syrup of Orange)—A nearly saturated solution of cane sugar in water with or without added flavour and drug.

Tablets—Tabellae—(e.g. Phenacetin Tablets)—Pharmacopoeial tablets are of two types—(1) compressed (C.T.); (2) moulded tablets or tablet triturates (T.T.).

The making of compressed tablets is a factory process involving expensive machinery. Tablet triturates are more simply made by pressing moistened material into a perforated plate but even these are not made by the retail pharmacist, so that the doctor when prescribing must know the sizes available. It is not necessary as a rule when prescribing to specify C.T. or T.T., but only when ordering in bulk and when the catalogue shows the same drug in the two forms of tablet. Hypodermic tablets (H.T.) are small and designed to dissolve completely and rapidly in a small volume of water. They are often prescribed to be taken under the tongue and should be specified when required in a prescription.

Tincture—Tinctura—(from the Latin tinctus, coloured)—An alcoholic solution of non-volatile drugs extracted by maceration or percolation and usually containing 45-70% of alcohol. When a liquid extract of the same drug exists, it is stronger than the tincture. The tinctures usually can be diluted with water without the formation of a precipitate and are more commonly used than liquid extracts in mixtures. The U.S.P. still retains the name Iodine Tincture for what is really a solution but was long ago misnamed on account of its colour and alcoholic content.

Standardized Tinctures and Extracts are ones with potent active principles which must show on assay—either chemical or biological—a concentration of active principle within specified limits.

Vinegar B.P.—Acetum—A solution of a drug in dilute acetic acid (e.g. Vinegar of Squill).

Toxins, Toxoids, Sera and Vaccines are listed and specified in the B.P. and U.S.P.

Sutures, Absorbent Cotton, Gauze, Bandages and qualities of Glass Containers are specified in the U.S.P.

Non-Official Preparations

Cachet or Konseal—A container of thin rice paper in which a nauseous powder can be swallowed. Two dish-like pieces of paper containing the powder are stuck together by moistening their rims with water. A far bigger dose can be swallowed in a cachet than in a gelatin capsule.

Drops—In common language reference is made to nose drops, ear drops and eye drops; all may be translated as guttae. Nose drops or nasal sprays are often translated as nebulae.

Enema or Clyster—A liquid preparation for injection into the rectum. It may be bland, medicated or nutrient.

Eye Wash—Collyrium—A dilute solution usually adjusted to be isotonic with tears or with the aqueous humour.

Gargle—Gargarisma—A liquid preparation for application to the pharynx by gargling or by irrigation.

Linctus—Linctus—A thick sweet liquid tending to cling to the tongue and pharynx; originally a medicine intended to be licked.

Mouth Wash—Collutorium—A solution for rinsing the mouth.

Nasal Douche—Collunarium—A solution for irrigating the nose.

Pastille—A small medicated disc or roll to be held in the mouth or cheek and allowed to dissolve slowly, e.g. penicillin pastilles.

Perles—Originally referred to small gelatin capsules but now designate small glass capsules covered with fabric and containing a volatile drug. The perles are crushed and the fumes of the volatile drug are inhaled.

Pigment or Paint—Pigmentum—A preparation for swabbing on the skin or mucous membrane with the object of producing a relatively prolonged action.

Solution Tablets B.P.C.—Solvellae—Tablets generally intended to be dissolved in water to make solutions for external use.

Tampon—A plug of plain or medicated cotton or wool for insertion into a natural cavity of the body or into a wound, often for purpose of arresting haemorrhage.

Three

Incompatibility

INCOMPATIBILITY IS SAID TO EXIST BETWEEN DRUGS if an undesirable reaction occurs when they are prescribed in the same preparation or administered at the same time. Incompatibilities may be classified as pharmacological or pharmaceutical. The occurrence of a reaction does not constitute an incompatibility; only the occurrence of an undesirable reaction.

Drugs with opposite pharmacological actions may be prescribed together purposely. For example, atropine is frequently prescribed with morphine to oppose the tendency of the latter to produce contractions of the stomach, pyloric sphincter, sphincter of Oddi, and the ureters. If, however, atropine were given before meals, say to prevent asthmatic attacks, and if the doctor were at the same time trying to improve the appetite of the patient by some other medication, a pharmacological incompatibility would exist, since the atropine would seriously impair the appetite.

Pharmaceutical incompatibilities were at one time classified as chemical or physical but such a distinction is often difficult and generally pointless. It is the privilege of the doctor to prescribe any combination of drugs which he believes will benefit his patient. He should realize, however, that it is extremely easy to prescribe combinations which will react to his embarrassment and sometimes to endanger the life of his patient. Deaths have occurred from a powerful alkaloid such as strychnine precipitating slowly from an improperly designed mixture and almost the whole amount in the bottle being swallowed in the last dose.

Incompatibilities may be avoided by prescribing drugs singly in simple form, by using well-tried formulae, by giving careful study to any innovations and by consulting a competent pharmacist when in doubt.

Some examples of incompatibility are listed below. Most of them have been committed at one time or another.

(*a*) Carbonates with acids—e.g. Ammonium Carbonate—with Syrup of Squill which contains acetic acid, will cause effervescence.

(*b*) Carbonates with salts of Calcium or Magnesium will precipitate.

(*c*) Salts of Iron with carbonates and phosphates precipitate. With tannins, as in Compound Tincture of Gentian, they will produce unsightly inks.

(*d*) Acids with salts of insoluble weak acids—e.g. Sodium Phenobarbitone with Syrup of Lemon, which contains citric acid—will cause precipitation of phenobarbitone.

(*e*) Alkalis with salts of alkaloids may cause precipitation of free alkaloid. Many alkaloids will precipitate with carbonates, phosphates and particularly iodides. Sometimes precipitation can be prevented by the judicious addition of alcohol.

(*f*) Glycosides in watery solution tend to hydrolyze slowly, with loss of activity and the liberation of a reducing sugar. This process is greatly hastened by the presence of acids or alkalis.

(*g*) Certain solids when triturated together will not form a powder but a soft sticky mass—e.g. Any two of these rubbed together: Camphor, Phenol, Thymol, Chloral, or any one of them with Phenazone or Phenacetin.

(*h*) Gums—e.g. Acacia, Starches and Dextrins—in aqueous solution will precipitate on dilution with alcohol.

(*i*) Resins, oleoresins, oils, etc. in alcoholic solution will precipitate on dilution with water. In some cases the precipitate is unimportant and may be filtered off—e.g. when Liquid Extract of Nux Vomica is diluted with water an unimportant waxy material separates.

(*j*) Strong aqueous solutions of salts—e.g. half saturated Potassium Citrate—are not miscible with alcohol. A tincture added to such a solution will collect as a supernatant layer. The addition of sufficient water will make the solutions miscible.

Whenever possible clear solutions should be prescribed. If an unimportant precipitate is likely to form, the patient should be warned, otherwise he may worry about it. Sometimes suspensions are ordered and it is well in such cases to increase the viscosity of the liquid with a mucilage or with Bentonite to delay settling. A "Shake Well" label should be put on the bottle. A potent drug like strychnine or hyoscyamine should never be allowed to precipitate.

Four

The Administration of Drugs

THE PURPOSES FOR WHICH DRUGS are given and the effects which they produce are discussed briefly in Chapter VIII. The following paragraphs deal with elementary and practical points concerned with the forms in which drugs are given.

Tablets. The popularity of tablets is well justified by their convenience and the accuracy of dosage they provide. They can easily be crushed in a spoon and swallowed with water by those who cannot swallow them whole. Smaller than average doses can be given with sufficient accuracy by dividing the tablets into halves or quarters. Some tablets are manufactured with grooves for this purpose. Tablet triturates are softer than compressed tablets and tend to powder when kept for long. Some drugs are customarily put up in this form, e.g. Codeine Phosphate and Nitroglycerin, presumably with the object of insuring faster disintegration in the stomach and hence faster action. Compressed tablets can now be made to disintegrate very rapidly, e.g. in a few seconds even in cold water. The B.P. sets a limit of 15 minutes as the time for disintegration in water at 37°C., when not otherwise specified.

Hypodermic tablets dissolve with extraordinary rapidity. To administer, boil about 1.5 cc. of water in a spoon; drop in a tablet, stir with a sterilized needle, draw the solution into a sterilized syringe and inject. If you wish to give only a fraction of a tablet (e.g. 1/3), measure the volume of the solution after it is drawn into the syringe. Expel the appropriate fraction (e.g. 2/3) and inject the remainder. Hypodermic tablets are very useful for sublingual administration. Many drugs, such as morphine or nitroglycerin, can be absorbed almost as completely and rapidly by holding them under the tongue as by injection.

Tablets of sodium chloride, potassium permanganate or chloramine and many others are very handy for making up solutions of known strength. Such tablets are called Solvellae in the B.P.C.

Mixtures. Liquid preparations for oral administration, though waning in popularity, have, for certain purposes, special points in their favour. They allow scope for variation and innovation which is sometimes useful to the physician. Certain important drugs such as paraldehyde, chloral hydrate, liquid paraffin, hydrochloric acid and alcohol, can hardly be given any other way. If palatability can be achieved with a mixture, less persuasion is needed to get the medicine taken with proper regularity. An attractive-looking preparation makes a surprisingly favourable impression on some patients. It is a good principle to avoid, when possible, prescribing murky liquids with ugly precipitates.

Flavours. The most important element of flavouring in a mixture is sweetness. If there is no reason for avoiding the use of sugar, one of the syrups should be used; otherwise saccharin may be used in sufficient quantity to provide a final concentration of about 1:10,000 in the medicine as it is to be taken. Syrups are customarily prescribed to constitute one quarter of the volume of the mixture. Sometimes it is advantageous to dissolve the drug in pure syrup, e.g. chloral hydrate.

Mild flavours such as Syrup of Orange, Syrup of Lemon, and Syrup of Citric Acid are popular and suitable for use with relatively mild or tasteless drugs. They are less effective, however, than stronger flavours for "covering" unpleasant medicines such as salicylates, bromides and iodides. The Compound Syrup of Sassafras C.F. (or the Compound Syrup of Sarsaparilla U.S.P.) has a persistent flavour resembling root beer. Syrup of Squill contains free acid and should not be used with carbonates. Aromatic Elixir is a favourite with those who enjoy a little alcohol and the action of the latter is sometimes useful. Syrup of Ginger imparts a warm, pungent and persistent flavour which makes it acceptable in carminative mixtures or to cover such drugs as bromides. Spirit of Chloroform also imparts a warm sweet flavour but with some people induces chloroform-flavoured belching.

Some flavouring preparations have little or no sweetening value and should be prescribed with syrup in addition. Among these is the Liquid Extract of Liquorice which has great covering power. Because of its strength it should not constitute more than 10% of the mixture. The Waters of Anise, Dill, and Peppermint may be used freely in addition to syrup. The Spirit of Cinnamon should be used very sparingly (1 in 2,000). The Compound Tincture of Cardamom has a warm flavour which is appreciated by those with sophisticated taste. It may be used in a concentration of about 1:8 in a mixture.

A bitter taste is imparted by the Tinctures of Quassia and Calumba, the Compound Tincture of Gentian and the Tincture of Nux Vomica, in dilutions of about 1 in 100. The popularity of beer proves that many people appreciate a slightly bitter flavour. Bitters used to be thought to stimulate gastric secretion. They may do so for those who like them.

Colours. It is not worth while trying to modify the colour of mixtures containing deeply coloured drugs but clear and faintly coloured solutions can often be made more attractive by judicious colouring. The red colour of the Compound Tincture of Cardamom fades in an acid medium but Amaranth and Cumidine Red are stable in acid and alkaline solutions. These two, with Tartrazine (yellow) and Brilliant Blue, are official in the Canadian Supplement to the B.P. Amaranth and Cumidine Red impart adequate colour at a concentration of 1 in 10,000; Brilliant Blue and Tartrazine at 1 in 50,000. A grass green colour is given by equal parts of Tartrazine and Brilliant Blue; purple may be obtained by Brilliant Blue 1.5 and Amaranth 8.5; orange by Cumidine Red 4 and Tartrazine 6.

Pills. Prescriptions are no longer written for pills to be made by the pharmacist. Proprietary pills and pharmacopoeial laxative pills (e.g. Pilula Aloes, Pilula Rhei Co.) are used to some extent.

Powders. When drugs are not too unpleasant and the bulk to be given is large, powders are a useful mode of administration. Powders of small bulk and unpleasant taste are best given in *capsules*. A larger dose can be given by *cachet* if the patient is shown how to swallow it. Powders may also be used to enable patients to make up solutions of specified strength at home.

Applications to the Skin. Many drugs will penetrate intact skin, probably through sweat glands and hair follicles for the most part. Only a few drugs are ordinarily given for systemic effect by application to the skin. Mercury by inunction is used in the treatment of syphilis. BAL, a liquid which acts as a potent antidote for arsenic and mercury, may also be given by inunction. The base or vehicle may greatly influence the absorption of a drug but no very useful general rules can be stated. Poisoning by dilute solutions of phenol, e.g. 2%, can follow application to large areas of relatively intact skin.

Drugs which ionize can be driven through the skin by the application of a direct current (iontophoresis). Local vasodilation can be produced this way and so can local anaesthetic effects.

Ointments with soft paraffin as a base are most useful for persistent protective action. They often contain very bland medicaments such as starch and zinc oxide. Soft paraffin itself varies in consistency with temperature. *Simple Ointment*, which contains soft paraffin with a little hard paraffin and a little wool fat, has a desirable consistency over a wide range of temperatures and is an excellent general-purpose base. The *Ointment of Wool Alcohols* (Eucerin) is much the same but can be made to incorporate an almost equal volume of water or watery solution. This makes it an excellent base for holding a watery solution of penicillin as penicillin cream. Wool Fat (Adeps Lanae) has also the property of incorporating water to form a cream but will not hold as much water as Eucerin and its consistency is stickier.

Many different drugs are incorporated in ointments. For antibacterial action various salts of mercury are used. For fungus infections, salicylic acid, benzoic acid, undecylenic acid are effective. Phenol and menthol are useful to allay itching and so are certain penetrating local anaesthetics such as Tetracaine and Nupercaine. Dithranol and ichthammol are used for rubefacient and antiseptic action.

Much ingenuity has been directed in recent years to devising watery creams (hydrophilic creams). They can be washed off easily and so have some advantages for the application of drugs to the scalp and perhaps for first-aid treatment of burns. They are essentially rather thick emulsions of oil or greases in water. They should not be confused with cold cream which is an emulsion of water in oils and which is not so easily washed off. It is sometimes used to dilute thicker ointments.

Rectal Applications. To soften impacted faeces an injection of olive oil or (perhaps even better) normal saline, is used. A volume of 100 or 200 cc. is injected and left to soften the faecal mass, after which appropriate measures to empty the rectum may be taken.

The glycerin suppository or soap stick is useful for establishing regular habits of defaecation in young children. Suppositories for the symptomatic relief of bleeding haemorrhoids or thrombosed haemorrhoids are more often sold over the drug-store counter than prescribed, but they do give relief. The student would do well to

look into the varieties on the market. A combination of an astringent to decrease bleeding and a local anaesthetic to relieve
pain is effective. Tubes of ointment containing a local anaesthetic
and provided with tips for rectal injection are sold for the treatment
of haemorrhoids and pruritus ani. Digital application is probably
just as effective.

Vaginal Applications. A vaginal douche requires a volume of at
least one litre. The drugs required should be prescribed in concentrated form, e.g. in powders, and the patient instructed to
dissolve the contents of one powder in the required volume of
warm tap water.

Powdered preparations of acetarsone are applied to the vagina
by insufflation for the treatment of trichomonas vaginitis. Vaginal
suppositories (pessaries) may be used to apply oestrogenic drugs
locally for vulvovaginitis in children or for senile vaginitis. Absorption from vaginal mucosa is very considerable. Systemic poisoning
from bichloride of mercury has resulted from the use of strong
solutions in the vagina with the object of inducing abortion.

Urethra and Bladder. Instillation of antiseptics and local
anaesthetics are sometimes made into the urethra and bladder.
Here again rapid absorption from the urethra is to be feared,
particularly in the case of local anaesthetics.

Conjunctiva. Eye washes and eye drops are customarily made
up to be isotonic with tears, i.e. with 1.4% of sodium chloride or
2% of boric acid. They are thus somewhat hypertonic to blood
and lymph. Hypertonicity of this degree is not too uncomfortable
and may be useful in promoting an outward drainage of fluid in
conjunctivitis. Antiseptic astringents such as zinc sulphate, lead
acetate and copper sulphate are often used but their concentration
should not exceed 1 in 500. Solutions of argentoprotein are not
irritant and are employed in strengths of 10 to 25%. For prevention of ophthalmia neonatarum, 1% of silver nitrate is instilled at
birth.

For their local effects on the pupillary muscle, mydriatics and
miotics may be applied in aqueous solutions, atropine sulphate 1%,
pilocarpine nitrate 1-2%, physostigmine salicylate 1/2%, homatropine hydrobromide 2%, cocaine hydrochloride 2-5%, butacaine
1%, tetracaine 1/2%. They may also be applied in lamellae or
oculenta. A 2% solution of soluble floruescein is used to show
small ulcers or injuries on the cornea.

Mouth and Pharynx. Mouth washes and gargles containing various astringents are much used but usually without much confidence in their effectiveness. A pigment containing glycerin, phenol and iodine, swabbed on the fauces and pharynx will often give appreciable relief in simple sore throats. Penicillin pastilles held in the cheek for long periods will relieve certain infections by organisms sensitive to penicillin. Infections of the gums are often treated with the application of antiseptic packs around the gingival margins.

Small ulcers in the mouth are effectively treated by touching with a crystal of copper sulphate, alum, or toughened caustic (Argenti Nitras Induratus).

Nasal Passages. Six or eight drops of solution in each nostril can be brought into effective contact with nearly all the nasal and post-nasal mucous membrane by proper movements of the head. This mode of application is even more efficient than an atomizer. Isotonic aqueous solutions are now used in preference to oily solutions for the majority of applications. The persistent use of oily solutions has resulted in oil-pneumonia. Ephedrine sulphate and ephedrine hydrochloride are most commonly used as nasal decongestants in concentrations of $1/2$ to 1% for symptomatic relief. More transient relief may be obtained from inhalation of certain volatile amines (amphetamine). Prolonged effects are given by the proprietary solutions of Neosynephrine and Tuamine. Ordinary antiseptics seem to be of little value in the nose. Prolonged use of silver preparations may lead to argyrism, a permanent bluish discoloration of the skin.

Absorption from the nasal mucous membranes is rapid. Effective control of diabetes inspidus can be maintained by the application of pitressin to the nasal mucosa, even though the hormone is a protein. For symptomatic relief of nasal discharge atropine by mouth is effective and the basis of some popular proprietary remedies for colds.

Trachea and Bronchi. A useful procedure for the relief of bronchitis is the inhalation of the vapours of Friars' Balsam poured on boiling water. The steam may rationally be supposed to have a soothing effect on the irritated bronchi, dry cold air certainly adds to the irritation. It would be interesting to know whether the Friar's Balsam contributed anything but an impressive odour. Very fine sprays of particle size less than 5 micra will reach the terminal bronchioles and are used to secure local effects of epinephrine (1 in 100) and penicillin.

Injections. A hypodermic injection is made into the areolar tissue under the skin. A volume of 1 cc. is usually given but 2 cc. or even 3 may be given if necessary, though likely to be uncomfortable. A needle 1/2- to 3/4-inch in length and of 25- or 27-gauge is used. The solution should be neutral and close to isotonic. Water freshly boiled in a spoon is used to dissolve a hypodermic tablet. The pharmacopoeial injections put up in ampuls are required to be made with pyrogen-free water, though this is probably not very important for injections of small bulk.

Intradermal injections are often made at the start of an infiltration of local anaesthetic and in various tests such as the Dick test and tuberculin test.

Somewhat irritant drugs such as bismuth salicylate and even very irritant drugs, at times, e.g. the mercurial diuretics, are injected intramuscularly. A 23- or 21-gauge needle at least 1 ½ inches long is used. The gluteal muscles are customarily used but the lateral aspect of the quadriceps femoris may be better. Syringes and needles must, of course, always be sterilized and the skin cleansed with alcohol before an injection. Oily vehicles are sometimes used for injections, usually to delay absorption, e.g. penicillin in beeswax and oil, or epinephrine in oil. Allergic reactions to the oil are not uncommon. The systemic effects of drugs given by hypodermic or intramuscular injection in aqueous solution are usually manifest in 10 to 20 minutes. If an injection is made into an extremity when the patient is severely chilled or in a state of circulatory collapse, the drug may not act for a long time, viz. several hours. If rapid action is essential an intravenous injection should be given.

Five

Posology

THE BRITISH PHARMACOPOEIA makes the following statement in regard to the doses as given in it.

It must be clearly understood that the "doses" mentioned in the Pharmacopoeia are not authoritatively enjoined, as binding on prescribers. They are intended merely for general guidance and represent, unless otherwise stated, the average range of quantities which are generally regarded as suitable for adults when administered by mouth. The oral doses mentioned may, in many cases, be repeated three or four times in twenty-four hours. It must not be assumed, however, that they indicate the greatest amounts of drugs that may be given. The medical practitioner will exercise his own judgement and act on his own responsibility in respect of the amount of any therapeutic agent he may prescribe or administer or the frequency of its administration. When however, an unusually large dose appears to have been prescribed, it shall be the duty of the pharmacist or dispenser to satisfy himself that the prescriber's intention has been correctly interpreted.

This statement is a very important one and should be thoroughly understood by every medical practitioner. In deciding what dose to order, certain factors should be considered:

Weight. The larger and more robust the individual the larger is the dose of most drugs that may be given to him. Small and weakly individuals should always receive small doses of any remedy at first.

Sex. Women are often said to be less resistant to the action of drugs than men but as a rule little distinction is made between the sexes. It must, however, be borne in mind that at the time of pregnancy or menstruation any drugs that bring about changes in the blood supply to the uterus or that would set up movements in its musculature should be either entirely avoided or given in very small doses and with caution. Also it must be remembered that many drugs are excreted in the milk and may make the milk unpalatable or even dangerous to a suckling child. Amongst the drugs excreted by the mammary glands are the oils of anise and dill, turpentine, copaiba; the purgative principles of rhubarb, senna and castor oil; opium, iodine, also some of the metals, antimony, arsenic, lead, and mercury.

Susceptibility. Every person differs from all others; and biochemically as well as physically there is a wide range of variation. Some individuals show marked effects from a small dose of a drug that does not produce an observable effect in most other persons. Just as persons range from very short to very tall, so in reaction to drugs they range from the susceptible (easily affected) to the resistant.

Idiosyncrasy. Persons who react in a quite abnormal way to a drug, e.g. are excited by morphine, are said to show idiosyncrasy to the drug.

Some of the manifestations of idiosyncrasy resemble allergic reactions, e.g. urticaria and rashes. It is often impossible to say how or when sensitization occurred. It could, of course, happen *in utero*. In some cases it is possible to observe sensitization develop, e.g. to sulphonamides. A rare but serious manifestation of idiosyncrasy is oedema of the glottis after taking iodides. Agranulocytosis after amidopyrine or after sulphonamides is another example. Other drugs which sometimes elicit idiosyncrasy are bromides, mercury, acetylsalicylic acid, procaine and diphenylhydantoin.

Tolerance. The continued use of certain drugs may make a person less susceptible to their actions and may necessitate the use of larger doses. Such drugs are said to induce tolerance.

Increased susceptibility to the action of a drug may also occur on continued administration. It is particularly liable to occur with drugs such as digitalis and mercury, which may be excreted more slowly than they are absorbed and thus tend to show *cumulation*. Disease may alter the absorption, excretion or destruction of some drugs and thus change the susceptibility of the patient. Liver disease, for example, increases susceptibility to the toxic effects of chloroform and carbon tetrachloride. Nephritis with anuria may cause retention of magnesium salts so that oral doses of magnesium sulphate can lead to a toxic accumulation of magnesium in the blood.

Pharmacopoeial doses are for adults; children require smaller doses. Several rules have been proposed for calculating the dose for a child. They usually err on the safe side and are chiefly useful when specific experience is lacking, or to check the reasonableness of a recollected dose. Children are particularly susceptible to morphine and its derivatives. It is a good rule not to use any opiates for infants less than one year old. On the other hand, children are relatively tolerant to alcohol, atropine and pheno-barbitone. With certain drugs which are given in doses to maintain a certain concentration in the blood, e.g. salicylates and sulphonamides, proportionately larger doses are required for children since metabolism and renal excretion are relatively large.

Young's rule is one which is very commonly used for calculating doses for children. The average adult dose is multiplied by the fraction, age/age + 12. For example, the average adult dose of Hexylresorcinol is 1 Gm. Applying Young's rule for a child of three gives: $\dfrac{1 \times 3}{12 + 3} = 0.2$ Gm. Actually, 0.3 Gm. may be given safely.

Clark's rule is to multiply the average adult dose by the weight of the child in lbs. and divide by 150. For a child of three weighing 30 lbs., the calculated dose of Hexylresorcinol would be $\dfrac{1 \times 30}{150}$ = 0.2 Gm.—i.e. the same as by Young's rule. Clark's rule gives larger doses than Young's rule at ages under 3 years.

Persons above the age of sixty are usually more affected by drugs than are younger persons. Doses for adults are intended for persons between 20 and 60 years of age. Persons over sixty should receive roughly 3/4 and persons over eighty-five roughly 1/2 of the adult dose, but this again is a rough guide and there are many exceptions, for example, purgatives.

The frequency of repetition makes a great difference in the size of dose to be administered. The more frequently the drug is to be administered the smaller the dose should be.

The time of day makes, as a rule, little difference, except with drugs meant to bring on or increase a normal daily condition. For example a larger dose of a hypnotic such as chloral would be necessary to produce sleep during the day than at night. Purgatives also can best be given at such a time that they will take effect at the hour of the patient's daily defaecation. For this purpose calomel and aloes must be given some eight hours in advance, while purgative salts act within two hours, if taken with plenty of water, on an empty stomach.

The presence or absence of food in the stomach may make a great difference in the rapidity with which drugs are absorbed and in the quantity coming in contact with the wall of the stomach and so irritating it, and as a consequence any drug irritant to the stomach may be given in larger quantities immediately after meals than before meals.

Synergists are drugs having the same main effects, though the manner of action may be slightly different. For example, colocynth, aloes and potassium sulphate are synergists, as they are all purgatives. All of these occur in the Compound Pill of Colocynth. It is sometimes an advantage and is a common practice in the administration of purgatives to include in a prescription two or more synergists, as in the instance mentioned above. When synergists are administered together it is necessary to give any one drug in only a fraction of its full dose.

Finally, the pharmacopoeial doses are not enjoined and the practitioner must use his own judgement. In many cases it is quite allowable to exceed the pharmacopoeial dose if the effects wished for are not achieved by its administration; the physician should watch carefully each and every patient and convince himself that the drugs given are really producing the wished-for action. In other words, he must not take it for granted that because he gives a pharmacopoeial dose of any drug he must as a consequence get the described pharmacological action.

The doses of the Pharmacopoeia are, unless otherwise stated, for administration by mouth. Many drugs can, however, be administered with advantage by hypodermic, intramuscular or intravenous injection. Owing to the more rapid absorption as a rule of drugs given by these methods and to the certainty that they will be absorbed in their entirety, it is usually unnecessary that such large doses be given. In those cases in which drugs are given by intravenous injection usually only a fraction of the oral dose is used. For drugs given subcutaneously (hypodermically) about one-half of the dose is given that would be used if taken by mouth. Drugs given by inunction must be given in larger doses than would be used if they were taken by mouth. As a rule the same is usually true for drugs given by the rectum if they are intended to have a general action.

Six

Prescription Writing

A PRESCRIPTION IS A WRITTEN DIRECTION and authority to a pharmacist to dispense medicine to a patient. The ownership of the prescription is debatable. Usually the prescription is kept and filed by the pharmacist. It seems wisest to adopt the attitude that the patient is not entitled even to a copy of the prescription except as a favour. This favour should not be granted in the cases where the prescription includes a narcotic drug or any drug which may be sold only on prescription, because the prescription can be used legally only once. To save subsequent arguments, the doctor should explain to the patient that he has no proprietary interest in the prescription, particularly when, for any reason, the doctor thinks it advisable to mark *ne repetatur* on the prescription.

All derivatives of opium (including codeine except in certain preparations), cocaine and cannabis come under the regulations of the Opium and Narcotic Drug Act (of Canada), which should be read and digested by all doctors. Its penalties are very severe. The pharmacist may fill a prescription for a narcotic as defined under the Act only if the prescription is *signed* and *dated* by a duly authorized and practising physician, veterinary surgeon or dentist whose signature is known to him. Since the pharmacist must record in his order book the prescriber's address, this should be included as a courtesy on the prescription. In the U.S.A. the prescriber's narcotic registration number must be shown as well. A number of other drugs may be sold only on prescription, by regulations under the Food and Drugs Act. The list includes Aminopyrin and its salts and derivatives, Barbiturates, Amphetamine, Benzedrine, (Isomyn) and their salts, Cinchophen and Neocinchophen, Dilantin Sodium, Orthodinitrophenol, Sulphonamides, Thyroid, Streptomycin, Penicillin except for oral use, in doses not more than 3000 units Tetraethylthiuram disulphide (antabuse), Aureomycin, Urethane, ACTH, and Cortisone.

The use of Latin for prescription writing is dearly cherished by

many physicians and pharmacists, and with some justification.
The arguments in its favour would carry more weight if physicians, as
a group, were well educated in Latin.   Since they are not, the regular
use of English will save many an unnecessary display of ignorance.
Many Latin abbreviations have become so strongly entrenched
that their use may be condoned on the same grounds that we
permit A.M. and P.M. in everyday English.   For example, the
symbol ℞ stands for *recipe*—take thou—and its use may be
justified in that it immediately designates a slip of paper as a
medical prescription and hence subject to the safeguards imposed
by law.

A typical prescription in English and Metric System is shown
below.   The traditional names for each part of the prescription are
shown in italics.   The vertical line represents the decimal point
for **Gm. or cc.**

Superscription	℞		
Inscription	Sodium Iodide		3|0
	Camphorated Tincture of Opium		
	Compound Syrup of Sassafras C.F.	a̅a̅	15|0
	Water to		60|0
Subscription	M. Sig.		
Signature	One teaspoonful as required for		
or Label	cough, not oftener than every two hours.		
Prescriber's	J. P. Jones, M.D.		
Signature (and	22 Blunt St.		
address)			

Abbreviations.   The names of ingredients are often abbreviated
but the practice is not admirable, and indeed hard to justify.
The Latin abbreviations which may be considered so well established
as to warrant use in an English prescription, are the following:

a̅a̅—*ana*—of each—applied to ingredients of which the same
quantity is required.   Must not be used to
couple a solid with a liquid.

ad lib.—*ad libitum*—as much as may be desired.

ex aq.—*ex aqua*—in water or with water.

M.—*misce*—Compound, combine or mix.

Mit.—*mitte*—send.

N. rep.—*ne repetatur*—Do not repeat.

t.i.d.—*ter in die*—three times a day.

p.c.—*post cibos*—after meals.

a.c.—*ante cibos*—before meals.

p.r.n.—*pro re nata*—as required.

q.s.—*quantum sufficiat*—a sufficient quantity.

q.3 h.—*quaque tertia hora*—every three hours.

q.4 h.—*quaque quarta hora*—every four hours.

s. or sig.—*signa* (or *signetur*)—Label or let it be labelled.

s.n.p.—*signa nomine proprio*—Label with its proper name.

General Directions

Superscription. Always write the patient's name and the date. The patient's address is a courteous addition on prescriptions for narcotics. The druggist must find it somehow.

Inscription. Capitalize names of all ingredients. They are proper names of preparations of specified quality, not just any material that might be known by the same name. Avoid abbreviations which might be ambiguous, e.g. Sulph. or Hydroc. Ac. Use a vertical line as a decimal point for Gm. or cc. whenever two or more ingredients are written. No other indication of weight or measure is necessary. Solids will be weighed and liquids measured. *With a single ingredient* write the quantity, followed by Gm., cc. or mg. in the conventional manner. The decimal point should always have figures (or zero) both before it and after it.

Subscription. If the ingredients are to be combined write M. If it cannot be done, the pharmacist will probably let you know. Other directions may be necessary, such as: Divide into twenty powders, or capsules; or, Send twenty such in powders, or capsules; or, Send twenty such tablets, or, twenty of each tablet; or, Make an emulsion; or, Filter; etc.; and finally, write Sig.

Signature or Label. It seems to be the prerogative of the busy practitioner to use abbreviations and put the responsibility of translating them into sensible English on the pharmacist. For example, the label for the foregoing prescription might have read mils 4, q. 2 h. p.r.n. for cough. It is surely more reasonable, however, to write on the prescription exactly what you wish the patient to read on the label. Always write enough to let the pharmacist know how the medicine is to be used. Never be content with "Use as directed."

An excellent practice is to make a carbon copy of every prescription you write and file it with the patient's history card.

Tablets. Tablets are prescribed by their denomination, or drug content, and the available denominations (usually called sizes) must be known.

℞ Sulphaguanidine Tablets   0.5 Gm.
    Send 150.
    Sig. Take twelve tablets immediately and then six tablets every
        four hours, five times daily for four days.

or

℞ Hyoscine Hydrobromide   0.3 mg.
    (Hypo. Tabs.)
    Send 25.
    Sig. Take one or two tablets by mouth not oftener than every
        four hours, for airsickness.

In the last prescription hypodermic tablets were specified because they come in a small tube of 25, which is very convenient to carry.

Confusion sometimes arises when two or more tablets are prescribed to be taken at the same time, for example, two tablets of Sulphadiazine and three tablets of Sodium Bicarbonate every six hours. It is best to separate the prescriptions and designate one as (*a*) and the other as (*b*).

℞ (*a*)
    Sulphadiazine Tablets.   0.5 Gm.
    Send 20.
℞ (*b*)
    Sodium Bicarbonate Tablets.   0.3 Gm.
    Send 30.
    Sig. Two tablets of (*a*) and three tablets of (*b*) every six hours.

If the tablets do not look too much alike, the pharmacist may send all in one box with a partition between the two halves, and one label as above. If the tablets look alike he will send them in separate boxes with an appropriate label in each.

Prescribing a Mixture. A number of considerations demand attention and are probably best dealt with in the following order— (1) the drug or drugs; (2) the dose or doses; (3) the volume per dose which involves looking up the solubility of the drug; (4) the flavouring agent; (5) the number of days the medicine is to be taken and the number of doses per day; (6) the size of bottle; (7) the label.

Suppose that the patient has symptoms of peptic ulcer and pylorospasm, and is under considerable nervous stress. You decide to give phenobarbitone and atropine. The doses you choose are

0.3 mg. of Atropine Sulphate and 30 mg. of Soluble Phenobarbitone. The doses are small and can easily be held in solution in 1 teaspoonful (4 cc.). The drugs are not very unpleasant, a mild flavour will suffice, but it must not contain acid which would be incompatible with the Soluble Phenobarbitone. You decide on Aromatic Elixir, perhaps with the thought that a little alcohol in the solution would be some protection against the possibility of precipitation of atropine by the somewhat alkaline preparation of phenobarbitone. The volume of flavouring is usually one-quarter of the dose. In this case you might make it one-half or the whole of the volume. You decide to try the medicine for one week, at the end of which time you wish to see the patient for further examination. The doses, you think, might best be taken at lunch-time, supper-time and bed-time, i.e. three times a day. The total number of doses will be 3 times 7, or 21. The total volume will be 4 × 21, or 84 cc.

Bottle sizes. The common bottle sizes are 15, 30, 60, 90, 120, 180, 240, 360 and 480 cc., corresponding to 1/2, 1, 2, 3, 4, 6, 8, 12 and 16 fluid ounces. Smaller bottles or vials of 2, 4 and 8 cc. are also available.

To return to the prescription, 90 cc. is the closest bottle size. It is considered poor practice to dispense an unfilled bottle. The patient may think he has been cheated. So instead of ordering 21 doses you order 22½ or even 30 doses to fill a 120 cc. bottle, on the chance that you may continue the therapy. The prescription may now be written for 30 doses, starting with the smallest or most potent ingredient.

	For William Brown	Aug. 12
℞	Atropine Sulphate	0|009
	Soluble Phenobarbitone	0|900
	Aromatic Elixir C. F.	60|000
	Water to	120|000
	M.	

Sig. One teaspoonful with water at 1, 6 and 10 p.m.

PRESCRIBING IN LATIN

Traditionally, the prescription was written mainly in Latin with the older systems of weights and measures. There is no reason why the metric system may not be used with the prescription in Latin, but to save space the two older practices will be illustrated together below, with an interlinear translation. Note the use of the genitive case.

```
For Arthur Henry                                        July 14
℞ (Recipe)
Take thou
        Ferri et Ammonii Citratis                       ℥ i
        of the Citrate of Iron and Ammonium             one ounce
        Tincturae Nucis Vomicae                         ℨ vi
        of the Tincture of Nux Vomica                   six drachms
        Syrupi                                          ℥ i
        of Syrup                                        one ounce
        Elixir Aromatici          ad                    ℥ iv
        of Aromatic Elixir    sufficient to make
                              the volume to             four ounces
        Misce.    Fiat mistura.    Signa
        Mix.     Let a mixture be made.     Label
        Drachmam unam ex aqua capiat, ter in die post cibos.
        Let him take one teaspoonful with water three times
        a day after meals.
```

In the inscription the quantities are in the accusative case, as
they are the objects of the verb *recipe*, e.g. ℥ i above would be written
out *unciam unam*. The ingredients are in the genitive case, e.g.
one ounce *of* syrup. It is this genitive which so often embarrasses
the prescriber and prompts him to use abbreviated Latin titles.
Abbreviations have sometimes led to serious misunderstanding.
A good rule to avoid ambiguity is to use the full stem of the Latin
word and omit only the changeable ending.

Note that in the subscription *misce* is followed by *Fiat mistura*.
This looks redundant but is not. *Mistura* means a preparation to
be swallowed. Phrases like *Fiat mistura, Fiat collyrium, Fiat
oculentum*, are warnings to the pharmacist of the intended use of
the prescription which may not be entirely clear from the label.
It was a good practice, but it has not been carried over into English
prescriptions. In the latter it is thus particularly important to
make the label fully informative.

A glossary of Latin words, with accepted abbreviations, follows.

NOUNS—with abbreviations for the genitive case

Acetas,-atis, m.	Acet.	an acetate
Acidum,-i, n.	Ac.	an acid
Adeps, Adipis, m.	Adip.	lard
Capsula,-ae, f.	Cap.	capsule
Ceratum,-i, n.		a waxy ointment
Cerevisia,-ae, f.		beer
Charta,-ae, f.		a paper (powder wrapped in paper)

Cibus,-i, m.		food
Cochleare,-is,-ia, n.	Coch.	spoonful
Collunarium,-i, n.	Collun.	nasal wash or douche
Collutorium,-i, n.	Collut.	a mouth wash
Collyrium,-i, n.	Collyr.	an eye wash or eye drops
Cyathus,-i, m.	Cyath.	drinking cup or glass
Dosis,-is, f.	Dos.	a dose
Emplastrum,-i, n.	Empl.	a plaster
Emulsio,-onis, f.	Emuls.	an emulsion
(*Emulsum,-i*, n. U.S.P.)		
Enema,-atis, n.	Enem.	an enema or clyster
Gutta,-ae, f.	Gtt.	a drop
Haustus,-us, m.	Haust.	A draught (the whole to be taken at one time)
Hora,-ae, f.	H. or Hor.	hour
Lac, Lactis, n.		milk
Linctus,-us, n.		a viscous liquid for oral use
Linimentum,-i, n.	Lin.	a liniment
Liquor,-oris, m.	Liq.	official solution
Lotio,-onis, f.	Lot.	a lotion
Mistura,-ae, f.	Mist.	a mixture
Mucilago,-aginis, f.	Mucil.	a mucilage
Nitras,-atis, m.	Nitrat.	a nitrate
Nitris,-itis, m.	Nitrit.	a nitrite
Numerus,-i, m.	Num.	a number
Oleum,-i, n.	Ol.	an oil
Pars,-tis, f.		a part
Pasta,-ae, f.	Past.	a paste
Pulvis,-eris, m.	Pulv.	a powder
Prandium,-i, n.		dinner
Sapo,-onis, m.	Sap.	a soap
Semis,-issis, m.	s̅s̅	a half
Solutio,-onis, f.	Sol.	a solution
Spiritus,-us, m.	Sp.	a spirit
Sulphas,-atis, m.	Sulphat.	a sulphate
Sulphidum,-i n.	Sulphid.	a sulphide
Suppositorium,-i, n.	Supp.	a suppository

Syrupus,-i, m.	Syr.	a syrup
Tinctura,-ae, f.	Tinct.	a tincture
Unguentum,-i, n.	Ung.	an ointment

ADJECTIVES

Acidus,-a,-um	Acid.	acid
Albus,-a,-um	Alb.	white
Amarus,-a,-um	Amar.	bitter
Aromaticus,-a,-um	Aromat.	aromatic
Compositus,-a,-um	Comp.	compound
Destillatus,-a,-um	Dest.	distilled
Dilutus,-a,-um	Dil.	diluted
Dimidius,-a,-um		half
Dulcis,-is,-e	Dulc.	sweet
Durus,-a,-um	Dur.	hard
Flavus,-a,-um	Flav.	yellow
Fortis,-is,-e	Fort.	strong
Levis,-is,-e	Lev.	light
Liquidus,-a,-um	Liq.	liquid
Mitis,-is,-e	Mit.	weak
Mollis,-is,-e	Moll.	soft
Ponderosus,-a,-um	Pond.	heavy
Simplex (gen. *-icis*)	Simpl.	simple
Solubilis,-is,-e	Solub.	soluble
Viridis,-is,-e	Vir.	green

VERBS AND OPERATIVE EXPRESSIONS

Agite, 2nd sing. imperative	Agit.	shake
Agite bene		shake well
Cape, 2nd sing. imperative		take thou
Capiat, 3rd sing. subj.		let him take
Divide, 2nd sing. imperative	Div.	divide
Fiat, 3rd sing. pres. pass. subj.		letthere be made
Fiat lotio		let a lotion be made
Fiat pulvis et mitte		
tales XX		let a powder be made and send twenty such
Fiat pulvis et divide in		let a powder be made
partes aequales XX		and divide into 20 equal parts

Fiant, 3rd pl. pres. pass. subj.

     Fiant pulveres tales XX   let twenty such powders be made

Misce, 2nd sing. imperative	M.	mix
Mitte, 2nd sing. imperative	Mit.	send
Ne repetatur	N. rep.	not to be repeated
Signa, 2nd sing. imperative	Sig.	label
Signetur, 3rd sing. pres. pass. subj.	Sig.	let it be labelled
Sumat, 3rd sing. pres. subj.		let him take
Sumendus, gerundive of *sumo*		to be taken

WEIGHTS AND MEASURES

Cochleare amplum / *magnum* / *plenum*	℥ ss̄	a tablespoonful
Cochleare medium / *modicum*	℥ ii	a dessertspoonful
Cochleare minimum / *parvum* / *parvulum*	℥ i	a teaspoonful
Congius,-ii, m.	C	a gallon
Drachma,-ae, f.	℥ i	a drachm
Fluidrachma,-ae, f.	℥ or f℥ (U.S.A.)	a fluid drachm
Fluiduncia,-ae, f.	℥ of f℥ (U.S.A.)	a fluid ounce
Granum,-i, n.	gr.	a grain
Libra,-ae, f.	lb.	a pound
Minimum,-i, n.	*m* or min.	a minim
Octarius,-ii, m.	0	a pint
Scrupulus,-i, m.	℈	a scruple
Uncia,-ae, f.	oz.	an ounce

OTHER WORDS AND PHRASES

Ad, prep. accus.	ad	to, up to
Ad libitum	Ad lib.	as much as desired
Alternis diebus	Alt. dieb.	every other day
Alternis horis, alterna hora	Alt. hor.	every other hour
Ana, indeclin.	āā	of each
Ante cibos	a.c.	before meals

Bis indies		twice daily
Cum, prep. abl.	c.	with
Cum cibis		with meals
Cum semisse	s̄s̄	and a half
Ex aqua	Ex aq.	in water
Febri durante		while fever lasts
Hora decubitus }	hor. decub.	} at bedtime
Hora somni }	h.s.	}
Indies		daily
Mane		in the morning
Mane nocteque		morning and night
primo mane		on rising
Per, prep. accus.		by
Per os		by mouth
Pro re nata	p.r.n.	as required
Post, prep. accus.		after
Post cibos	p.c.	after meals
Quantum sufficiat	q.s.	a sufficient quantity
Quaque	q.	each
Quaque tertia hora	q. 3 h.	every third hour
Quaque quarta hora	q. 4 h.	every fourth hour
Quotidie		daily
Tales		such
Ter in die	t.i.d.	three times a day

Numerals

1. *unus, -a, -um* (one)	5. *quinque*
2. *duo, -ae, -o*	6. *sex*
3. *tres, tria*	7. *septum*
4. *quattuor*	8. *octo*
9. *novem*	20. *viginti*
10. *decem*	21. *unus et viginti* or *viginti unus*
11. *undecim*	24. *viginti quattuor*

Ordinals

1st. *primus* (first)
2nd. *secundus*
3rd. *tertius*
4th. *quartus*

Adverbs

1. *semel* (once)
2. *bis* (twice)
3. *ter* (thrice)
4. *quater* (four times)

Seven

Dispensing

IT IS A GOOD RULE THAT A DOCTOR should not do his own dispensing. Dispensing or Magistral Pharmacy is an art and science which requires training in addition to the proper temperament. It is extremely easy to make serious, and even fatal, errors. The dispenser who understands his business can be of great help to the doctor. He can and should examine the prescription for inadvertent errors, and the doctor who resents queries or suggestions from a pharmacist regarding his prescriptions is very foolish.

The physician should know some of the elements of dispensing because he may not always have the services of a qualified pharmacist and may have to do his own dispensing or supervise a relatively untrained person.

General. First read the prescription and check doses to see that they are reasonable. Then write the label: it can be drying while the prescription is being made up. Take down the various ingredients from the shelves and line them up on the work table. Check the labels and examine the contents critically. Materials sometimes get mysteriously into the wrong bottle. When the prescription is finished, and not before, recheck all ingredients before replacing them on the shelves. Pentobarbitone can easily be misread for Phenobarbitone.

Solids are weighed and liquids measured. Some materials, e.g. iron and ammonium citrate, are best dissolved in the bottle. Other materials such as sodium carbonate are best ground up in a mortar with the solvent to hasten solution. Filtration may be required to remove particles of insoluble material. Replace all stoppers from stock bottles immediately. In fact, it is a good rule never to lay the stopper down. Interchange of stoppers can lead to most peculiar complications. Always pour from the back of a bottle to save the label. Select the proper size of bottle to suit the prescription and see that the bottle is well filled.

Tablets. Avoid, as much as possible, touching tablets while counting them.

Capsules. In filling capsules the fingers must be perfectly dry and clean. An empty capsule and a weight corresponding to the quantity to be dispensed in each capsule are placed in one scale pan. The weight of each capsule is checked in the other scale pan as it is filled and its contents are adjusted if necessary to the proper weight.

While watery solutions cannot be dispensed in capsules, some oils or alcoholic solutions can be. With such liquid fillings the two halves must be sealed together by moistening the end of the narrower capsule with water.

Capsules are made in eight sizes ranging from 3/8 to one inch in length and are numbered respectively from No. 5 to No. 000. The number of grains or of grammes which can be put into any size of capsule depends in part on the closeness of packing and on the specific gravity of the substance. The following Table gives some approximate figures in grammes for the various sizes:

	00	0	1	2	3	4	5
Reduced Iron	3.2	2.3	1.6	1.3	1.1	0.8	
Barbitone	0.53	0.46	0.29	0.24	0.1	0.07	
Quinine Sulphate	0.6	0.4	0.25	0.2	0.13	0.1	0.06
Acetylsalicylic Acid	0.8	0.5	0.37	0.3	0.26	0.15	0.1
Bismuth Carbonate	1.3	0.9	0.75	0.6	0.4		
Sodium Bicarbonate	1.0	0.7	0.5	0.4	0.3	0.2	
Powdered Digitalis	0.6		0.19	0.14	0.09	0.07	

No. 000 is too large for most persons to swallow.

Powders. If a very small quantity of an active drug like atropine is to be distributed in a much larger bulk of powder it is very important that it be distributed uniformly. This may best be done by triturating at first with twice its bulk of powder. Then that amount is triturated again with twice its volume and this process is repeated till distribution in the final quantity has been accomplished.

Ointments. When an insoluble solid such as zinc oxide or starch is to be incorporated in an ointment, it should be so finely powdered that no grittiness may be detected when the ointment is rubbed between the fingers, or in the case of oculenta, even when rubbed into the eyes. The powder is piled on an ointment slab and mixed with a spatula with a small quantity of the base. More base is added in small portions and worked in till the whole quantity has been incorporated. The pharmacopoeial ointments are made up by drug manufacturers and only modifications or special formulae are made by the retail pharmacist. Water or watery solutions can be incorporated into the Ointment of Wool Alcohols. The latter gives a less sticky and more pleasant smelling preparation than Wool Fat. These creams are essentially water in oil emulsions. On standing they sometimes "crack" with the formation of drops of water. The so-called hydrophilic ointments or creams are analogous to oil-in-water emulsions. They have been made possible by the newer emulsifying agents such as sodium lauryl suphate. They are easily made and should be made shortly before use because unless kept hermetically sealed they dry out quickly. The outstanding useful property of the group is that they are easily removed with water which makes them suitable for applying drugs such as sulphur to the scalp.

For most purposes the Simple Ointment of the B.P. is a more useful base than soft paraffin, since it contains a small quantity of wool fat and of hard paraffin, which confer stability of consistency over a wider range of temperatures.

After an ointment has been made and packed into a box or jar, a smooth professional-looking finish is given by warming a spatula and drawing it over the surface of the ointment.

Cachets. About twice as much powder can be swallowed in a single cachet as can be swallowed in a single capsule. To fill one and seal it requires either a special machine or a simple improvisation consisting of two ointment jars about one inch in diameter. A half cachet is set like a pie plate on the open mouth of the jar, i.e. resting with its rim on the rim of the jar. The required dose of powder is put into it. The upper side of the rim is moistened with a wet brush and the empty half-cachet is inverted over it. Even pressure is applied by means of a second ointment jar to make the two halves stick together.

Emulsions. Skill in making emulsions used to be a matter of some pride among pharmacists. There is little call nowadays for making them extemporaneously. The much-used emulsions of liquid paraffin and of benzyl benzoate are factory-made, although they are easy enough to make with the electric stirrers now common in every pharmacy.

Bottles. Clear glass bottles with bakelite screw-caps and with graduations in fluid ounces and in cc. are widely available. The sizes available commonly are 2, 4, 8, 15, 30, 60, 90, 120, 180, 240, 360, and 480 cc. The smallest sizes are sometimes called vials.

The keeping qualities of some dilute solutions, e.g. Physostigmine Salicylate, depend on the quality of the glass container. The U.S.P. specifies four types of glass which are acceptable for different purposes. The specifications hinge on the amount of alkali or other soluble material which can be leached out of the glass. The U.S.P. also specifies acceptable methods of measuring the light-transmission of coloured glasses which are used to protect certain solutions from inactivation by light. It is a good practice to put poisons in coloured bottles of distinctive shape so that they may be recognized by touch in dim light.

Ointment Containers. The wide-mouthed jars or boxes for ointments come in sizes known as ½, 1, 2, 3, 4, 6 and 8 oz. These would correspond in capacity to 15, 30, 60, 90, 120, 180 and 240 cc. They are made of metal, glass or paper treated with silica.

Eight

Description & Discussion of Drugs

Dᴿᵁᴳˢ ᴿᴱᴄᴼᴳᴺᴵᶻᴱᴰ by the British Pharmacopoeia, the United States Pharmacopoeia, and certain other authorities are presented in this section mainly in alphabetical order. Certain exceptions have been made to save duplication. For example, all local anaesthetics having the ending -aine, are presented together under L. All derivatives of opium and its alkaloids, including codeine and papaverine, are presented under Opium. Atropine is presented under Belladonna, and Strychnine under Nux Vomica. Vitamins and synthetic drugs of similar action are under V. Sex hormones and their derivatives and analogues are under S. Until the organization of this section becomes familiar the student will usually save time by looking first in the Index.

The arrangement has been designed to facilitate comparisons between British and United States nomenclature and standards. Whenever the same title is used in the B.P. and the U.S.P. and the specifications are essentially the same in both, no distinguishing initials (B.P. or U.S.P.) are used after the title of the drug. Synonyms are given in brackets and include those recognized by the B.P. and the U.S.P. and other common names. Trade names in the sense of trade-marked names, are preceded by the initials T.N. It should not be assumed that substances sold under such names are always identical with those sold under the corresponding official names. New drugs, or preparations not described in any pharmacopoeia or formulary are followed by the letter N. The letters P.I. (International Protocol) and I.A. (International Agreement) refer to nomenclature suggested at a conference in Brussels in 1925.

Doses are given only for drugs or preparations which are administered internally and follow the various names and synonyms. For a number of drugs the U.S.P. states that the dose is "to be determined by the physician according to the needs of the patient." This has been shortened to "as prescribed," or "as determined by the physician."

42

Formulae, molecular weights, melting points in degrees centigrade, etcetera, follow when they are available. Solubilities, specific gravities, and analogous data are given for 25°C., unless otherwise stated. This is in accordance with the practice of the Canadian Supplements to the B.P. and of the U.S.P. The B.P. gives solubilities usually at 15.5°C. Figures preceded by the expression Gm./cc. are taken from the B.P. and refer to density uncorrected for weight in air, at 20°C.

Figures for solubility follow the letter S, and mean the least volume of solvent (cc.) which will dissolve 1 Gm. of the solute at 25°C., unless otherwise stated. The letters W, A, B, E, C, and G stand for water, alcohol (95%), benzol, ether, chloroform, and glycerin respectively. The figures for solubility are approximate only.

Abbreviations may be used instead of numbers to indicate solubility. Their interpretation according to the U.S.P. is given in the following table:

Term	Abbreviation	Parts of Solvent Required to Dissolve 1 Part of Solute
Very soluble	vs.	less than 1 part
Freely soluble	fs.	from 1 to 10 parts
Soluble	sol.	from 10 to 30 parts
Sparingly soluble	sps.	from 30 to 100 parts
Slightly soluble	ss.	from 100 to 1000 parts
Very slightly soluble	vss.	from 1000 to 10,000 parts
Practically insoluble	ins.	more than 10,000 parts

Descriptions of drugs are not necessarily quoted verbatim from the B.P. or U.S.P. or any other source but have been composed with the particular purpose of this book in mind.

Regarding *tablets*, *capsules*, *injections*, and similar preparations, a difference in the practice of the B.P. and the U.S.P. should be noted. The U.S.P. lists sizes or strengths commonly available. They may not, however, be available in Canada but it would not be unreasonable to ask a pharmacist to try to obtain them. The B.P., on the other hand, usually gives only one size or strength which is to be supplied if no size is specified on a prescription. It thus represents a commonly used size.

Since the construction of Latin titles for such preparations as capsules, tablets, and injections, is readily deducible, these titles have been omitted to save space.

In deference to what seems to be universal usage among medical men on this continent, the abbreviation cc. is used instead of ml. If in any circumstance the small difference between the cubic centimetre and millilitre is of importance, cc. is to be read as meaning millilitre (see chapter I).

Acacia. *Acacia.* (Gum Acacia, Gum Arabic)

S: 2W, ins. A, forms a viscid, slightly acid solution in water. A gum exuded from *Acacia Senegal* and other species, having a bland mucilaginous taste; supplied in flakes, lumps, or powder. Acacia in aqueous solution is precipitated by alcohol in concentrations of 30% or over.

Powdered Acacia B.P. *Acaciae Pulvis.* A white powder.

Acacia Mucilage U.S.P. *Mucilago Acaciae.* (Mucilage of Gum Arabic)

Dose: 15 cc. (4 fl. dr.). Acacia 350, Benzoic Acid 2, Water to make 1,000 cc.

Mucilage of Acacia B.P. *Mucilago Acaciae*

Acacia 40, Chloroform Water 60.

Acacia Syrup U.S.P. *Syrupus Acaciae.*

Acacia 100, Sodium Benzoate 1.0, Sucrose 800, Vanilla Ticture 5, and Water to make 1000 cc.

⟨ Acacia and its preparations are used for their colloidal properties, e.g. to delay the settling of suspensions, to emulsify oils, and to make pills and lozenges. The use of Acacia for intravenous injection to increase the volume and colloidal osmotic pressure of blood has been largely abandoned. See Tragacanth.

Acetanilid U.S.P. *Acetanilidum.* (Antifebrin, N-phenylacetamide)

Dose: 0.2 Gm. (3 gr.). $CH_3CONHC_6H_5$. Mol.wt. 135.16. M.p. 114-116°. S: 190 W, 20 W 100°, 3.5 A, 0.6 A 78°, 4 C, 17 E, 5 G. White crystals or a white crystalline powder; odourless; taste pungent.

Acetanilid Tablets U.S.P.

Sizes, 200 and 300 mg. (3 and 5 gr.).

⟨ Acetanilid lowers the temperature in fever and relieves pain of the less intense varieties. Although a common ingredient of proprietary headache powders, it is little used medically. Prolonged use, or large doses, cause methaemoglobinaemia and consequent cyanosis.

Acetic Acid. *Acidum Aceticum*
Sp.gr. 1.045, 25°C. Gm./cc. 1.039-1.040. S: misc. W, A, G.
A clear colourless liquid having a strong characteristic odour and
sharp acid taste. Contains 32.5-33.5% (B.P.), 36-37% (U.S.P.)
w/w CH_3COOH.

Dilute Acetic Acid B.P. *Acidum Aceticum Dilutum*
A colourless liquid containing 5.7-6.3% w/w CH_3COOH.

Glacial Acetic Acid. *Acidum Aceticum Glaciale*
$CH_3.COOH$. Mol.wt. 60.05. B.p. 118°. Gm./cc. 1.048-1.051.
S: misc. W, A, G. A clear colourless liquid with a pungent
characteristic odour; *caution* caustic. Contains not less than
99% (B.P.), 99.4% (U.S.P.), of CH_3COOH.

Acetone B.P. (1932). *Acetonum.* (Dimethyl Ketone)
$CH_3.CO.CH_3$. Mol.wt. 58.08. B.p. 56°. S: misc. W, A, E, C
and with most volatile oils. A transparent, colourless, mobile,
volatile liquid, having a characteristic odour; inflammable.

℘ Acetone is used as a solvent, or for cleansing the skin or for
drying syringes and pipettes.

Acetophenetidin U.S.P. *Acetophenetidinum.* **Phenacetin B.P.**
Phenacetinum. (Acetophenetidin, Acetyl-p-phenetidine, Aceto-
p-phenetidine)
DOSES: B.P. 0.3-0.6 Gm. (5-10 gr.); U.S.P. 0.3 Gm. (5 gr.).
$CH_3.CO.NH.C_6H_4.OC_2H_5$. Mol. wt. 179.21. M.p. 134-136°. S:
1,300 W, 85 W 100°, 15 A, 3 A 78°, 15 C, 130 E. White glistening
crystalline scales or a fine white crystalline powder; odourless;
taste slightly bitter.

Acetophenetidin Tablets U.S.P.
Sizes, 120, 200, 300 mg. (2, 3, 5 gr.)

Tablets of Phenacetin B.P. (Acetophenetidin Tablets)
Size, 0.3 Gm. (5 gr.).

℘ Taken orally, phenacetin relieves pain of less severe kinds and
reduces fever. Large doses or prolonged administration will cause
methaemoglobinaemia. It is, however, considered a safe drug to
use in moderation as an alternative to, or in combination with,
acetylsalicylic acid.

Acetylsalicylic Acid. *Acidum Acetylsalicylicum.* (Aspirin)

DOSES: B.P. 0.3-1 Gm. (5-15 gr.); U.S.P. 0.3 Gm. (5 gr.). $CH_3.CO_2.C_6H_4.COOH$. Mol.wt. 180.15. M.p. 135-138°. S: 300 W, 5 A, 17 C, 10-15 E; sol. in strong solutions of ammonium acetate. Small, colourless, needle-shaped or tabular crystals or a white crystalline powder; odourless; taste slightly acid.

Acetylsalicylic Acid Capsules U.S.P.

Size, 300 mg. (5 gr.).

Acetylsalicylic Acid Tablets U.S.P. (Aspirin Tablets)

Sizes, 60 and 300 mg. (1 and 5 gr.).

Tablets of Acetylsalicylic Acid B.P.

Size, 0.3 Gm. (5 gr.). *Note: in Canada, Aspirin is a trade name.*

Compound Tablets of Codeine B.P. (Tablets of Aspirin, Phenacetin and Codeine)

Each tablet contains: Acetylsalicylic Acid 0.26 Gm. (4 gr.), Phenacetin 0.26 Gm. (4 gr.), Codeine Phosphate 0.008 Gm. (1/8 gr.).

Tablets of Acetylsalicylic Acid and Phenacetin B.P. (Aspirin and Phenacetin Tablets)

Each tablet contains: Acetylsalicylic Acid 0.23 Gm. (3½ gr.), Phenacetin 0.16 Gm. (2½ gr.).

❡ Acetylsalicylic acid relieves pain if it is not too severe and lowers the temperature in fever. Large doses (5-10 Gm. per day in divided doses) are commonly given for long periods to control the symptoms of rheumatic fever, often with an equal weight or double its weight of sodium bicarbonate. Acetylsalicylate is rapidly converted to salicylate in the body but the acetylated form while it lasts is thought to have a stronger analgesic action. It is doubtful whether salicylate influences the processes of rheumatic disease in any way.

Overdosage gives rise to salicylism characterized by ringing in the ears, nausea, vomiting, dyspnoea, coma (acidotic), and death. Hypoprothrombinaemia is a regular effect of intensive therapy with salicylates and may lead to haemorrhages.

Idiosyncrasies to acetylsalicylic acid are fairly common and may vary from nausea with small doses to severe allergic manifestations.

Acetylsalicylic acid is frequently prescribed with codeine to obtain a greater degree of analgesic action. A maximum effect seems to be obtained with 0.3 Gm. of acetylsalicylic acid and 30 mg. of codeine.

Acetylsalicylic acid is used for its analgesic effect in dentistry. Claims have been made for its local anaesthetic effect when applied as a powder or paste for relief of pain in connection with peridontal diseases or when employed as a gargle and mouth rinse, but without convincing evidence of its usefulness.

Aconite B.P. *Aconitum.* (Aconite Root)
Dried root of *Aconitum Napellus Linn.*

Powdered Aconite B.P. *Aconiti Pulvis.* A greyish-brown powder.

⟨The actions of aconite are due to the very poisonous alkaloid aconitine, once a common ingredient of arrow poisons. Aconitine acts on nerve endings to produce at first tingling and later numbness and anaesthesia. With adequate doses by mouth the heart rate is decreased. With overdoses, death may ensue from cardiac and circulatory failure. A dose of about 5 Gm. of aconite or 5 mg. of aconitine is usually fatal.

There is little to recommend the internal or external use of aconite in medical practice. It is sometimes used in dentistry in a liniment with iodine, applied to the gums as a counter-irritant.

Liniment of Aconite B.P. *Linimentum Aconiti*
An alcoholic extract representing 50% w/v of aconite. Contains Camphor 3% and 75-85% v/v of C_2H_5OH.

Adrenal Cortex Extract N.N.R.
Doses: 50-100 cc. by intravenous or subcutaneous injection, initially; 10 cc. daily by subcutaneous injection for maintenance. An extract of adrenal glands of domesticated animals used as food by man, containing adrenal cortical steroids but little or no epinephrine. The final product is an aqueous solution containing 0.9% NaCl and 10% of C_2H_5OH. Each cc. contains 50 dog units or 2.5 rat units. The assay depends on the maintenance of life in adrenalectomized dogs, and the maintenance of growth in young adrenalectomized rats. Available in 10 cc. and 50 cc. vials. The Connaught Medical Research Laboratories supply Adrenal Cortical Extract in 25 cc. vials (30 dog units per cc.).

Lipo-Adrenal Cortex N.N.R.
Doses: 1-2 cc. daily by intramuscular injection for maintenance. Adrenal cortical steroids extracted from the adrenal

glands of hogs, and dissolved in a vegetable oil.   Each cc. contains
40 rat units, the equivalent of 2 mg. of 11-dehydro-17-hydroxy-
corticosterone (Cortisone) or 1 mg. of compound F.   Preserved with
chlorobutanol 0.5 %.   Available in 1 cc. and 5 cc. vials.

Adrenocorticotrophic Hormone N.   (T.N. Acthar, ACTH)

Doses: 80-120 mg. daily in divided doses by intramuscular
injection; for investigational use only.   ACTH is protein material
obtained from pituitary glands of hogs.   It is purified to remove
oxytocic and vasopressor principles of the posterior lobe and certain
active principles of the anterior lobe.   It is assayed biologically by
its effect of decreasing the ascorbic acid content of the adrenal
cortex of hypophysectomized rats.   The usual dose of 20 mg. is
supplied as a sterile dry powder in a vial, to be dissolved in 2 cc.
of Water for Injection immediately before use.

Cortisone Acetate N.   (T.N. Cortone Acetate)

Doses: 100-200 mg. daily by intramuscular injection; 11-
dehydro-17-hydroxycorticosterone-21-acetate. S: 50,000 W. Supplied in 20 cc. vials as a sterile suspension in isotonic saline solution,
containing 1.5% of benzyl alcohol as a preservative.   Each cc. contains 25 mg. of Cortisone Acetate.   Cortisone is also effective when
given orally and is available in tablets each containing 25 mg.
Cortisone Acetate.

⟪ More than 25 steroid substances have been isolated from the
adrenal cortex.   Of these, only a few are capable of maintaining
adrenalectomized animals in good health.   The most active ones
are Cortisone (Kendall's Compound E) and Kendall's Compound F.
The latter is 17-hydroxy-corticosterone.   It differs from cortisone
in having an OH group instead of a keto group at the 11 position.
There is some reason to think that Compound F may be the principal hormone produced by the human adrenal cortex.   The adrenal
cortex extracts presumably owe their activity to the presence of
Compounds E or F or related substances.   Another closely related
substance is deoxycortone (DCA, or Doca), a steroid prepared synthetically from stigmasterol.   Deoxycortone can maintain life in
adrenalectomized animals but does not restore full vigour or normal
resistance to stresses.   It is deficient in certain important actions
of Compounds E and F, which are described below.

The main use of adrenal cortex extracts is in the treatment of adrenal insufficiency (Addison's disease).   They have also been recommended for alleviation of withdrawal symptoms of alcohol addiction.   The aqueous preparations are used when rapid effects are needed.   The oily extract is used for slower and more prolonged effects in maintenance.   The adrenal cortex extracts are very expensive and it has been customary to eke them out with the less expensive deoxycortone.   The latter sometimes suffices by itself provided the patient lives very carefully and succeeds in avoiding infections.   When cortisone becomes plentiful and less expensive it may well supplant entirely the cortical extracts and deoxycortone. Very small doses, e.g. 5 mg. a day, are sufficient for the maintenance of patients with Addison's disease.   Much larger doses, e.g. 100-300 mg. a day, have been shown to modify dramatically the course of rheumatoid arthritis, rheumatic fever, and a large number of other so-called diseases of adaptation, such as lupus erythematosus, nonspecific iritis, and bronchial asthma.

⟪ Cortisone has many actions; or to put it another way, no single fundamental action has yet been discovered which will explain all of the diverse effects which it produces.   The sodium retaining action of cortisone is less prominent than that of deoxycortone. Small doses of cortisone are effective in correcting the excessive loss of sodium and retention of potassium which are characteristic of Addison's disease.   However, large doses of cortisone do not have as much tendency to cause excessive retention of sodium as do large doses of deoxycortone.   Cortisone is much more effective than deoxycortone in correcting the muscle weakness and the deficiency of liver glycogen in adrenalectomized animals.   In large doses, cortisone raises the blood sugar, decreases circulating eosinophiles and in experimental animals causes spleen and thymus gland to decrease in weight. After several weeks of administration to humans, in daily doses of 100 mg. or more, it causes some growth of facial hair in women, rounding of facial contour and the appearance of livid striations on the sides of the abdomen.   The three effects last mentioned are characteristic of Cushing's syndrome.   Cortisone also retards the healing of wounds by depression of granulation tissue; it also interferes with the action of hyaluronidase.   Another action of importance is the augmentation of diuresis in response to water intake.   All these apparently unrelated, but important, actions have potential value in the treatment of disease.

Adrenocorticotrophic hormone can produce all the effects of Compounds E or F if injected into patients with normal adrenal glands. In addition, it causes depletion of ascorbic acid and cholesterol in the adrenal cortex. Presumably the depletion of ascorbic acid is connected with the liberation of adrenal cortical hormone. ACTH is sometimes injected to test the functional state of the adrenal cortex.

Acriflavine B.P. *Acriflavina*

A mixture of hydrochlorides of 2:8-diamino-10-methylacridinium chloride, and 2:8-diaminoacridine. S: 3 W (may precipitate on dilution or on standing), 500 physiological solution of sodium chloride at 15.5°; sol. A 90%, G; almost ins. E, C, fixed and volatile oils and liquid paraffin. An orange-red to red crystalline powder; odourless; taste acid.

⁅ Acriflavine is bactericidal at 1:1000 dilution and bacteriostatic at much higher dilutions, even in the presence of pus and serum. A solution of 1:1000 may be used to treat wounds and impregnate dressings to prevent infection. See also Proflavine.

Agar. *Agar.* (Agar-Agar)

Dose: U.S.P. 4 Gm. (1 dr.). S: slowly sol. hot W; ins. cold W· A dried gelatinous material obtained from *Gelidium cartilagineum* and other red algae. Translucent, pale strips or sheets, or greywhite flakes, or a coarse powder.

Agar Powder B.P.

Doses: 4-16 Gm. (60-240 gr.).

⁅ Agar consists largely of the hemicellulose, gelose. It passes through the intestinal tract without destruction but it absorbs water and increases greatly in bulk, which gives it laxative properties.

Normal Human Serum Albumin U.S.P. *Albuminum Seri Humanum Normale*

Dose: intravenous, 25 Gm. (100 cc. of 25% solution). A sterile solution of the serum albumin component of the blood from healthy donors prepared by a fractionation process. It must be free from harmful substances detectable by animal inoculation and may or may not contain a preservative.

Alcohol U.S.P.   Alcohol 95% B.P.   *Alcohol.   (Spiritus Vini Rectificatus)*

$C_2H_5.OH$.   Mol.wt. 46.07.   B.p. 78°.   Sp.gr. 0.816 at 15.5°. S: misc. W, E, C.   A transparent, colourless, mobile, volatile liquid; odour characteristic; taste burning.   Burns with a blue, smokeless flame.   Contains not less than 94.9% v/v or 92.3% w/w of C_2H_5OH (U.S.P.) at 15.56°, or 94.7-95.2% v/v (B.P.)

Dilute Alcohols B.P.

A series is described containing 90, 80, 70, 60, 50, 45, 25, 20% C_2H_5OH by volume.

Diluted Alcohol U.S.P.   *Alcohol Dilutum.*   (Diluted Ethanol)

Alcohol U.S.P. 500, Water 500.   Contains 48.4-49.5% by volume of C_2H_5OH at 15.56°.

Alcohol 90% B.P.   *Spiritus Rectificatus.*   (Rectified Spirit)

Sp.gr. 0.832-0.835 at 15.5°.   Alcohol 95% 947, Distilled Water to make 1000 cc.

Proof Spirit N.   *Spiritus Tenuior*

Content of C_2H_5OH: British,—49.3% w/w or 56.9% v/v; U.S.A.—42.5% w/w or 50.0% v/v.

℄ Ethyl Alcohol 70% w/w or 76.9% v/v at 15.5° is bactericidal but does not kill spores.   Bactericidal potency decreases rapidly with concentrations below 76.9% v/v.   Concentrations as low as 18% v/v are still bacteriostatic and fungistatic and thus have a value as a preservative.

Moderate doses by mouth have effects popularly described as "stimulating."   They probably result from depression of cerebral inhibition.   Such doses are also analgesic, i.e. they dull sensations of pain; they also cause vasodilation in the skin and increased gastric secretion, particularly on an empty stomach.   Motor skill and judgement are impaired from the onset.   A concentration of 150 mg. per 100 cc. of blood is widely accepted as evidence of alcoholic intoxication.

Alcohol applied externally cools and hardens the skin and protects against bedsores.   For trigeminal neuralgia and other forms of intractable pain, alcohol may be injected around the affected nerve trunk.   Wallerian degeneration ensues and gives relief from pain for many months.

In dentistry alcohol may be used as a desiccant in the preparation of cavities and in root canal therapy.   Weaker concentrations (about 75% by volume) are useful for sponging out cavities and removing debris from pulp chambers. It is employed as a solvent for antiseptics such as thymol, phenol, and camphor.

Almond Oil B.P. *Oleum Amygdalae*. **Expressed Almond Oil U.S.P.**
Oleum Amygdalae Expressum. (Sweet Almond Oil)
DOSES: B.P. 15-30 cc. ($\frac{1}{2}$-1 fl.oz.). Sp.gr. 0.910-0.915. S: ss. A, misc. E, C, B, and petroleum benzin. The oil expressed from the kernels of varieties of *Prunus Amygdalus* Batsch. A clear, straw-coloured, oily liquid, with a bland taste; almost odourless.

⟪Almond Oil has had a variety of uses. It has been given internally as a laxative and applied externally as an emollient for chapped hands. It has also been used as a vehicle for injections and is a common ingredient of cold creams.

Purified Volatile Oil of Bitter Almond B.P. *Oleum Amygdalae Volatile Purificatum*
Not less than 95% benzaldehyde C_6H_5CHO. S: 2 A 70% at 15.5°. Gm./cc. 1.040-1.044.
Prepared by distillation from the cake left after pressing out the fixed oil from almond, peach, or apricot kernels. A colourless or pale-yellow liquid; odour and taste those of bitter almonds.

⟪A flavouring agent used in the Emulsion of Cod-liver Oil.

Aloe U.S.P. **Aloes B.P.** *Aloe*
DOSE: U.S.P. 0.25 Gm. (4 gr.). Aloes is the dried juice from the cut leaves of various species of *Aloe;* dark-brown or greenish-brown masses having a characteristic odour and bitter nauseous taste; almost entirely soluble in 60% alcohol.

Powdered Aloes B.P. *Aloes Pulvis*
DOSES: 0.12-0.3 Gm. (2-5 gr.).

Pill of Aloes B.P. *Pilula Aloes*. (Aloes Pill)
DOSES: 0.25-0.5 Gm. (4-8 gr.). Aloes 58% w/w with Hard Soap, Oil of Caraway, and Syrup of Liquid Glucose.

⟪Aloes or aloin is a common ingredient of "vegetable laxative" pills. The laxative action is attributed to emodin and other anthracene derivatives, acting for the most part on the large intestine to promote peristalsis. The pill is usually taken at night and soft stools are passed in the morning. Some of the drug may be excreted in the urine, giving it a red or violet colour if alkaline, or brownish-yellow if acid.   Aloes has the reputation of producing griping and hence belladonna is often combined with it to reduce this effect.   Aloes is also reputed to stimulate uterine contractions and cause abortion, consequently it is wise to avoid prescribing it for constipation during pregnancy.

Aloin. *Aloinum*
   DOSES: B.P. 15-60 mg. ($\frac{1}{4}$-1 gr.);   U.S.P. 15 mg. ($\frac{1}{4}$ gr.). S: sol. W, A, acetone; ss. E.   A yellow micro-crystalline powder; odourless or with a slight odour of aloes; taste intensely bitter; a partially purified preparation representing the active constituents of aloes.

Alum B.P.   *Alumen.*   (Ammonium Alum or Potassium Alum)
   $AlNH_4(SO_4)_2 12H_2O$ (mol.wt. 453.32); $AlK(SO_4)_2 12H_2O$ (mol.wt. 474.38).   S: ammonium alum, 7 W, 0.3 W at 100°; potassium alum 7.5 W, 0.3 W at 100°; both almost ins. A, sol. G.   Colourless crystals; taste sweet and astringent.

   ℂAlum precipitates protein, is germicidal in 5% solution and bacteriostatic in 1% solution.   The powder is sometimes applied to ulcers in the mouth or to stop bleeding from tooth sockets.   For astringent action, a 2% solution may be used as a vaginal douche and a 1% solution as a mouth wash or eye wash.   To produce emesis 1 Gm. may be given in syrup every 15 minutes.   It acts by local irritation and produces no depression.

Aluminum Acetate Solution U.S.P.   *Liquor Alumini Acetatis.*
   (Burow's Solution)
   Made from Aluminum Subacetate Solution, Glacial Acetic Acid and Water.   Contains 4.8-5.8% w/v of Aluminum Acetate.   For external use.   Dilute with 9 vols. of water.

Aluminum Subacetate Solution U.S.P.   *Liquor Alumini Subacetatis*
   Made from Aluminum Sulfate 16 Gm. with Acetic Acid, Precipitated Calcium Carbonate and Water to make 100 cc.   For external use.   Dilute with 9 vols. water.

Aluminum Hydroxide Gel U.S.P.   *Gelatum Alumini Hydroxidi.*
   (Colloidal Aluminum Hydroxide)
   DOSE: 8 cc. (2 fl.dr.).   A white viscous suspension, translucent in thin layers.   Flavouring oils or saccharin may be added.

Dried Aluminum Hydroxide Gel U.S.P. *Gelatum Alumini Hydroxidi Siccum*

DOSE: 0.6 Gm. (10 gr.). S: ins. W, A; sol. dil. mineral acid and in solutions of fixed alkali. A white, tasteless, odourless, amorphous powder. 1 Gm. combines with not less than 250 cc. of N/10 HCl.

Aluminum Phosphate Gel U.S.P. *Gelatum Alumini Phosphatis*

DOSE: 8 cc. (2 fl.dr.). A white viscous suspension which may show some settling out on standing. Flavouring oils, sugar, or saccharin may be used.

℥ Aluminium hydroxide reacts with hydrochloric acid in the stomach to form aluminium chloride. The free acidity is reduced. The pH does not rise to 7.0 but stays well on the acid side. The amount of hydrochloric acid secreted is also reduced, perhaps because of the astringent action of the aluminium chloride. Very little aluminium is absorbed. Most of it is excreted in the faeces as phosphate. The absorption of phosphate is prevented and may lead to phosphate deficiency. Aluminium phosphate has been used in place of the hydroxide to avoid the adverse effect on phosphate absorption. Aluminium phosphate is used for the symptomatic as well as systematic treatment of peptic ulcer.

Aluminum Sulfate U.S.P. *Alumini Sulfas*

$Al_2(SO_4)_3 . 18 H_2O$. Mol. wt. 666.43. S: 1 W; ins. A. White crystalline powder or shining plates; odourless; taste sweetish, becoming mildly astringent. See Alum.

Amaranth U.S.P. *Amaranthum*

$C_{20}H_{11}N_2O_{10}S_3Na_3$. Mol.wt. 604.48. S: 15 W; ss. A. A dark brown powder. A dark-red colour is imparted when the concentration of this dye is 1:10,000. The colour is stable in acids and alkalis.

℥ This dye may be used to colour medicines for oral administration.

Amaranth Solution U.S.P. *Liquor Amaranthi*

Amaranth 1, Distilled Water to make 100.

Amidopyrine B.P. *Amidopyrina.* **Aminopyrine U.S.P.** *Aminopyrina* (Dimethylaminophenazone)

DOSES: B.P. 0.3-0.6 Gm. (5-10 gr.); U.S.P. 0.3 Gm. (5 gr.). $C_{13}H_{17}N_3O$. Mol.wt. 231.29. M.p. 107-109°. S: 18 W, 1.5 A, 1 C, 13 E. Colourless crystals or white powder; odourless; almost tasteless.

⟨Amidopyrine is an effective antipyretic and analgesic agent. Its use, however, is hard to justify because of the risk of producing granulocytopenia in susceptible persons. It is true that this risk is small but it is unnecessary, since other drugs are available which are just as effective.

Aminacrine Hydrochloride B.P. *Aminacrinae Hydrochloridum*. (5-aminoacridine. T.N. Acramine Yellow, Monacrine) $C_{13}H_{10}N_2.HCl.H_2O$. Mol.wt. 248.71. S: 300 W at 20°; sol. A 90%, G; almost ins. E, C. Pale-yellow, crystalline, odourless powder; taste bitter.

⟨Aminacrine is an effective antiseptic in concentrations of 1:1000 and has little damaging effect on living tissues. It causes less staining of tissues and of linen than do other acridine antiseptics such as acriflavine.

Aminophylline U.S.P. *Aminophyllina*. (Theophylline Ethylenediamine). **Theophylline with Ethylenediamine B.P.** *Theophyllina cum Aethylenediamina*

DOSES: B.P. 0.1-0.5 Gm. (1½-8 gr.); U.S.P. oral 0.2 Gm. (3 gr.), intramuscular or intravenous 0.25 Gm. (4 gr.). $C_{16}H_{24}N_{10}O_4.2H_2O$, Mol.wt. 456.46. S: 5 W (solution becomes turbid on standing); ins. A, E. A white or slightly yellowish powder having a bitter taste and a slight ammoniacal odour. Contains about 80% of anhydrous theophylline and about 13% of ethylenediamine.

Aminophylline Injection U.S.P.

DOSE: 0.25 Gm. (4 gr.) intravenously or intramuscularly. Strengths: 250 mg. (4 gr.) in 10 cc., or 500 mg. (7½ gr.) in 2 cc., or 500 mg. (7½ gr.) in 20 cc.

Injection of Theophylline with Ethylenediamine B.P.

DOSES: intravenous or intramuscular 0.1-0.5 Gm. (1½-8 gr.). Strengths: (a) 0.25 Gm. in 10 cc. for intravenous use, (b) 0.5 Gm. in 2 cc. for intramuscular use. Solution (a) is to be supplied if strength and route of administration are not stated.

⟨The principal active ingredient of Aminophylline is theophylline. Ethylenediamine serves to increase the solubility of the theophylline. Whether it contributes in any other way to the action of theophylline is doubtful. Sodium acetate also increases the solubility of theophylline but Theophylline and Sodium Acetate, although an official preparation, has not achieved the popularity of Aminophylline. The actions of theophylline which are most useful are: relaxation of bronchiolar musculature, coronary dilation, stimulation of the myocardium, diuresis, and stimulation of respiration.

Aminophylline may be given orally, rectally, or intravenously to relieve bronchial asthma. It is also effective in pulmonary oedema (left ventricular failure). It is sometimes given in congestive failure of the heart to augment the action of mercurial diuretics.

A number of sudden deaths have been reported following the intravenous injection of Aminophylline. In certain cases of asthma, only intravenous injections of Aminophylline will afford relief, and consequently some risk is justified.

Aminophylline Suppositories U.S.P.
Each suppository contains 500 mg. (7½ gr.) of Aminophylline.

Aminophylline Tablets U.S.P.
DOSE: 0.2 Gm. (3 gr.). Sizes 100 and 200 mg. (1½ and 3 gr.).

Dilute Solution of Ammonia B.P. Diluted Ammonia Solution U.S.P. *Liquor Ammoniae Dilutus.* (Ammonia Water, Diluted Ammonium Hydroxide Solution, Solution of Ammonia)
Contains about 10% of NH_3 by weight.

⟪Solutions of ammonia are employed in liniments for their rubefacient effect on the skin. Serious poisoning can occur by inhalation of ammonia vapour. About 30 cc. of the strong, or 90 cc. of the dilute solution by mouth are usually fatal.

Strong Solution of Ammonia. *Liquor Ammoniae Fortis.* (Stronger Ammonia Water, Stronger Ammonium Hydroxide Solution)
Gm./cc. 0.880-0.886. Sp.gr. U.S.P. about 0.9. A clear colourless liquid; odour strongly pungent and characteristic. Contains about 27-30% by weight (U.S.P.) or 31.5-33.5% by weight (B.P.) of ammonia.

Aromatic Ammonia Spirit U.S.P. *Spiritus Ammoniae Aromaticus*
DOSE: 2 cc. (30 min.). Ammonium Carbonate 3.4%, Diluted Ammonia Solution 9%, with Lemon Oil, Lavender Oil, Myristica Oil, Alcohol, and Distilled Water. Contains 62-68% v/v of C_2H_5OH.

Aromatic Spirit of Ammonia B.P. *Spiritus Ammoniae Aromaticus.*
(Spirit of Sal Volatile)
DOSES: 1-4 cc. (15-60 min.). Ammonium Bicarbonate 2.5%,
Strong Solution of Ammonia 6%, with Oil of Lemon, Oil of Nutmeg,
Alcohol, and Distilled Water. Contains 65-70% v/v of C_2H_5OH.

₡ Aromatic Spirit of Ammonia has a popular reputation as a
stimulant. Inhalation of its vapour irritates the nose and reflexly
increases respiration and heart rate. Diluted with about 15 times
its volume of water and swallowed, it produces a sensation of
warmth. It is hard to think of any rational use for it except to
encourage the faint-hearted.

Ammonium Bicarbonate B.P. *Ammonii Bicarbonas*
DOSES: 0.3-0.6 Gm. (5-10 gr.). NH_4HCO_3. Mol.wt. 79.06.
S: 5.5 W at 15.5°; ins. A 90%. White crystals or a fine white
crystalline powder; odour slightly ammoniacal; taste pungent.

Ammonium Carbonate U.S.P. *Ammonii Carbonas*
DOSE: 0.3 Gm. (5 gr.). S: 4 W. Decomposes in hot water.
A mixture of Ammonium Bicarbonate and Ammonium Carbamate
$NH_4NH_2CO_2$. Translucent, hard, crystalline masses; odour
strongly ammoniacal; taste pungent and ammoniacal.

₡ Ammonium Bicarbonate and Carbonate are used as components
of cough mixtures to stimulate bronchial secretion in unproductive
cough. Larger doses are emetic by irritating the gastric mucosa.
The irritation is due mostly to free ammonia which is readily
liberated.

Ammonium Chloride. *Ammonii Chloridum.* (Muriate of Ammonia,
Sal Ammoniac)
DOSES: B.P. 0.3-4 Gm. (5-60 gr.); U.S.P. expectorant, 0.3 Gm.
(5 gr.); diuretic, daily, 4 Gm. (60 gr.). NH_4Cl. Mol.wt. 53.5.
S: 2.6 W, 100 A, 8 G, 1.4 W at 100°. White, crystalline, granular
powder; odourless; taste saline and cooling; somewhat hygroscopic.

₡ Ammonium Chloride in small doses (e.g. 0.6 Gm.) may be
used as an expectorant instead of Ammonium Carbonate. Large
doses are given to produce systemic acidosis, e.g. in the treatment
of lead poisoning or to acidify the urine (see Hexamine). It is
also used as a diuretic by itself or to augment the action of mercurial
diuretics.

Ammonium Chloride Capsules U.S.P. *Capsulae Ammonii Chloridi*
Average daily dose 4 Gm. (60 gr.). Sizes, 0.3 and 0.5 Gm.
(5 and 7½ gr.).

Dilute Solution of Ammonium Acetate B.P. *Liquor Ammonii*
Acetatis Dilutus. (Solution of Ammonium Acetate)
Doses: 8-30 cc. (¼-1 fl.oz.). Contains 7.2% w/v $NH_4C_2H_3O_2$.

ℂ The Dilute Solution of Ammonium Acetate has been used in
fever mixtures to promote sweating and diuresis.

Strong Solution of Ammonium Acetate B.P. *Liquor Ammonii*
Acetatis Fortis
Doses: 1-4 cc. (15-60 min.). Contains 55-60% w/v of Ammonium
Acetate. Made from Glacial Acetic Acid, Ammonium Carbonate,
and Strong Solution of Ammonia. A thin syrupy liquid with the
odour of ammonia and acetic acid. A stock solution.

Ammonium Mandelate Tablets U.S.P. See Mandelic Acid
Size, 300 mg. (5 gr.).

Amphetamine. *Amphetamina.* (T.N. Benzedrine)
$C_6H_5CH_2CHNH_2.CH_3$. Mol.wt. 135.2. S: ss. W, A, E; readily
sol. in acids. A colourless mobile liquid; odour unpleasant and
characteristic; taste acrid; volatilises slowly at ordinary temperatures.

Amphetamine Inhalant U.S.P.
Contains not less than 90% of labelled amount of Amphetamine
in a suitable inhaler.

ℂ Amphetamine resembles ephedrine in its actions but has more
stimulating effect on the central nervous system. It is used as a
nasal decongestant by inhalation.

Amphetamine Sulphate *Amphetaminae Sulphas.* (T.N. Ben-
zedrine Sulphate)
Doses: 2.5-10 mg. (1/24-1/6 gr.); U.S.P. 5 mg. (1/12 gr.).
$(C_9H_{13}N)_2H_2SO_4$. Mol. wt. 368.5. S: 8.8 W, 515 A at 20°; ins. E.
A white odourless powder; taste slightly bitter followed by a sen-
sation of numbness.

Amphetamine Sulphate Tablets U.S.P.
Sizes, 5 and 10 mg. (1/12 and 1/6 gr.).

℄ Tablets of amphetamine sulphate are used to reduce sleepiness in the narcolepsies and often for combatting ordinary sleepiness from fatigue. Appetite is decreased and consequently the drug may be used as an adjunct to dietary restriction in the treatment of obesity. Some persons become anxious and tremulous under its influence and may have an increased pulse rate and blood pressure. A more potent analeptic is d-Amphetamine (Dexedrine) with less effect on the heart and circulation, in the sense that pounding of the heart or a rapid pulse is experienced less frequently with ordinary doses.

Amylene Hydrate. *Amyleni Hydras.* (Tertiary Amyl Alcohol)
DOSES: B.P. 2-4 cc. (30-60 min.). $(CH_3)_2(C_2H_5)COH$. Mol.wt. 88.15. Sp.gr. 0.803-0.807. Gm./cc. 0.808-0.811. B.p. 97-103°. S: 8 W; misc. A, C, E, G. A clear colourless liquid; odour camphoraceous; taste burning, pungent; volatile at ordinary temperatures. See Bromethol.

Amyl Nitrite. *Amylis Nitris.* (Isoamyl Nitrite)
DOSES: B.P. 0.12-0.3 cc. (2-5 min.) by inhalation; U.S.P. 0.2 cc. (3 min.) by inhalation. $CH_3.CH(CH_3)CH_2.CH_2NO_2$. Mol.wt. 117.15. Sp.gr. 0.865-0.875. S: almost ins. W; misc. A, E. A mixture of nitrites of some of the isomers of amyl alcohol. A clear yellowish liquid; odour ethereal, fragrant; taste pungent and aromatic; volatile at low temperatures and inflammable.

℄ Single doses of amyl nitrite are dispensed in glass capsules (perles) which may be crushed in a handkerchief and the vapour inhaled. Within a minute the face and neck flush and a violent throbbing is felt in the head. The pulse rate is usually increased. The effects usually pass off in a few minutes but headache may persist longer. The drug produces a general vasodilation, most evident in the blush area. Relief of pain in angina pectoris is produced by dilatation of the coronary arteries and also by a reduction in the work of the heart, resulting from reduced venous return. The blood pressure is usually lowered by a small dose but may be raised by a larger one, probably as a reflex effect of the irritant vapour in the nose. Nitroglycerine is another substance often prescribed for angina pectoris, in hypodermic tablets which are dissolved under the tongue. The effects produced resemble those of amyl nitrite but are usually slower in onset.

Anise Oil U.S.P. Oil of Anise B.P. *Oleum Anisi.* (Oil of Aniseed)
DOSES: B.P. 0.06-0.2 cc. (1-3 min.). S: almost ins. W, 3 A. Sp.gr. 0.978-0.988. A colourless or pale-yellow oil having the characteristic odour and taste of anise. Distilled from *Pimpinella Anisum* or *Illicium verum.* A carminative flavour.

TABLE OF ANTIHISTAMINIC DRUGS

Proprietary Names	*Non-proprietary Names and Common Dosage Units*
Anthisan	Mepyramine Maleate B.P.N.*
(May and Baker)	Tablets, 50 gm.
Antistine	Antazoline Hydrochloride N.N.R.
(Ciba)	Tablets, 100 mg.
Benadryl	Diphenhydramine Hydrochloride U.S.P.
(Parke Davis)	Capsules, 25, 50 mg.
Decapryn	Doxylamine Succinate N.N.R.
(Merrell)	Tablets, 12.5, 25 mg.
Diatrin	Thenylpyramine Hydrochloride N.N.R.
(Warner)	Tablets, 50 mg.
Dramamine	Dimenhydrinate N.N.R.
(Searle)	Tablets, 100 mg.
Gravol	Dimenhydrinate N.N.R.
(Horner)	Tablets, 50 mg.
Histadyl	Methylpyraline Hydrochloride N.N.R.
(Lilly)	Tablets, 50 mg.
Neoantergan	Pyranisamine Maleate N.N.R.
(Poulenc)	Mepyramine Maleate B.P.N.
	Tablets, 50 mg.
Neohetramine	Thonzylamine Hydrochloride N.N.R.
(Wyeth)	Tablets, 25, 50, 100 mg.
Perazil	Chlorcyclizine Hydrochloride B.P.N.*
(Burroughs and Wellcome)	Tablets, 50 mg.
Tagathen	Chlorothen Citrate N.N.R.
(Lederle)	Tablets, 25 mg.
Phenergan	Promethazine Hydrochloride B.P.N.*
(Poulenc)	Tablets, 25 mg.

*Name assigned by the British Pharmacopoeia Commission.

Pyribenzamine   Tripelennamine Hydrochloride U.S.P.
  (Ciba)   Tablets, 50 mg.

Thenylene   Methapyrilene Hydrochloride N.N.R.
  (Abbott)   Tablets, 50 mg.

Thephorin   Phenindamine Tartrate N.N.R.
  (Hoffmann-LaRoche)   Tablets, 25 mg.

Trimeton   Prophenpyridamine N.N.R.
  (Schering)   Tablets, 25 mg.

ℭ Antihistaminic drugs suppress or diminish many, but not all, of the effects of histamine. The stimulation of gastric secretion of hydrochloric acid by the administration of histamine is not suppressed by any of the antihistaminic drugs presently available. Asthma induced experimentally in guinea pigs (or in human subjects) by the inhalation of nebulized histamine, is diminished. Ordinary asthmatic attacks are, more often than not, resistant to these drugs.

Reactions to histamine introduced into human skin by iontophoresis can be suppressed by oral administration of these drugs. The effects of histamine on blood pressure and its action of producing contractions of isolated smooth muscle from the gut or uterus, can be suppressed by antihistaminics. Their mode of action is thought to be competitive inhibition, i.e. by combining with the cell receptors which are attacked by histamine. In addition to antagonizing histamine, these drugs have other important actions, e.g. anticholinergic, local anaesthetic, antiseptic, and convulsant. Many are strongly hypnotic or sedative in ordinary doses, although in overdoses many are convulsant. Fatalities have been reported from suicidal and accidental overdosage.

It is probable that the anticholinergic (or atropine-like) action of these drugs is quite important, for example in relieving the symptoms of ordinary head colds. The greatest usefulness of the antihistamines is for the relief of hay fever and urticaria.

Benadryl, Dramamine, Gravol and Antistine are reported to alleviate motion sickness and pernicious vomiting of pregnancy. It is not known how many antihistaminic drugs share this action.

A few cases of agranulocytosis have been reported following the use of an antihistaminic. This should be kept in mind as a possible consequence of frequent use.

Antimony Potassium Tartrate U.S.P. *Antimonii Potassii Tartras.*

Potassium Antimonyl Tartrate B.P. *Antimonii et Potassii Tartras.*
(Tartarated Antimony, Tartar Emetic)

DOSES: B.P. oral, expectorant, 2-8 mg. (1/32-1/8 gr.), emetic 30-60 mg. ($\frac{1}{2}$-1 gr.), intravenous 30-120 mg. ($\frac{1}{2}$-2 gr.); U.S.P. oral, expectorant, 3 mg. (1/20 gr.), intravenous for tropical diseases 30 mg. increasing to 150 mg. ($\frac{1}{2}$-2$\frac{1}{2}$ gr.). $K(SbO)C_4H_4O_6.\frac{1}{2}H_2O$. Mol.wt. 333.95. S: 12 W, 15 G; 3 W at 100°; ins. A. Colourless transparent crystals or a white granular powder; odourless; taste sweet; efflorescent.

Injection of Potassium Antimonyl Tartrate B.P.

DOSES: intravenous, 30-120 mg. ($\frac{1}{2}$-2 gr.). Strength, 20 mg. per cc. (1/3 gr. in 15 min.).

℘ Sodium and Potassium Antimonyl Tartrates are interchangeable. The emetic effect is produced reflexly by irritation of the gastro-intestinal tract. The same action is probably the basis of the expectorant effect of smaller doses, i.e. the bronchial secretions are increased reflexly.

Tartar emetic is given intravenously for the treatment of tropical trypanosome infections. Antimony sodium thioglycollate is less toxic and irritating than tartar emetic and may be given intramuscularly as well as intravenously.

Bal is an effective antidote for antimony poisoning.

Sodium Antimonyl Tartrate B.P. *Antimonii et Sodii Tartras.*
(Antimony Sodium Tartrate)

DOSES: as for preceding. $C_4H_4O_7SbNa$. Mol.wt. 308.84. S: 1.5 W; ins. A 90% at 15.5°. Colourless and transparent or whitish scales or powder; odourless; taste sweetish; hygroscopic.

Injection of Sodium Antimonyl Tartrate B.P.

DOSES: intravenous, 30-120 mg. ($\frac{1}{2}$-2 gr.). Strength, 60 mg. per cc. (1 gr. in 15 min.).

Antimony Sodium Thioglycollate U.S.P. *Antimonii Sodii Thioglycollas*

DOSE: 50 mg. ($\frac{3}{4}$ gr.). $C_4H_4O_4NaS_2Sb$. Mol. wt. 324.95. S: freely sol. W; ins A. A white or pink powder having no odour or a slight mercaptan odour.

Antimony Sodium Thioglycollate Injection U.S.P.
DOSE: 50 mg. ($\frac{3}{4}$ gr.) intramuscularly or intravenously. Sizes, 50 mg. ($\frac{3}{4}$ gr.) in 10 cc., 100 mg. ($1\frac{1}{2}$ gr.) in 20 cc.

Aromatic Elixir U.S.P. *Elixir Aromaticum.* (Simple Elixir)
Contains Compound Spirit of Orange 1.2%, Syrup 37.5%, Alcohol and Distilled Water. Contains 22-24% v/v of C_2H_5OH.

The Aromatic Elixir of the *Canadian Formulary* is approximately the same except that it contains about 16% v/v of C_2H_5OH, and so is Red Aromatic Elixir C.F. which contains in addition a red dye, Cudbear (*Persio*).

Arachis Oil B.P. *Oleum Arachis.* **Peanut Oil U.S.P.** *Oleum Arachidis.* (Ground Nut Oil, Nut Oil)
Sp.gr. 0.912-0.920. S: vss. A; misc. E, C, CS_2. Pale-yellow or colourless oily liquid; taste bland; expressed from seeds of *Arachis hypogaea.* A vehicle for oily injections.

Arsenic Trioxide B.P. *Arseni Trioxidum.* (Arsenious Acid, Arsenious Anhydride, Arsenious Oxide, White Arsenic)
Doses: 1-5 mg. (1/60-1/12 gr.) As_2O_3. Mol.wt. 197.8 S: 65 W at 15.5°; ss. A, E; fs. G; sol. HCl, alkali hydroxides and carbonates. A heavy, white, tasteless, odourless powder; extremely poisonous.

℃ Arsenic is an intracellular poison which interferes with cellular oxidations, presumably by combining with sulphur containing enzymes. Symptoms depend on the mode of administration. Enteritis, with intense congestion of the intestinal tract, is a frequent manifestation of toxic doses taken by mouth. Neuritis, dermatitis, and blood dyscrasias may occur with prolonged intake of small quantities. Bal is an effective antidote.

Arsenic in small doses was thought at one time to have beneficial effects in anaemia and in some skin diseases but its value is very questionable. Veterinarians use arsenic to improve the growth of hair in cattle and increase subcutaneous fat.

Arsenic was once used in dentistry as a caustic to devitalize tooth pulp but has been practically abandoned as too dangerous.

Arsenic poisoning may occur in industry. In cases of chronic arsenical poisoning the metal may be found in abnormal amounts in hair and cuticle. It is slowly excreted in the urine and examination of the urine may be necessary to establish a diagnosis.

Charlatans have used arsenical pastes to treat external cancers. Extensive neuritis often results.

Arsenical Solution Can. Gaz. *Liquor Arsenicalis.* (Fowler's Solution)

DOSES: 0.12-0 5 cc. (2-8 min.). Arsenic Trioxide 1%, Glycerin 10%, with Amaranth and Chloroform Water.

Arsenical Solution B.P. *Liquor Arsenicalis.* (Fowler's Solution, *Solutio Arsenicalis seu Fowleri* P.I.)
Doses: B.P. 0.12-0.5 cc. (2-8 min.) Arsenic Trioxide 0.95-1.05% w/v.

℃ The arsenical solutions were once used extensively as mouth washes in trench mouth. Their use should not be prolonged for fear of poisoning. Penicillin lozenges or packs are now used in preference to the arsenical solutions. Note that both versions of Fowler's Solution contain about 1% of arsenic trioxide, but differ in method of preparation.

ORGANIC ARSENICALS

Acetarsol B.P. *Acetarsol.* (Acetarsone, T.N. Stovarsol)
DOSES: 60-250 mg. (1-4 gr.). 3-acetylamino-4-hydroxy-phenyl arsonic acid. $CH_3.CONH.C_6H_3(OH)AsO(OH)_2$. Mol.wt. 275.1 M.p. about 245° S: almost ins. cold W, moderately in W 100°, ins. A, sol. dil. alkalis. A white crystalline powder; odourless; taste faintly acid.

Solution Tablets of Acetarsol B.P.C. *Solvellae Acetarsolis*
Size, 0.25 Gm. (4 gr.).

℃ Acetarsol is a pentavalent arsenical given orally for amoebic dysentery. For trichomonas vaginitis it is applied in the form of a powder by means of an insufflator or as a solution tablet. Carbarsone, a similar compound, is said to be safer and more effective for the treatment of amoebic dysentery.

Carbarsone. *Carbarsonum.* (T.N. Amabevan, Leucarsone, p-carbamidophenylarsonic acid)
DOSES: B.P. 0.12-0.2 Gm. (2-3 gr.); U.S.P. 0.25 Gm. (4 gr.). $C_7H_9O_4N_2As$. Mol.wt. 260.07. M.p. about 190°. S: ss. W, A; nearly ins. C, E; sol. in solutions of alkali hydroxides and carbonates. A white, almost odourless powder; taste slightly acid.

Carbarsone Capsules U.S.P.
Size, 250 mg. (4 gr.).

Carbarsone Suppositories U.S.P.

Each suppository contains 130 mg. (2 gr.) Carbarsone.

℃ Carbarsone is given by mouth, usually in capsules of 0.25 Gm. (4 gr.) thrice daily for the treatment of amoebic dysentery. While safer than acetarsone, cumulation can occur and so can the usual manifestations of poisoning by arsenicals, such as exfoliative dermatitis and hepatitis.

Dichlorophenarsine Hydrochloride U.S.P. *Dichlorophenarsinae Hydrochloridum.* (T.N. Clorarsen, Dichlor-mapharsen)

DOSE: intravenous, 45 mg. ($\frac{3}{4}$ gr.). $C_6H_6AsCl_2NO.HCl$. Mol. wt. 290.41. S: sol. W, solutions of alkali hydroxides and carbonates and in dilute mineral acids. A white odourless powder.

℃ Dichlorophenarsine Hydrochloride may be administered intravenously in buffered solution for the treatment of syphilis.

Neoarsphenamine B.P. *Neoarsphenamina.* (Novarsenobenzol, Novarsenobenzene)

DOSES: intravenous, 0.15-0.6 Gm. ($2\frac{1}{2}$-10 gr.); S: vs. W; ss. A; almost ins. C, E, and dehydrated A. A yellow powder almost free from odour; unstable as a powder or solution in air.

℃ Neoarsphenamine was for many years the drug of choice for the treatment of syphilis by intravenous arsenical therapy. It is simpler to use than arsphenamine (not requiring neutralization) and safer. It has been replaced to a large extent by Oxophenarsine.

Oxophenarsine Hydrochloride U.S.P. *Oxophenarsinae Hydrochloridum.* 3-amino-4-hydroxyphenylarsinoxide hydrochloride. (T.N. Mapharsen)

DOSE: intravenous, 45 mg. ($\frac{3}{4}$ gr.). $C_6H_6AsO_2N.HCl$. Mol.wt. 235.49. S: sol. W, solutions of alkali hydroxides and carbonates and in dilute mineral acids. A white or nearly white odourless powder.

℃ Oxophenarsine Hydrochloride is one of the most effective arsenicals for the treatment of syphilis by intravenous injection.

Sulpharsphenamine B.P. *Sulpharsphenamina.* (Sulpharsenobenzene)

DOSES: subcutaneous or intramuscular, 0.1-0.6 Gm. ($1\frac{1}{2}$-10 gr.). S: sol. W; ins. A, E. A yellow dry powder; odourless; contains approximately 20% As.

Injection of Sulpharsphenamine B.P.

DOSES: subcutaneous or intramuscular, 0.1-0.6 Gm. (1½-10 gr.).
Supplied dry in sealed containers. Fresh solutions in Water for
Injection are made immediately before use.

⟪ Sulpharsphenamine has the actions of arsphenamine. It is,
however, given intramuscularly, *not* intravenously. It is useful in
treating congenital syphilis in infants.

Tryparsamide. *Tryparsamidum*

DOSES: B.P. subcutaneous, intramuscular or intravenous,
1-2 Gm. (15-30 gr.); U.S.P. intravenous, 2 Gm. (30 gr.).
$C_8H_{10}AsN_2O_4Na.\frac{1}{2}H_2O$. Mol.wt. 305.09. S: 2 W; ss. A; ins. E,
C, B. A white or colourless, odourless, crystalline powder; slowly
affected by light.

Injection of Tryparsamide B.P.

DOSES: subcutaneous, intramuscular or intravenous, 1-2 Gm.
(15-30 gr.). Supplied in sealed containers. Fresh solutions are to
be made up with Water for Injection immediately before use.

⟪ Tryparsamide is a pentavalent arsenical compound, unlike
the preceding compounds in which the arsenic is trivalent. For
reasons not well understood, tryparsamide is effective against
syphilis in the central nervous system but not against other forms
of syphilis.

Aspidium U.S.P. *Aspidium.* **Male Fern B.P.** *Filix Mas*

The dried rhizome of *Dryopteris Filix-mas*, known in commerce
as American Aspidium or Marginal Fern. Odour disagreeable;
taste sweetish and astringent, then bitter and nauseous.

Powdered Male Fern B.P. *Filicis Pulvis*

A brown powder used for the preparation of the Extract of Male
Fern.

Extract of Male Fern B.P. *Extractum Filicis.* (Aspidium Oleoresin)

DOSES: 3-6 cc. (45-90 min.). Gm./cc. not less than 0.995. A
dark-green ethereal extract containing much oil from which the
ether has been evaporated. Standardized to contain 25% of filicin.
Frequently contains a sediment.

Aspidium Oleoresin U.S.P. *Oleoresina Aspidii.* (Oleoresin of
Male Fern, Oleoresin of Marginal Fern)

DOSE: *Caution*—single dose, 4 Gm. (60 gr.).

A dark-green thick liquid frequently depositing a sediment. Contains 24% of crude filicin.

❦ Male Fern is particularly effective against tapeworms. The active principle is probably filicic acid, which changes readily into an inactive material, filicin. The extract is best given as a freshly prepared emulsion in the morning on an empty stomach and followed in two hours by a saline purge. The treatment should not be repeated for four weeks. Toxic effects include colic, diarrhoea, headache, yellow vision, and sometimes temporary blindness.

Aureomycin Hydrochloride U.S.P. *Aureomycini Hydrochloridum.* (T. N. Duomycin)

DOSES: 5-10 mg. per kg. body weight, orally, every four hours. S: 75 W, 560 A; ins. C, E, dioxane, acetone; sol. in sols. of alkali hydroxides and their carbonates. A yellow crystalline antibiotic, a product of *Streptomyces aureofaciens*. Available for oral use in capsules of 50 or 250 mg.; also, for ophthalmic use, in vials containing 25 mg. with a suitable buffer, to be dissolved in 5 cc. of distilled water; also in vials containing 50 mg., each with a vial containing 10 cc. of 0.75% solution of sodium carbonate as diluent, for intravenous injection. Subcutaneous or intramuscular injections may cause severe local reactions.

Aureomycin Hydrochloride Capsules U.S.P.

Size, 250 mg. (4 gr.).

❦ Aureomycin is an antibiotic agent which is potent against a very wide range of gram-positive and gram-negative micro-organisms, and also against rickettsial infections such as Rocky Mountain Spotted Fever, Q Fever, Typhus, Lymphogranuloma Venereum, Rickettsialpox, Tularaemia and Psittacosis. Primary Atypical Pneumonia of unknown origin often responds favourably to aureomycin. True viral infections do not respond well as a rule.

BARBITURATES AND THIOBARBITURATES

Amytal N.N.R. (Amobarbital N.F.)

DOSES: 20-40 mg. (1/3-2/3 gr.), 3 times daily as a sedative; 0.1-0.3 Gm. (1½-5 gr.) as a hypnotic. $C_{11}H_{18}O_3N_2$. Mol.wt. 226.27. S: ss. W; sol. A, E, alkali hydroxides. A white powder or crystals; odourless; taste slightly bitter.

Amytal Tablets N.N.R.
Sizes, 8, 16, 32, 48, and 96 mg. ($\frac{1}{8}$, $\frac{1}{4}$, $\frac{1}{2}$, $\frac{3}{4}$, and $1\frac{1}{2}$ gr.).

Elixir Amytal N.N.R.
0.44 Gm. and 0.88 Gm. per 100 cc.

Amytal Sodium N.N.R. (Amobarbital Sodium N.F.)
DOSE: 0.2 Gm. (3 gr.) hypnotic or sedative. $C_{11}H_{17}O_3N_2Na$.
Mol.wt. 248.26. S: vs. W, 1 A; ins. E. A white, odourless, hygroscopic powder; taste bitter.

Amytal Sodium Capsules (Pulvules) N.N.R.
Sizes, 100 and 200 mg. ($1\frac{1}{2}$ and 3 gr.).

⟨ Amytal and its sodium salt resemble barbitone in their actions. The duration of action is definitely less than that of barbitone, so that amytal may be classed as a barbiturate of moderate duration or action (4-8 hrs.). The sodium salt is sometimes given intravenously to suppress convulsions or to subdue unruly patients.

Barbital U.S.P.   *Barbitalum.*   **Barbitone B.P.**   *Barbitonum.*
(Diethylbarbituric Acid, Diethylmalonylurea, T.N. Veronal)
DOSES: B.P. 0.3-0.6 Gm. (5-10 gr.);   U.S.P. 0.3 Gm. (5 gr.).
$(C_2H_5)_2C.CO.NH.CO.NH.CO.$ Mol.wt. 184.19.   M.p. 188-192°.
S: 130 W, 15 A, 75 C, 35 E; 13 W 100°; sol. acetone and ethyl acetate. Colourless or white crystals; odourless; taste slightly bitter.

Barbital Sodium U.S.P.   *Barbitalum Sodicum.*   **Barbitone Sodium B.P.**   *Barbitonum Sodium.* (Soluble Barbitone, Soluble Barbital, Sodium Diethylbarbiturate, Sodium Diethylmalonylurea, T.N. Medinal)
DOSES: B.P. 0.3-0.6 Gm. (5-10 gr.);   U.S.P. 0.3 Gm. (5 gr.).
$(C_2H_5)_2.C.CO.NH.CO.NNa.CO.$ Mol.wt. 206.19. S: 5 W; 2.5 W at 100°; ss. A; ins. E, C. White crystalline powder; odourless; taste bitter.

Barbital Tablets U.S.P.   **Tablets of Barbitone B.P.**
Size, 0.3 Gm. (5 gr.).

Tablets of Barbitone Sodium B.P.   **Barbital Sodium Tablets U.S.P.**
Size, 0.3 Gm. (5 gr.).

❡ Barbitone was the first of the barbiturate sedatives used in medical practice. It is cheap and considered by many to be a very useful hypnotic. It is rather slow in acting—an oral dose may take an hour to produce definite drowsiness. Its action is prolonged, which may sometimes be desirable but at other times a handicap if it leads to dullness the next day. The sodium salt is soluble and probably acts more rapidly than the acidic form when taken by mouth. Any barbiturate may produce mental confusion, even in ordinary dosage. This may result in the patient taking large overdoses and poisoning himself. Consequently not more than 12 doses should be prescribed at a time. A dose of 5 Gm. is often fatal. Serious poisoning is characterized by deep prolonged coma; ephedrine, picrotoxin, and metrazol (leptazol) are effective antidotes.

Dial N.N.R. Allobarbitone B.P.C. (5,5-diallylbarbituric acid, Diallyl Malonylurea)

Doses: 0.1-0.2 Gm. (1½-3 gr.). $C_{10}H_{12}O_3N_2$. Mol.wt. 208.11. M.p. 171-173°. S: 300 W (cold), 50 W at 100°; moderately sol. A, E, ethyl acetate, acetone. A white crystalline powder.

❡ Dial belongs to the group of barbiturates with long duration of action. It is used as a hypnotic or sedative.

Dial Tablets N.N.R.

Sizes, 30 and 100 mg. (½ and 1½ gr.).

Elixir Dial N.N.R.

4 cc. contain 50 mg. (¾ gr.) in 25% alcohol.

Hexobarbitone B.P. *Hexobarbitonum.* (Hexobarbital, T.N. Evipan, Evipal)

Doses: 0.25-0.5 Gm. (4-8 gr.). $C_{12}H_{16}O_3N_2$. Mol.wt. 236.3. M.p. 145-147°. S: 3000 W 20°; sol. dehydrated A, methyl A, B, C, E. Colourless prismatic crystals; odourless and tasteless.

Hexobarbitone Sodium B.P. *Hexobarbitonum Sodium.* (Soluble Hexobarbital, T.N. Evipal Sodium, Evipan Sodium)

Doses: 0.2-1 Gm. (3-15 gr.) by intravenous or intramuscular injection; 2-4 Gm. (30-60 gr.) by rectal injection. $C_{12}H_{15}O_3N_2Na$. Mol.wt. 258.3. S: vs. W, A, methyl A, acetone; ss. C, E; ins. B. A white, very hygroscopic powder; odourless; taste bitter; precipitates in solutions made acid with CO_2.

Injection of Hexobarbitone Sodium B.P.

DOSES: intravenous or intramuscular, 0.2-1 Gm. (3-15 gr.). Supplied dry in sealed containers. Fresh solutions in Water for Injection are made immediately before administration.

℆ Hexobarbitone is an ultra-short acting barbiturate. It is almost all destroyed in the liver. Although an oral dose is given, it is mostly used in the form of the sodium salt for intravenous anaesthesia. Post-anaesthetic stupor or depression is longer than after soluble thiopentone (Pentothal Sodium).

Methylphenobarbitone B.P. *Methylphenobarbitonum.* (T.N. Phemitone)

DOSES: 60-200 mg. (1-3 gr.). $C_2H_5(C_6H_5)CCON(CH_3)CONHCO$. Mol.wt. 246.3. M.p. 178-181°. S: almost ins. W; sol. A 90%, E, C, aqueous solutions of alkali hydroxides. A white, crystalline, odourless, and tasteless powder.

℆ Phemitone, in chemistry and in action, resembles phenobarbitone. It has been used increasingly in recent years to control both *grand mal* and *petit mal* in epilepsy. The hypnotic effect of anticonvulsive doses of phemitone is said to be less marked than that of phenobarbitone.

Pentobarbitone Sodium B.P. *Pentobarbitonum Sodium.* Pentobarbital Sodium U.S.P. *Pentobarbitalum Sodicum.* (Soluble Pentobarbitone, Soluble Pentobarbital, T.N. Nembutal)

DOSES: B.P. 0.1-0.2 Gm. (1½-3 gr.); Can. Supp. 30-100 mg. (½-1½ gr.) oral, 0.2 Gm. (3 gr.) for pre-operative use; U.S.P. 0.1 Gm. (1½ gr.). $C_{11}H_{17}O_3N_2Na$. Mol.wt. 248.3. S: vs. W; fs. A; ins. E. A white crystalline powder; odourless; taste slightly bitter.

Sterile Pentobarbital Sodium U.S.P. *Pentobarbitalum Sodicum Sterile.*

DOSE: intravenous, 0.1 Gm. (1½ gr.).

Pentobarbital Sodium Capsules U.S.P. (Soluble Pentobarbital Capsules)

Sizes, 50 and 100 mg. (¾ and 1½ gr.).

Pentobarbital Sodium Tablets U.S.P. (Soluble Pentobarbital Tablets)

Sizes, 30, 50 and 100 mg. (½, ¾, 1½ gr.).

ℭ Pentobarbitone is classed as a barbiturate of relatively short and rapid action, and is particularly suited for use as a hypnotic or pre-operative sedative. Ordinary doses by mouth produce drowsiness in about half an hour and act for 5 to 7 hours. Pentobarbitone is largely destroyed in the liver. Cases of delirium and excitement under the influence of pentobarbitone have been reported fairly often, usually when the drug is given when pain or fever is present.

Phenobarbital U.S.P. *Phenobarbitalum.* **Phenobarbitone B.P.**
Phenobarbitonum. (Phenylethylmalonylurea. T.N. Luminal)
DOSES: B.P. 30-120 mg. ($\frac{1}{2}$-2 gr.); U.S.P. 30 mg. ($\frac{1}{2}$ gr.). $C_{12}H_{12}O_3N_2$. Mol.wt. 232.23. M.p. 173-178°. S: 1000 W, 10 A, 40 C, 15 E; sol. in solutions of fixed alkali hydroxides and carbonates. White small crystals or a white crystalline powder; odourless; taste slightly bitter.

Sterile Phenobarbital Sodium U.S.P. *Phenobarbitalum Sodicum Sterile.*

Phenobarbital Tablets U.S.P.
Sizes, 15, 30, 100 mg. ($\frac{1}{4}$, $\frac{1}{2}$, $1\frac{1}{2}$ gr.).

Tablets of Phenobarbitone B.P.
Size, 30 mg. ($\frac{1}{2}$ gr.).

Phenobarbital Elixir U.S.P. *Elixir Phenobarbitali*
DOSE: 4 cc. (1 fl.dr.) which contains 16 mg. ($\frac{1}{4}$ gr.) of Phenobarbital, with Sweet Orange Peel Tincture, Amaranth Solution, Alcohol, Glycerin, Syrup, and Distilled Water. Contains 12-15% v/v of C_2H_5OH.

Phenobarbital Sodium U.S.P. *Phenobarbitalum Sodicum.* **Phenobarbitone Sodium B.P.** *Phenobarbitonum Sodium.* (Soluble Phenobarbital. T.N. Luminal Sodium)
DOSES: B.P. oral, 0.03-0.12 Gm. ($\frac{1}{2}$-2 gr.), 0.06-0.2 Gm. (1-3 gr.) single by injection; U.S.P. 30 mg. ($\frac{1}{2}$ gr.). $(C_2H_5)(C_6H_5)CCO.NH$ CONNaCO. Mol.wt. 254.22. S: vs. W; sol. A; ins. E, C. Flaky crystals or a white crystalline powder; odourless; taste bitter.

Injection of Phenobarbitone Sodium B.P.
DOSES: Single intravenous or intramuscular, 60-200 mg. (1-3 gr.), supplied dry in sealed containers. Solutions in Water for Injection are to be made immediately before use.

Tablets of Phenobarbitone Sodium B.P.
Size, 30 mg. ($\frac{1}{2}$ gr.).

Phenobarbital Sodium Tablets U.S.P. (Soluble Phenobarbital Tablets)
Sizes, 30 and 100 mg. ($\frac{1}{2}$ and $1\frac{1}{2}$ gr.).

⓵ Phenobarbitone resembles barbitone in being slow in onset of action and very prolonged in effect. Unlike barbitone it has a marked anti-convulsant effect in doses which are not anaesthetic or even very hypnotic. Accordingly one of its main uses is to treat epilepsy. Combination with diphenylhydantoin is said to increase its effectiveness. If it is used as a hypnotic it should be given early in the evening or it may fail to act that night and keep the patient drowsy the next day. In small doses it may be given three times a day to relieve emotional tension which may be aggravating hypertension or peptic ulcer. Phenobarbitone is almost all excreted unchanged in the urine over a period of several days. Examination of the urine is important if poisoning by phenobarbitone is suspected. Poisoning by taking large overdoses of phenobarbitone is not uncommon. Death has been reported with 1.7 Gm. (27 gr.) and recovery has been reported after 9 Gm. Doses of 6-9 Gm. are commonly fatal. The most prominent effect of overdosage is deep coma with loss of reflexes, fall in blood pressure, and finally respiratory failure. The body temperature is usually low at the onset but may rise to a fever before death. Analeptics have proved useful in treating cases of poisoning. Of these, picrotoxin and metrazol are probably most effective.

Seconal Sodium N.N.R. (Secobarbital Sodium)
DOSES: 0.1-0.2 Gm. ($1\frac{1}{2}$-3 gr.). $C_{12}H_{17}N_2NaO_3$. Mol.wt. 260.27.

Pulvules Seconal Sodium (Capsules) N.N.R.
Sizes, 50 and 100 mg. ($\frac{3}{4}$ and $1\frac{1}{2}$ gr.).

Seconal Sodium Elixir N.N.R.
100 cc. contain 0.44 Gm. of Seconal.

⓵ The action of seconal sodium is rapid and relatively brief. It is effective for the type of insomnia in which difficulty is experienced in getting to sleep rather than staying asleep. The drug is destroyed in the liver and little or none can be found in the urine.

Vinbarbital Sodium N.N.R. (Sodium 5-ethyl-5-(1-methyl-butenyl) barbiturate. T.N. Delvinal Sodium)
DOSES: 0.1-0.2 Gm. (1½-3 gr.).

Capsules Delvinal Sodium N.N.R.
Sizes, 0.03, 0.1, and 0.2 Gm. (½, 1½ and 3 gr.).

Elixir Delvinal Sodium N.N.R.
30 cc. contain 0.26 Gm. of Vinbarbital Sodium.

⚌ Delvinal is relatively rapid and brief in its action. The duration of action seems to be between that of pentobarbitone and of seconal, possibly 5 or 6 hours, for ordinary doses.

Thiopentone Sodium B.P. *Thiopentonum Sodium.* **Thiopental Sodium U.S.P.** *Thiopentalum Sodicum.* (Thiopentone Soluble, Sodium 5-ethyl-5-(1-methyl-butyl) thiobarbituric acid, T.N. Pentothal Sodium)
DOSES: B.P. intravenous, 0.1-0.5 Gm. (1½-8 gr.).
$C_{11}H_{17}N_2O_2SNa$. Mol.wt. 264.32. S: sol. W, A; ins. E, B, and petroleum benzin. Solutions decompose on standing. A yellowish-white hygroscopic powder having a disagreeable odour and a bitter taste.

Injection of Thiopentone Sodium B.P.
DOSES: intravenous, 0.1-0.5 Gm. (1½-8 gr.). Supplied dry in sealed containers. Fresh solutions in Water for Injection are to be made immediately before use.

⚌ Soluble Thiopentone is given almost exclusively by intravenous injection to produce anaesthesia of short duration. Two or three cc. of 5% are injected slowly, that is in about 15 seconds. Additional amounts may be given by continuous drip under constant control by the anaesthetist. Two common hazards are laryngeal spasm and excessive respiratory depression. Five per cent solutions of thiopentone are damaging to tissues and should not be allowed to get outside the vein.

Sterile Thiopental Sodium U.S.P. *Thiopentalum Sodicum Sterile.* (Sterile Thiopentone Soluble)
DOSE: to be determined by the physician. Sizes, 0.5, 1.0, 5 Gm. (7½, 15, 75 gr.).

Barium Sulphate. *Barii Sulphas*

BaSO₄. Mol.wt. 233.4. S: ins. W, aqueous solutions of acids and alkalies and organic solvents. A heavy, white, amorphous powder; odourless and tasteless. *When this drug is prescribed, the name should be written out in full to avoid confusion with Barium Sulphide*, which is very poisonous.

◖ The main use of Barium Sulphate is for radiography of the intestinal tract.

Belladonna Herb B.P. *Belladonnae Herba.* **Belladonna Leaf U.S.P.** *Belladonnae Folium.* (Deadly Nightshade Leaf)

The leaves and other aerial parts of *Atropa Belladonna* (or *Atropa acuminata* B.P.). Contains not less than 0.3% of alkaloids calculated as hyoscyamine.

Powdered Belladonna Herb B.P. *Belladonnae Herbae Pulvis*

Coarsely powdered herb.

Prepared Belladonna Herb B.P. *Belladonna Praeparata*

DOSES: 30-200 mg. (½-3 gr.). Finely powdered herb adjusted to contain 0.28-0.32% of alkaloids calculated as hyoscyamine. Green; odour slight; taste somewhat bitter and acrid.

Belladonna Root B.P. *Belladonnae Radix.* (Deadly Nightshade Root)

The dried roots of *Atropa Belladonna* Linn. or *Atropa acuminata*. Contains not less than 0.4% of alkaloid calculated as hyoscyamine.

Powdered Belladonna Root B.P. *Belladonnae Radicis Pulvis*

A grey to light-brown powder.

Dry Extract of Belladonna B.P. *Extractum Belladonnae Siccum*

DOSES: 15-60 mg. (¼-1 gr.). An extract of Belladonna Herb containing 0.95-1.05% of alkaloids. The maximum dose contains 0.6 mg. (1/100 gr.) of the alkaloids calculated as hyoscyamine.

Liquid Extract of Belladonna B.P. *Extractum Belladonnae Liquidum*

An alcoholic extract of Belladonna Root standardized to contain 0.70-0.80% of alkaloids calculated as hyoscyamine. Contains 48-66% v/v of C₂H₅OH.

Liniment of Belladonna B.P. *Linimentum Belladonnae*

Contains 0.35-0.40% of the alkaloids of Belladonna Root and 5% w/v of camphor in 50-60% v/v of C₂H₅OH.

Belladonna Extract U.S.P. *Extractum Belladonnae*
Made from leaf and contains 1.15-1.35% of alkaloids.

Pilular Belladonna Extract U.S.P.
An extract of Belladonna Leaf, adjusted with liquid glucose to make a plastic mass containing 1.25% of alkaloids.

Powdered Belladonna Extract U.S.P.
DOSE: 15 mg. ($\frac{1}{4}$ gr.). An extract of Belladonna Leaf adjusted with dried starch to contain 1.25% of alkaloids.

Belladonna Suppositories B.P. *Suppositoria Belladonnae*
Each suppository contains 1 mg. (1/60 gr.) of the alkaloids from the Liquid Extract of Belladonna.

Belladonna Tincture U.S.P. **Tincture of Belladonna B.P.**
Tinctura Belladonnae
DOSES: B.P. 0.3-1 cc. (5-15 min.); U.S.P. 0.6 cc. (10 min.). Contains about 0.03% w/v of alkaloids. The maximum B.P. dose contains about 0.3 mg. (1/200 gr.) of alkaloids calculated as hyoscyamine. The Tinctures, both B.P. and U.S.P., contain about 64-70% v/v of C_2H_5OH.

⟪ The galenical preparations of Belladonna have no obvious advantage over Atropine but may be used, for example in laxative pills, with some saving in cost.

Belladonna Ointment and Plaster have some numbing effect on exposed nerve endings but none on intact skin. Their use for local anaesthetic effects is declining. It should be kept in mind that the alkaloids of the galenical preparation are mostly in the laevo form and hence are more active than the equivalent weight of atropine. See Atropine.

Atropine. *Atropina*
DOSE: U.S.P. 0.4 mg. (1/150 gr.). $C_{17}H_{23}O_3N$. Mol.wt. 289.36. M.p. 114-116°. S: 460 W, 2 A, 27 G, 1 C, 25 E; 90 W at 80°. Colourless, odourless, bitter crystals; *extremely poisonous*. An alkaloid; optically inactive dl-hyoscyamine obtained from *Atropa Belladonna* Linn. and species of *Datura* and *Hyoscyamus*, or produced synthetically.

Atropine Sulphate. *Atropinae Sulphas*

Doses: B.P. ¼-1 mg. (1/240-1/60 gr.); U.S.P. 0.5 mg. (1/120 gr.). $(C_{17}H_{23}O_3N)_2H_2SO_4.H_2O$. Mol.wt. 694.82. M.p. not lower than 188°. S: 0.5 W, 5 A, 2.5 G; 2.5 A at 78°. Colourless crystals or a white crystalline powder; odourless; taste bitter; efflorescent; *extremely poisonous*.

Atropine Sulphate Tablets U.S.P.

Sizes, 0.3, 0.4, 0.5, 0.6, 1.2 mg. (1/200, 1/150, 1/120, 1/100 1/50 gr.).

Tablets of Atropine Sulphate B.P.

Size, 0.6 mg. (1/100 gr.).

Injection of Atropine Sulphate B.P.

Doses: subcutaneous, 0.25-1 mg. (1/240-1/60 gr.). Strength, 0.6 mg. per cc. (1/100 gr. in 15 min.).

Lamellae of Atropine B.P. *Lamellae Atropinae*

A gelatin disc, 1.3 mg. (1/50 gr.), containing 0.013 mg. (1/5000 gr.) of Atropine Sulphate. For insertion in the conjunctival sac to produce a local effect on the eye.

Ointment of Atropine for the Eye B.P. *Oculentum Atropinae*

Contains 0.25% Atropine Sulphate.

Ointment of Atropine and Yellow Oxide of Mercury for the Eye B.P. *Oculentum Atropinae cum Hydrargyri Oxido*

Contains 0.125% Atropine Sulphate and 1% of Yellow Oxide of Mercury.

⟪ Atropine is a racemic mixture of d- and l-hyoscyamine. Most of its activity is due to the laevo-isomer. The fundamental action may be described as anticholinergic. It blocks, or partly blocks, depending on concentration, the action of acetylcholine, which is believed to transmit nerve impulses at certain synapses and nerve endings. It thus depresses or inhibits the actions of cholinergic nerves. It is much less effective, however, at the synapse between pre-ganglionic and post-ganglionic fibres than at other cholinergic nerve endings such as the endings of secretory nerves to the salivary glands and sweat glands, of cholinergic nerve endings in the intestinal tract and of vagus endings in the heart. It presumably acts at synapses in the central nervous system but these actions are not well analyzed.

A therapeutic dose of 0.6 mg. decreases nasal, salivary, and bronchial secretion and may decrease sweating. It decreases the tone of bronchiolar muscle and smooth muscles in the intestinal tract, including the pylorus. It may also decrease tonus in the bladder to some extent. The pulse rate is usually *decreased* by a few beats per minute. This effect is attributed to a central action, usually described as stimulation of the cardio-inhibitory vagus centre. Larger doses *increase* the heart rate by inhibiting transmission of impulses at the vagal endings in the heart. Doses of 2-4 mg. of atropine may increase the resting pulse rate by 40-50 beats per minute by abolition of tonic vagal control of the sinus node. Such doses may cause some dilatation of pupils. Still larger doses stimulate breathing, cause flushing, a rise in body temperature, dryness of the mouth and skin, tremors, hallucinations and sometimes convulsions, and finally death by respiratory paralysis. A fatal dose is about 0.1 Gm. for adults and 0.01 Gm. for children.

Instilled into the eye, a 0.1% solution will produce dilatation of the pupil (mydriasis); 1% solutions will paralyze accommodation (cycloplegia), an effect which may last for 3-7 days. It is well to remember that 0.5 cc. of a 1% solution contains 5 mg. Too free application to the eye may thus produce systemic effects and even toxic effects. Atropine increases intraocular pressure and hence should not be applied if glaucoma is suspected.

Atropine may be used to produce prolonged dilatation of the pupil, e.g. in iritis, or prior to anaesthesia to lessen salivary and bronchial secretions, to prevent or alleviate asthmatic seizures, to decrease pylorospasm in peptic ulcer, to alleviate bladder spasm in cystitis, to treat motion sickness, and to treat Parkinsonian syndromes. See also Homatropine and Syntropan. In dentistry atropine may be used to decrease excessive salivary flow during the taking of dental impressions.

Bentonite U.S.P. *Bentonitum*

S: ins. W. Native colloidal hydrated aluminium silicate. Swells in water to approximately 12 times its volume to form a suspension or opalescent paste.

Bentonite is frequently used to stabilize suspensions, e.g. Calamine Lotion. It is also used in creams of high water content to keep the water from separating.

Bentonite Magma U.S.P. *Magma Bentoniti*
Bentonite 50, Distilled Water to make 1000 cc.

Benzalkonium Chloride U.S.P. *Benzalkonii Chloridum.* (Alkyl-dimethyl-benzylammonium Chloride)
S: vs. W, A, acetone; almost ins. E; ss. B. A white or yellowish-white amorphous powder or gelatinous pieces; odour aromatic; taste very bitter.

Benzalkonium Chloride Solution U.S.P. *Liquor Benzalkonii Chloridi.* (T.N. Zephiran Chloride)
A clear, colourless liquid having an aromatic odour and a bitter taste. Available solutions are 0.1% aqueous, 12.8% aqueous, and 0.1% in alcohol 50cc., acetone 10 cc., with water to make 100 cc. The 12.8% solution must be diluted before use as it will damage tissues.

℈ Benzalkonium Chloride is a cationic detergent, or cleansing agent. It is powerfully germicidal. For disinfecting skin or surgical instruments strengths of 1:1000 to 1:5000 may be used. For bladder irrigations 1:40,000 is suitable. For eye washes or vaginal douches strengths of 1:10,000 to 1:20,000 may be used.
Soap is an anionic detergent. Its anions will combine with the benzalkonium cations and render them inactive. Soap should be thoroughly removed before applying a cationic detergent.

Benzoic Acid. *Acidum Benzoicum*
C_6H_5COOH. Mol.wt. 122.12. M.p. 121-123°. S: 275 W, 3 A, 5 C, 3 E. White crystals, usually scales or needles; odourless or may have a slight odour of benzaldehyde or benzoin.

℈ Benzoic Acid is bacteriostatic and fungistatic. Sodium Benzoate is inactive in this respect but in acid solution liberates enough benzoic acid to be an effective preservative for foods. Large doses can be taken by mouth without apparent harm and the small percentages permitted by law for the preservation of food are considered to be entirely harmless.

Benzoin. *Benzoinum*
A dried balsamic resin from *Styrax Benzoin* Dryander, or *Styrax paralleloneurus* Brans (Sumatra benzoin), or *Styrax tonkinensis* (Siam benzoin). Contains not less than 12.5% of benzoic acid (U.S.P.). Brittle masses; odour agreeable and balsamic.

Benzoin Tincture U.S.P. *Tinctura Benzoini*
A macerate of Benzoin, 20 Gm to make 100 cc.
Contains 75-83% of C_2H_5OH.

Compound Benzoin Tincture U.S.P. Compound Tincture of Benzoin B.P. *Tinctura Benzoini Composita.* (Friars' Balsam)
U.S.P.—Benzoin 10, Aloe 2, Storax 8, Tolu Balsam 4, all extracted to make 100 cc.; 74-80% v/v C_2H_5OH. B.P.—Sumatra benzoin 10, with Aloes, Storax, and Balsam of Tolu, all extracted to make 100 cc.; contains 70-77% v/v C_2H_5OH.

℃ A teaspoonful of Friars' Balsam may be added to a pint of hot water and the fumes inhaled for laryngitis or bronchitis. It was at one time a favourite dressing for wounds and sores of all kinds. All the preparations of benzoin have a reputation for promoting healing.

Benzyl Benzoate. *Benzylis Benzoas*
$C_{14}H_{12}O_2$. Mol.wt. 212.2. S: ins. W, G; misc. A, E, C. Sp.gr. 1.116-1.120. Gm./cc. 1.115-1.119. F.p. not below 17°. B.p. about 323°. Colourless crystals or a colourless oily liquid, having a faint aromatic odour and a burning taste.

Benzyl Benzoate Lotion U.S.P. *Lotio Benzylis Benzoatis*
Benzyl Benzoate 25%, with Triethanolamine, Oleic Acid, and Water; or Saponated Benzyl Benzoate 27.5% in Water.

Benzyl Benzoate Chlorophenothane Lotion U.S.P. *Lotio Benzylis Benzoati et Chlorophenothani*
Chlorophenothane (D.D.T.) 10, Benzyl Benzoate 115, Ethyl Aminobenzoate 20, Polysorbate (80) 25, Water to make 1000 cc.

℃ The preparations of Benzyl Benzoate are used to treat scabies and pediculosis.

Benzyl Alcohol. B.P. *Alcohol Benzylicum*
$C_6H_5.CH_2OH$. Mol.wt. 108.13. B.p. 200-210°. Gm./cc. 1.040-1.050. S: 25 W at 15.5°; misc. A, C, E. A colourless, almost odourless liquid; taste sharp and burning.

℃ Benzyl Alcohol may be used in ointments (10%) to allay itching. It has some antiseptic action.

Betanaphthol B.P.   *Betanaphthol.*   (Naphthol)

DOSES: 0.3-0.6 Gm. (5-10 gr.); $C_{10}H_7OH$. Mol.wt. 144.16. M.p. 120-122°. S: 1000 W, 1 A, 17 C, 1.5 E; 80 W at 100°; sol. G, olive oil and solutions of alkali hydroxides. White or slightly buff-coloured shining leaflets or a white or yellowish-white crystalline powder; odour faint and resembling phenol; darkens on exposure to light.

⟪ An ointment containing 1-2% of Betanaphthol is used for its antiseptic and antipruritic action. A 10% ointment will cause peeling of the skin and persistent pigmentation. It may also cause nephritis. It has been used internally in capsules with some effect as an anthelmintic for hookworm but is said to be inferior to thymol and more dangerous.

Bishydroxycoumarin U.S.P.   *Bishydroxycoumarinum.*   **Dicoumarol B.P.**   *Dicoumarol.*   (Dicoumarin)

Doses: 50-300 mg. (¾-5 gr.) daily. $C_{19}H_{12}O_6$. Mol.wt. 336.3. M.p. 285-293°. S: ss. W; sol. in solutions of strong alkalis. White or creamy-white crystalline powder; odour slight and pleasant; taste slightly bitter.

Bishydroxycoumarin Capsules U.S.P.

Size, 50 mg. (¾ gr.).

⟪ Dicoumarol is an anticoagulant. It is active by mouth but only after a lapse of 24 hours. It inhibits the production of pro-thrombin by the liver and may be used to combat emboli or throm-boses. Its use should be controlled by frequent determinations of prothrombin time. It is antagonized by vitamin K.

Bismuth Carbonate B.P.   *Bismuthi Carbonas.*   **Bismuth Sub-carbonate U.S.P.**   *Bismuthi Subcarbonas.*   (Bismuth Oxy-carbonate, Basic Bismuth Carbonate)

DOSES: B.P. 0.6-2 Gm. (10-30 gr.); U.S.P. 1 Gm. (15 gr.). S: ins. W, A; sol. nitric and hydrochloric acids. A heavy white or creamy white powder; odourless and tasteless.

⟪ Bismuth Carbonate is a poor antacid by reason of low efficiency per unit weight, and cost. It is, however, useful for the treatment of diarrhoea and gastritis and possibly peptic ulcer. The clinging quality of the fine powder makes it stick to eroded spots on mucous membranes and form a protective coating. If a small amount of soluble salt is formed locally, an astringent and antiseptic action is added. Small amounts of Bismuth Carbonate, combined with other antacids, can hardly have much protective action.

Bismuth Oxychloride B.P. *Bismuthi Oxychloridum.* (Bismuth Subchloride)
DOSES: oral, 0.6-2 Gm. (10-30 gr.).; intramuscular, 60-200 mg. (1-3 gr.). S: ins. W; sol. dilute hydrochloric acid. White or nearly white amorphous or finely crystalline powder; odourless and tasteless. Contains 79-81% of Bi.

Bismuth Potassium Tartrate U.S.P. *Bismuthi Potassii Tartras.* (Potassium Bismuthyl Tartrate)
DOSE: 0.1 Gm. (1½ gr.) intramuscular. S: 2 W; ins. A, C, E. A granular, white, odourless powder having a sweetish taste; darkens on exposure to light. Contains 60-64% of Bi.

Sodium Bismuthyl Tartrate B.P. *Bismuthi et Sodii Tartras*
DOSES: intramuscular, 60-200 mg. (1-3 gr.). S: in less than 1 W. A white powder or slightly yellow scales. Contains 35-42% of Bi.

Precipitated Bismuth B.P. *Bismuthum Praecipitatum*
DOSES: intramuscular, 60-200 mg. (1-3 gr.). S: ins. W. Bismuth metal in fine powder. Contains not less than 98.5% of Bi.

Bismuth Salicylate B.P. *Bismuthi Salicylas.* **Bismuth Subsalicylate U.S.P.** *Bismuthi Subsalicylas.* (Basic Bismuth Salicylate)
DOSES: B.P. oral, 0.6-2 Gm. (10-30 gr.); intramuscular, 60-200 mg. (1-3 gr.); U.S.P. oral, gastrointestinal, 1 Gm. (15 gr.); antisyphilitic, intramuscular in oil, 0.1 Gm. (1½ gr.). S: ins. W. A white or nearly white amorphous powder; odourless and tasteless.

INJECTIONS OF BISMUTH

Injection of Bismuth B.P. *Injectio Bismuthi*
DOSES: intramuscular, 0.5-1 cc. (8-15 min.). Precipitated Bismuth 20%, Dextrose 5%, with Chlorocresol in Water for Injection. The maximum dose (1 cc.) contains 200 mg. of Precipitated Bismuth.

Injection of Bismuth Oxychloride B.P. *Injectio Bismuthi Oxychloridi*
DOSES: 1-2 cc. (15-30 min.). Bismuth Oxychloride 10%, Dextrose 5%, with Chlorocresol in Water for Injection. Maximum dose (2 cc.) contains 200 mg. (3 gr.) of Bismuth Oxychloride.

Bismuth Potassium Tartrate Injection U.S.P.

DOSE: 100 mg. (1½ gr.) intramuscular. A sterile aqueous solution or a sterile suspension in a suitable fixed oil. Sizes, aqueous 30 mg. (½ gr.) or 50 mg. (¾ gr.) in 2 cc.; sizes in oil, 100 mg. (1½ gr.) or 200 mg. (3 gr.) in 2 cc.

Injection of Bismuth Salicylate B.P.

DOSES: intramuscular, 0.6-1.2 cc. (10-20 min.) . Contains 10% of Bismuth Salicylate with camphor and phenol in arachis oil.

Injection of Sodium Bismuthyl Tartrate B.P.

DOSES: intramuscular, 60-200 mg. (1-3 gr.). Strength, 60 mg. per cc. (1 gr. in 15 min.).

Bismuth Subsalicylate Injection U.S.P. *Injectio Bismuthi Subsalicylatis*

DOSE: 100 mg. (1½ gr.) intramuscular. A sterile suspension of Bismuth Subsalicylate in suitable fixed oil. Sizes, 100 mg. (1½ gr.) in 1 cc.; 120 mg. (2 gr.) in 1 cc.

℀ The various injections of bismuth are given intramuscularly in the treatment of syphilis. Injections are usually made once a week, into the gluteal muscles, during and between courses of intravenous therapy with organic arsenicals. The substances most often used in Canada are Bismuth Salicylate and Bismuth Oxychloride. Some soreness at the site of injection is common and occasionally systemic toxic effects of bismuth are seen, namely, gingivitis, stomatitis, and nephritis.

Bismuth Subgallate B.P. *Bismuthi Subgallas.* (Bismuth Oxygallate, Basic Bismuth Gallate)

S: ins. W, A, E; sol. in hot mineral acids with decomposition. A yellow powder; odourless and tasteless.

℀ Bismuth Subgallate is used for the most part externally in dusting powders. It has some astringent properties. It may also be given internally in capsules or cachets to treat diarrhoea, or in suppositories for haemorrhoids.

Suppositories of Bismuth Subgallate B.P.

Each contains 0.3 Gm. (5 gr.) of Bismuth Subgallate.

Compound Lozenges of Bismuth B.P. *Trochisci Bismuthi Compositi*

Each lozenge contains 150 mg. (2¼ gr.) Bismuth Carbonate, with Heavy Magnesium Carbonate, Calcium Carbonate, Acacia, Sucrose, Oil of Rose, and Water q.s.

℃ An antacid lozenge. See Bismuth Carbonate.

Sobisminol Mass N.N.R.

DOSES: oral, 4.5-6.75 Gm. daily in divided doses. A brown, pasty mass prepared by the interaction of sodium bismuthate, triisopropanolamine, and propylene glycol. Exact chemical nature is not known. S: sol. W, A; partially sol. E, acetone. Taste bitter with a sweetish metallic after taste. Contains 19.25-20.25% of Bi.

Pulvules Sobisminol Mass N.N.R. (Capsules)

Size, 0.75 Gm. (containing 150 mg. of Bi).

Sobisminol Solution N.N.R.

DOSE: intramuscular, 2 cc. twice weekly. Each cc. contains about 20 mg. of Bi and 0.5 cc. of propylene glycol.

℃ Sobisminol Mass is intended for the oral treatment of syphilis. The patient should be watched carefully for several days for signs of bismuth poisoning and the dose should be adjusted according to the patient's tolerance. Untoward symptoms include nausea, vomiting, diarrhoea, and stomatitis. Sobisminol Solution is intended for intramuscular administration and is said to have the advantage of minimal discomfort at the site of injection.

Borax B.P. *Borax.* **Sodium Borate U.S.P.** *Sodii Boras.* (Purified Borax, Sodium Tetraborate)

DOSES: B.P. 0.3-1 Gm. (5-15 gr.). $Na_2B_4O_7.10H_2O$. Mol. wt. 381.43. S: 16 W, 1 G, 1 W 100°; ins. A. Colourless transparent crystals or a white crystalline powder; odourless; efflorescent in warm dry air; aqueous solutions are alkaline to litmus. See Boric Acid.

℃ Solutions of Borax are alkaline. A solution of 0.13% Sodium Borate and 1.24% Boric Acid has a pH 7.1 and makes a non-irritating eyewash.

Glycerin of Borax B.P. *Glycerinum Boracis*

Borax 12% w/w in Glycerin.

℀ Glycerin of Borax is used sometimes to swab inflamed or ulcerated throats.

Boric Acid. *Acidum Boricum.* (Boracic Acid)
DOSES: B.P. 0.3-1 Gm. (5-15 gr.). H_3BO_3. Mol. wt. 61.84. S: 18 W, 18 A, 4 G, 4 W at 100°, 6 A at 78°. Colourless crystals with a pearly lustre, slightly unctuous to the touch.

℀ Boric Acid and Sodium Borate are bacteriostatic in 2-4% solution but not bactericidal. They do not irritate wounds or sensitive tissue, hence their popularity for eye washes and dressings. Powdered Boric Acid should not be applied to large wounds or burns, as serious poisoning can occur from absorption of borate. Boric Acid Ointment (10%) has produced poisoning when applied to a very large burn.

Powdered Boric Acid is a useful dusting powder for the feet where it suppresses odorous bacteria or fungi.

Glycerin of Boric Acid B.P. *Glycerinum Acidi Borici*
Boric Acid 31% w/w in Glycerin: contains about 50% w/w of boroglycerin.

℀ Used sometimes to paint sore throats.

Ointment of Boric Acid B.P. *Unguentum Acidi Borici*
Boric Acid 1%, in Paraffin Ointment.

Boric Acid Ointment U.S.P. *Unguentum Acidi Borici*
Boric Acid 10%, with Liquid Petrolatum and White Ointment.

Brilliant Blue Can. Gaz. *Caeruleum Nitens.* (F.D. & C. Blue No. 1)
$C_{37}H_{34}N_2O_9S_3Na_2$. Mol.wt. 792.5. S: 7 W, 65 A. A dark-purple, bronzy powder.

℀ Brilliant Blue is a food dye which may be used to colour mixtures. A solution of 1: 50,000 gives adequate colouring.

Brilliant Green B.P. *Viride Nitens*
$C_{27}H_{34}O_4N_2S$. Mol.wt. 482.61. S: sol. W and A 90%. Small, glistening, golden crystals.

℀ Brilliant Green is a powerful antiseptic, killing staphylococcus and other forms at dilutions of less than 1:1,000,000. It is usually applied to skin in solutions of 1:2,000. A 5% solution has been used successfully in the treatment of erysipelas, by application locally.

Bromethol B.P. *Bromethol.* **Tribromoethanol Solution U.S.P.** *Liquor Tribromoethanolis.* (Tribromoethyl Alcohol Solution. Solution of Tribromoethyl Alcohol. T.N. Avertin with Amylene Hydrate)

DOSES: B.P. by rectal injection as a basal anaesthetic 0.075-0.1 cc. per kg. body weight ($\frac{1}{2}$-$\frac{2}{3}$ min. per lb. body weight); U.S.P. 0.06 cc. (1 min.) per kg. body weight. *Caution. The total amount administered should not exceed 8 cc. for women or 10 cc. for men regardless of body weight.*

Bromethol is diluted immediately before administration with 39 times its own volume of water at 40°C., with vigorous shaking. One cc. of Bromethol contains 1 Gm. of Tribromoethyl Alcohol.

℄ Bromethol is a general anaesthetic but is too depressant to respiration to be used alone. For this reason too, morphine should not be given with it. Induction by Bromethol *per rectum* is said to be very tranquil. Adequate anaesthesia for operation is then secured by giving sufficient nitrous oxide, with or without ether.

Butopyronoxyl U.S.P. *Butopyronoxyl.* (T.N. Indalone)

$C_{12}H_{18}O_4$. Mol.wt. 226.26. Sp. gr. 1.052-1.060. S: ins. W; misc. A, C, E, glacial acetic acid. An insect repellent for application to the skin.

Oil of Cade B.P. *Oleum Cadinum.* (Juniper Tar Oil)

Gm./cc. 0.970-1.045. Sp.gr. 0.950-1.055. S: ss. W, 9 A; misc. amyl alcohol, C, glacial acetic acid; partially sol. petroleum benzin; almost completely sol. 3 E. The empyreumatic volatile oil obtained from the woody portions of *Juniperus Oxycedrus* Linn. A dark brown, clear, thick liquid having a tarry odour and a warm, faintly aromatic, bitter taste.

℄ Juniper Tar has the antiseptic and irritant actions of other tars and is used for chronic skin diseases, usually in ointments at strengths of 2 to 25%.

Cacao U.S.P. *Cacao*

A powder prepared from the roasted cured kernels of the ripe seed of *Theobroma Cacao* Linn. A brown powder having a chocolate taste and odour.

Cacao Syrup U.S.P.., C.F. *Syrupus Cacao.* (Cocoa Syrup)
Cacao 175, Vanilla Tincture 50, Gelatin 10, Sucrose 800, Water to make 1000 cc.

Caffeine B.P. *Caffeina.* (Theine)
Doses: 0.3-0.6 Gm. (5-10 gr.). $C_8H_{10}O_2N_4.H_2O$. Mol.wt. 212.2. M.p. 235-237°. S: at 25°: 50 W, 70 A, 6 C, 600 E; 6 W 80°; 25 A 60°. Colourless, silky crystals; odourless; taste bitter; efflorescent in dry air. An alkaloid from the dried leaves of *Camellia sinensis.*

Caffeine U.S.P. *Caffeina*
Dose: 0.2 Gm. (3 gr.). $C_8H_{10}N_4O_2$. Mol.wt. 194.19. M.p. 235-237.5°. S: 50 W, 75 A, 6 C, 600 E; 6 W 80°; 25 A 60°. White, glistening crystals usually matted together; odourless; taste bitter.

Caffeine and Sodium Benzoate. *Caffeina et Sodii Benzoas.* (Caffeine with Sodium Benzoate)
Doses: B.P. oral, 0.3-1 Gm. (5-15 gr.); subcutaneous, 0.12-0.3 Gm. (2-5 gr.); U.S.P. oral or intramuscular, 0.5 Gm. (7½ gr.). S: 1.2 W, 30 A; ss. C. A white powder; odourless; taste slightly bitter. Contains 47-50% anhydrous caffeine.

Caffeine and Sodium Benzoate Injection U.S.P.
Sizes, 250 mg. (4 gr.) in 2 cc.; 500 mg. (7½ gr.) in 2 cc.

Injection of Caffeine and Sodium Benzoate B.P.
Doses: subcutaneous, 0.12-0.3 Gm. (2-5 gr.). Strength, 0.25 Gm. per cc. (3¾ gr. in 15 min.).

℃ Caffeine and its salts are generally described as stimulants but this tells little of their various effects on the human organism. A vast amount of information is available about the effects of caffeine but its medicinal uses are not very important. The main effects of therapeutic doses are wakefulness and diuresis. It has been used hopefully as a cardiac stimulant and coronary dilator without adequate evidence of effectiveness. Some headaches are said to be relieved by caffeine, hence its incorporation in many headache remedies. A cup of tea or of coffee may contain about 0.1-0.2 Gm. (1½-3 gr.) of caffeine, enough to have a definite effect on the central nervous system, promoting wakefulness and suppressing sensations of fatigue, also enough to produce a definite diuresis. Acute poisoning from caffeine is rare. Chronic poisoning from excessive use of tea and coffee is not uncommon. The symptoms may be indigestion, nervousness, palpitation, and sometimes skin rashes. Caffeine as such, or in the form of strong tea or coffee, is useful in the treatment of morphine poisoning.

Oil of Cajuput B.P. *Oleum Cajuputi*
 DOSES: 0.06-0.2 cc. (1-3 min.). Gm./cc. 0.913-0.923. S: 2 A 80% 15.5°. The oil distilled from the fresh leaves and twigs of *Melaleuca Leucadendron* and other species of *Melaleuca*. Contains 50-65% w/w cineole. A colourless or yellow oil; odour agreeable and camphoraceous; taste aromatic, bitter, and camphoraceous.

℃ Oil of Cajuput is antiseptic and irritant to the skin. It has been used for ringworm of the scalp and is sometimes given internally, one or two drops on sugar, as a carminative.

Spirit of Cajuput B.P. *Spiritus Cajuputi*
 DOSES: 0.3-2 cc. (5-30 min.). Oil of Cajuput 10% v/v in 80-82% v/v C_2H_5OH.

Calamine U.S.P., C.F. *Calamina.* (Calamina Praeparata, Prepared Calamine)
 S: ins. W. An amorphous impalpable pink or reddish-brown powder; 98% zinc oxide coloured with iron oxide. In the B.P. Calamine is described as a basic zinc carbonate coloured with ferric oxide.

℃ Applied to the skin in a lotion or an ointment, Calamine acts as a bland protective with a tendency to dry up exudative lesions.

Calamine Lotion. *Lotio Calaminae*
 B.P.—Calamine 15, Zinc Oxide 5, with Glycerin and Distilled Water to make 100 cc.
 U.S.P.—Calamine 8, Zinc Oxide 8, in 100 cc.

Calcium Carbonate B.P. *Calcii Carbonas.* **Precipitated Calcium Carbonate U.S.P.** *Calcii Carbonas Praecipitatus.* (Precipitated Chalk)
 DOSES: B.P. 1-4 Gm. (15-60 gr.); U.S.P. 1 Gm. (15 gr.). $CaCO_3$. Mol.wt. 100.09. S: ins. A, W; ss. water containing CO_2. A white micro-crystalline powder; odourless; tasteless; 2.1 Gm. (32 gr.) neutralize about 500 cc. N/10 HC1.

℃ Calcium Carbonate is commonly used as a gastric antacid and is slightly constipating. It should not be used to neutralize poisonous doses of acid in the stomach, for fear of excessive production of CO_2. It is used extensively in tooth powders.

Calcium Chloride. *Calcii Chloridum*

DOSES: B.P. oral. 0.6-2 Gm. (10-30 gr.)   *Note*—B.P. specifies anhydrous salt, while the U.S.P. calls for the dihydrate. $CaCl_2$. Mol.wt. 111.0 (B.P.); or $CaCl_2.2 H_2O$. Mol.wt. 147.03 (U.S.P.). S: anhydrous, 1.5 W at 15.5°; 3 A 90%; hydrate, 1.2 W, 10 A; 0.7 W at 100°, 2 A at 78°.   The hydrate consists of white, hard, odourless fragments or granules, the anhydrous of dry white granules or porous masses; taste warm and slightly acrid, bitter; very deliquescent.

Hydrated Calcium Chloride B.P. *Calcii Chloridum Hydratum*

DOSES: intravenous, 0.6-2 Gm. (10-30 gr.). $CaCl_2.6H_2O$. Mol.wt. 219.1. S: 0.25 W, 0.95 A 90% at 15.5°. Colourless crystals; odourless; taste slightly bitter; very deliquescent.

℃ The two actions of calcium chloride which are most useful medically are (1) production of systemic acidosis, and (2) raising of blood calcium. A 5% solution may be injected intravenously for tetany or lead colic. If any is injected outside the vein, severe pain and tissue damage result. One Gm. by mouth every 2 or 3 hours renders the urine acid and if continued leads to systemic acidosis. A large amount of the calcium ion is apparently excreted by the bowel in combination with fatty acid leaving chloride ions free to acidify the blood and urine. Calcium ions specifically antagonize the narcosis produced by magnesium ion.

Calcium Gluconate. *Calcii Gluconas*

DOSES: B.P. oral, 1-4 Gm. (15-60 gr.); U.S.P. oral, 5 Gm. (75 gr.); intravenous, 1 Gm. (15 gr.). $Ca(C_6H_{11}O_7)_2.H_2O$. Mol.wt. 448.39. S: 30 W; 5 W at 100°; ins. A, C, E. A white, crystalline or granular, odourless and tasteless powder.

Injection of Calcium Gluconate B.P.

DOSES: intravenous or intramuscular, 10-20 cc. (150-300 min.) of 10% solution.

Calcium Gluconate Injection U.S.P.

Strength, 1 Gm. (15 gr.) in 10 cc. for intravenous or intramuscular injection.

Calcium Gluconate Tablets U.S.P.
Sizes, 0.5 and 1.0 Gm. (7½ and 15 gr.).

℘ For raising blood calcium the gluconate is preferable to calcium chloride. It is tolerated better by mouth and is less injurious to tissue on injection. It has no acidifying action.

Calcium Hydroxide. *Calcii Hydroxidum.* (Slaked Lime, Calcium Hydrate)
Ca(OH)$_2$. Mol.wt. 74.1. S: 630 W; 1300 W at 100°; sol. G, syrup; ins. A. A soft, white crystalline powder; odourless; taste alkaline and slightly bitter.

Calcium Hydroxide Solution U.S.P. Solution of Calcium Hydroxide B.P. *Liquor Calcii Hydroxidi.* (Liquor Calcis, Solution of Lime, Lime Water)
DOSES: B.P. 30-120 cc. (1-4 fl. oz.); U.S.P. 15 cc. (4 fl. dr.). A clear, colourless liquid; taste and reaction alkaline; contains not less than 0.15% w/v Ca(OH)$_2$.

℘ Lime Water was once the standard treatment for indigestion and diarrhoea in infants. Dietary adjustments are now preferred in the majority of cases.

Calcium Lactate. *Calcii Lactas*
DOSES: B.P. 1-4 Gm. (15-60 gr.); U.S.P. 5 Gm. (75 gr.). Ca(C$_3$H$_5$O$_3$)$_2$.5H$_2$O. Mol.wt. 308.3. S: 20 W; ins. A; readily sol. hot W. A white powder; almost odourless and tasteless; contains about 13% Ca.

Calcium Lactate Tablets U.S.P.
Sizes, 300 and 600 mg. (5 and 10 gr.).

Tablets of Calcium Lactate B.P.
Size, 0.3 Gm. (5 gr.).

Calcium Mandelate—see Mandelic Acid.

Dibasic Calcium Phosphate U.S.P. *Calcii Phosphas Dibasicus.* (Dicalcium Orthophosphate)
DOSE: 1 Gm. (15 gr.). CaHPO$_4$.2H$_2$O. Mol.wt. 172.10. S: almost ins. W; readily sol. dil. hydrochloric and nitric acids; ins. A. A white, odourless, and tasteless powder; stable in air.

Calcium Phosphate B.P. *Calcii Phosphas.* (Tribasic Calcium Phosphate)

DOSES: 0.6-2 Gm. (10-30 gr.). S: ins. W, A; sol. dil. hydrochloric and nitric acids. A white, odourless, and tasteless powder; contains not less than 85% $Ca_3(PO_4)_2$.

℀ Calcium Phosphate may be used as a gastric antacid. It does not produce systemic acidosis or liberate gas. It may also be used to add bulk to powders or extracts.

Chlorinated Lime B.P. *Calx Chlorinata* (Calcium Chloride Hypochlorite, Bleaching Powder)

S; partly sol. A, W. A white powder with a characteristic odour: becomes moist and decomposes when exposed to air, liberating free chlorine; decomposition more rapid in water; contains not less than 30% w/w available chlorine.

℀ Chloride of Lime is used to disinfect sinks, urinals, etc. by the liberation of chlorine. It is also used for the preparation of the Surgical Solution of Chlorinated Soda (Dakin's Solution).

Aromatic Powder of Chalk B.P. *Pulvis Cretae Aromaticus*

DOSES: 0.6-4 Gm. (10-60 gr.). Chalk 25%, with Cinnamon, Nutmeg, Clove, Cardamom and Sucrose.

Aromatic Powder of Chalk with Opium B.P. *Pulvis Cretae Aromaticus cum Opio*

DOSES: 0.6-4 Gm. (10-60 gr.). Aromatic Powder of Chalk with Powdered Opium. Contains in 4 Gm. (60 gr.), 10 mg. ($\frac{1}{7}$ gr.) of anhydrous morphine.

Chalk B.P. *Creta.* **Prepared Chalk N.F.** *Creta Praeparata* (Drop Chalk)

DOSES: B.P. 1-4 Gm. (15-60 gr.); N.F. 1 Gm. (15 gr.). S: ins. W, A. A white or greyish-white micro-crystalline powder or masses; odourless and tasteless. Contains not less than 97% of $CaCO_3$ (mol.wt. 100.1) when dried.

Chalk Mixture C.F. *Mistura Cretae*

DOSE: 15-30 cc. (4-8 fl. dr.). Prepared Chalk 3% w/v, with Saccharin Sodium, Bentonite, Cinnamon Water, and Distilled Water.

℀ The preceding preparations of Chalk are intended for the symptomatic treatment of diarrhoea. The preparation containing opium is presumably the most potent.

Calumba B.P. *Calumba.* (Calumba Root)
Dried slices of the root of *Jateorhiza palmata*; contains a bitter principle but no tannin.

Powdered Calumba B.P. *Calumbae Pulvis*
A yellowish-grey powder.

Concentrated Infusion of Calumba B.P. *Infusum Calumbae Concentratum*
DOSES: 2-4 cc. (30-60 min.). Calumba 40 Gm. with Alcohol and Distilled Water to make 100 cc., by maceration. Contains 21-24% v/v of C_2H_5OH. When diluted with 7 volumes of distilled water it yields a product similar in strength, but not in flavour, to the fresh infusion.

Fresh Infusion of Calumba B.P. *Infusum Calumbae Recens*
DOSES: 15-30 cc. ($\frac{1}{2}$-1 fl. oz.). Calumba 5% w/v with cold Distilled Water. Should be dispensed within 12 hours of its preparation.

Tincture of Calumba B.P. *Tinctura Calumbae*
DOSES: 2-4 cc. ($\frac{1}{2}$-1 fl. dr.). Calumba 10 Gm. with Alcohol and water to make 100 cc., by maceration. Contains 57-60% v/v of C_2H_5OH.

⟪ Calumba is a simple bitter, i.e. it contains no tannic acid and hence can be used in mixtures containing iron. For some people bitters may stimulate appetite but for others they seem to be ineffective. Several hundred cc. of Recent Infusion may be given by enema to expel thread worms. See Quassia.

Camphor. *Camphora*
DOSES: B.P. oral, 0.12-0.3 Gm. (2-5 gr.); U.S.P. oral or intramuscular, 0.2 Gm. (3 gr.). $C_{10}H_{16}O$. Mol.wt. 152.23. S: 800 W, 1 A, 0.5 C, 1 E; fs. CS_2, petroleum benzin, fixed and volatile oils. A colourless solid, or colourless to white, translucent, tough masses; penetrating, characteristic odour; taste pungent. Obtained from *Cinnamomum Camphora* or made synthetically.

Ammoniated Liniment of Camphor B.P. *Linimentum Camphorae Ammoniatum*
Camphor 12.5% w/v with Strong Solution of Ammonia, Oil of Lavender, and Alcohol. Contains 54-58% v/v C_2H_5OH.

Camphor Liniment U.S.P. Liniment of Camphor B.P. *Linimentum Camphorae.* (Camphorated Oil)
B.P.—Camphor 20, Arachis Oil 80 Gm. U.S.P.—Camphor 20, Cotton Seed Oil 80 Gm.

Spirit of Camphor B.P. *Spiritus Camphorae*
DOSES: 0.3-2 cc. (5-30 min.). Contains Camphor 10% w/v and 80-82% v/v C_2H_5OH.

Camphor Water. *Aqua Camphorae*
DOSES: B.P. 15-30 cc. ($\frac{1}{2}$-1 fl.oz.). A saturated solution of Camphor in water (about 0.1% of Camphor).

Camphorated Opium Tincture. See Opium.

⟨ The popularity and variety of medicinal preparations of camphor must be due to a large extent to its impressive odour. In large doses, 1-10 Gm., camphor is a convulsant. Subconvulsant doses have effects on the heart, circulation, and respiration, but do not seem applicable to any useful purpose. On the skin, local application produces reddening but little irritation or burning. A saturated aqueous solution is bacteriostatic and fungistatic but has little or no germicidal action.

The Camphorated Tincture of Opium is a useful cough sedative. The pungent taste may contribute some expectorant action.

The various liniments provide varying degrees of rubefacient and counterirritant action.

Three parts of camphor and one part of phenol rubbed together produce a liquid known as Phenol and Camphor B.P.C., which has antiseptic and obtundent properties and which (with caution) may be applied to the skin for the treatment of fungus infections. Various combinations of camphor and phenol with or without liquid paraffin or alcohol have been called Camphorated Phenol or Campho-Phenique. They are used in dentistry as antiseptics in the treatment of root canals.

Capsicum B.P. *Capsicum*
The dried ripe fruit of *Capsicum minimum*; taste burning and pungent.

Powdered Capsicum B.P. *Capsici Pulvis*
Orange to brownish-red powder.

Tincture of Capsicum B.P.   *Tinctura Capsici*
DOSES: 0.3-1 cc. (5-15 min.).   Capsicum 5 Gm., with Alcohol and Water to make 100 cc., by maceration.   Contains 57-60% v/v C_2H_5OH.

Ointment of Capsicum B.P.   *Unguentum Capsici.* (Capsicum Ointment)
Capsicum 25 Gm. with 95 Gm. of Simple Ointment.   The capsicum is extracted in melted ointment and strained off.

℃ Capsicum ointment may be applied as a counterirritant to relieve the pain of arthritis, lumbago, or neuralgia.

Caraway.   *Carum.*   (Carui Fructus, Caraway Fruit, Caraway Seed)
The dried fruit of *Carum Carvi.*

Powdered Caraway B.P.   *Cari Pulvis*
A fawn to brown powder.

Oil of Caraway B.P.   *Oleum Cari.*   (Oleum Carui)
DOSES: 0.06-0.2 cc. (1-3 min.).   Gm./cc. 0.905-0.915.   S: 1 A 90%.
A colourless or pale-yellow liquid; odour and taste aromatic.

℃ Caraway has an exotic flavour acceptable to some people. It is said to be an excellent carminative.

Carbachol.   *Carbacholum.*   (Carbamylcholine Chloride.   T.N. Doryl, Lentin)
DOSES: B.P. oral 1-4 mg. ($\frac{1}{60}$-$\frac{1}{16}$ gr.); subcutaneous 0.25-0.5 mg. ($\frac{1}{240}$-$\frac{1}{120}$ gr.); U.S.P. oral 2 mg. ($\frac{1}{30}$ gr.); subcutaneous 0.25 mg. ($\frac{1}{240}$ gr.). $C_6H_{15}O_2N_2Cl$.   Mol.wt. 182.65.   M.p. 200-203° U.S.P. or 210-212° B.P.   S: vs. W; ss. A abs.; almost ins. acetone, E. Small white crystals or a crystalline powder; odour faint; markedly hygroscopic.

Carbachol Injection U.S.P.
Size, 0.25 mg. ($\frac{1}{250}$ gr.) in 1 cc.

Injection of Carbachol B.P.
DOSES: subcutaneous, 0.25-0.5 mg. ($\frac{1}{240}$-$\frac{1}{120}$ gr.).   Strength, 0.25 mg. per cc. ($\frac{1}{240}$ gr. in 15 min.).

Carbachol Tablets U.S.P.
Size, 2 mg. ($\frac{1}{30}$ gr.).

⟪ Carbachol produces all the peripheral effects of acetylcholine and is more suitable for administration as it is less rapidly destroyed by cholinesterase. It may be used in post-operative ileus and urinary retention. It may also be used to produce vasodilatation in Raynaud's disease or applied locally to the eye for a miotic action and to lower intraocular tension.

Carbon Dioxide. *Carbonei Dioxidum.* (Carbonic Acid Gas)

CO_2. Mol.wt. 44.01. S: 1 vol. in about 1.3 W. A heavy, colourless gas; taste in aqueous solution faintly acid; odourless; purity, not less than 99% v/v.

⟪ Carbon Dioxide is a physiological stimulant of respiration. A mixture containing 5% v/v of CO_2 not only stimulates breathing but also bronchial secretions. It has been used as an expectorant in the treatment of pulmonary tuberculosis. Five to 10% mixtures are given by inhalation post-operatively to stimulate breathing and prevent atelectasis. Concentrations above 15% may produce convulsions and coma. The use of CO_2 mixtures to combat respiratory failure, except of the kind due to over-ventilation, is not very effective or rational since in such states too much CO_2 may be in the blood stream already.

Carbon Tetrachloride B.P. *Carbonei Tetrachloridum.* (Tetrachloromethane)

DOSES: single oral, 2-4 cc. (30-60 min.). CCl_4. Mol.wt. 153.8. B.p. 76.5-77.5°. Gm./cc. 1.592-1.595. S: ins. W; misc. A abs., E, C. A clear, colourless, volatile liquid; odour characteristic; taste burning; non-inflammable.

⟪ Carbon Tetrachloride has anaesthetic properties like chloroform but is more toxic to the liver and consequently is never used as an anaesthetic. It may, however, be given by mouth (in capsules) for the treatment of hookworm, tapeworm, and threadworm. Like other anthelmintics, it is given on an empty stomach in the morning and followed in 2 hours by a saline purge. The treatment may be repeated in a week. Toxic symptoms are most likely to occur in alcoholics and in the undernourished. Preliminary treatment with a high carbohydrate, high calcium diet is recommended.

Carbromal B.P.C. *Carbromalum.* (Uradal)

DOSES: 0.3-1 Gm. (5-15 gr.). Bromodiethylacetylurea. $C_7H_{13}O_2N_2Br$. Mol.wt. 237.1. M.p. 116-118°. S: 3000 W, 18 A, 14 E, 3 C. A white crystalline powder; almost odourless and tasteless. Available in tablets of 0.3 Gm. (5 gr.).

℃ Carbromal is a sedative which is used to reduce excitement and favour sleep.   It is usually given about half an hour before bedtime. It is said to be less powerful than the barbiturates or chloral hydrate but singularly free from unpleasant side effects.

Cardamom Fruit B.P. *Cardamomi Fructus.* **Cardamom Seed U.S.P.** *Cardamomi Semen*

The dry ripe seeds of *Eletteria Cardamomum*; taste warm, aromatic, and slightly bitter; odour aromatic.

Compound Cardamom Tincture U.S.P. Compound Tincture of Cardamom B.P. *Tinctura Cardamomi Composita*

DOSES: B.P. 2-4 cc. (30-60 min.); U.S.P. 4 cc. (1 fl.dr.).   B.P· Cardamom 1.4, Caraway 1.4, Cinnamon 2.8, with Cochineal, Glycerin and Alcohol to make 100 cc., by percolation.   Contains 52-57% v/v of C_2H_5OH.   U.S.P.—Cardamom 2, Cinnamon 2.5, Caraway 1.2, with Cochineal, Glycerin, and Diluted Alcohol to make 100 cc., by maceration.   Contains 43-47% v/v of C_2H_5OH.

℃ Cardamom has a reputation as a carminative.   It is used as a flavour in mixtures containing iron.

Cascara Sagrada. *Cascara Sagrada.* (Rhamnus Purshiana)
The dried bark of *Rhamnus Purshiana*; taste persistent, bitter.

Powdered Cascara Sagrada B.P. *Cascarae Sagradae Pulvis*
A light yellowish-brown to olive-brown powder.

Cascara Sagrada Extract U.S.P. *Extractum Cascarae Sagradae.* (Powdered Cascara Sagrada Extract)

DOSE: 0.3 Gm. (5 gr.).   A dry, powdered, aqueous extract, adjusted with starch so that 1 Gm. of the extract represents 3 Gm. of Cascara Sagrada.

Cascara Sagrada Extract Tablets U.S.P. (Cascara Tablets)
Sizes, 0.12, 0.2, 0.3 Gm. (2, 3, 5 gr.).

Aromatic Cascara Sagrada Fluidextract U.S.P. *Fluidextractum Cascarae Sagradae Aromaticum*

DOSE: 2 cc. (30 min.).   Cascara Sagrada 100, Magnesium Oxide 12, with Pure Glycyrrhiza Extract, Saccharin, Oil of Anise, Oil of

Coriander, Methyl Salicylate, Alcohol, of each q.s., and Water to make 100. Contains 17-19% v/v of C_2H_5OH.

Cascara Sagrada Fluidextract U.S.P. *Fluidextractum Cascarae Sagradae.* (Rhamnus Purshiana Fluidextract). **Liquid Extract of Cascara Sagrada B.P.** *Extractum Cascarae Sagradae Liquidum* (Bitter Extract of Cascara)
Doses: B.P. 2-4 cc. (30-60 min.); U.S.P. 1 cc. (15 min.).
Both are aqueous extracts of Cascara Sagrada (1000 Gm. made up to a final volume of 1000 cc.). Alcohol is added as a preservative. B.P. contains 21-24% and U.S.P. 17-19% v/v of C_2H_5OH.

Dry Extract of Cascara Sagrada B.P. *Extractum Cascarae Sagradae Siccum*
Doses: 0.12-0.5 Gm. (2-8 gr.). A dried aqueous extract.

Elixir of Cascara Sagrada B.P. *Elixir Cascarae Sagradae*
Doses: 2-4 cc. (30-60 min.). Cascara Sagrada 100 Gm., Light Magnesium Oxide 15 Gm., with Liquorice, Saccharin Sodium, Oil of Coriander, Oil of Anise, Alcohol and Glycerin, and Distilled Water to make 100 cc. Contains 1-1.2% v/v of C_2H_5OH.

⟪ Cascara is a very popular laxative. The active principle is not known with certainty but is thought to be emodin (trioxy-methylanthraquinone) or some related derivative of anthracene. The action is mainly on the large intestine. A dose at bedtime gives rise to one or two soft stools the next morning. Cascara compares favourably with other laxatives for the treatment of chronic constipation. There seems to be no after constipation following a moderate dose. It is considered safe to prescribe cascara (with caution) for the treatment of constipation during pregnancy.

Some of the active principles are excreted in the urine, colouring it red or violet if alkaline, or brownish if acid.

The Elixir and the Aromatic Fluidextract are more pleasant to take than the other preparations of Cascara.

Castor Oil. *Oleum Ricini*
Doses: B.P. 4-16 cc. (60-240 min.); U.S.P. 15 cc. (4 fl.dr.). Gm./cc. 0.953-0.964. S: 3.5 A 90% 15.5°; misc. dehydrated A, C, E, and glacial acetic acid. The fixed oil obtained from the seeds of *Ricinus communis*. A pale yellowish or almost colourless, transparent, viscous liquid having a faint, mild odour and a bland and afterwards slightly acrid and usually nauseating taste.

ℭ In the small intestine castor oil is hydrolyzed with the liberation of ricinoleic acid which irritates the mucosa of the intestine, causing hyperactivity of the glands and musculature of the gastro-intestinal tract and copious soft stools in 4 or 5 hours. It is usually given before breakfast or at some other time on an empty stomach.

Castor oil is often given to induce labour at term. The mechanism of its influence on uterine contractions is not known but it is usually explained as a reflex consequence of intestinal irritation.

Castor oil is also used in rubbing alcohol to leave an oily film on the skin to protect it and prevent the development of bedsores. Drops of castor oil in the eye are soothing, and drugs for application to the eye are sometimes dissolved in it.

Oil of Cassia Can. Gaz. *Oleum Cassiae*
See Cinnamon Oil.

Catechu B.P. *Catechu.* (Pale Catechu, Gambir)
A dried aqueous extract from *Uncaria Gambier*; taste bitter, astringent, subsequently sweetish; odourless; contains a tannin.

Powdered Catechu B.P. *Catechu Pulvis*
A pale-brown powder.

Tincture of Catechu B.P. *Tinctura Catechu*
DOSES: 2-4 cc. (30-60 min.). Catechu 20, Cinnamon 5, with Alcohol and Water to make 100 cc., by maceration. Contains 37-40% v/v C_2H_5OH.

ℭ Catechu contains among other things a tannic acid. It is reputed to be a useful astringent for the treatment of diarrhoea or intestinal haemorrhage.

Oxidized Cellulose U.S.P. *Cellulosum Oxidatum.* (Absorbable Cellulose, Cellulosic Acid. T.N. Oxycel, Hemo-Pak).
Oxidized Cellulose dried in a vacuum over P_2O_5 for 18 hours. S: sol. in dil. alkalis; ins. acids, W.

ℭ Cellulosic acid acts on shed blood to produce an artificial clot; consequently oxidized cellulose packs are used for stopping haemorrhage from small blood vessels in situations where ligation of bleeding vessels is not practicable. Small pieces of oxidized cellulose need not be removed at the end of an operation but may be left in position, as they are absorbed, usually in less than a week. The material is not suitable for prolonged application as dressings for injuries involving the skin, for it interferes with epithelialization. The clot-forming action of cellulosic acid is not enhanced by thrombin. Thrombin is probably inactivated by the cellulosic acid. Consequently haemostatics containing thrombin should not be used with oxidized cellulose.

Cetrimide B.P. *Cetrimidum.* (T.N. Cetavlon, CTAB)

For external use only, in concentrations of 1:100 to 1:1000. Consists largely of cetyl-trimethyl ammonium bromide together with smaller amounts of other alkyltrimethyl ammonium bromides, and some sodium bromide. S: 50 W, fs. A. A white powder, with a fishy odour and a strong soapy taste.

⟪ Cetrimide is a typical cationic detergent. It is used for pre-operative cleansing of the skin in a strength of 1%. Repeated application may result in sensitization, which is indicated by excessive dryness of the skin.

Cetostearyl Alcohol B.P. *Alcohol Cetostearylicum*

M.p. not below 43°. S: ins. W; sol. E; ss. A 90% or in light petroleum. A white or cream-coloured unctuous mass or almost white flakes; odour faint and characteristic; taste bland. A mixture of solid aliphatic alcohols, mostly stearyl and cetyl alcohols. See Emulsifying Wax.

Cetyl Pyridinium Chloride N.N.R. (T.N. Ceepryn Chloride)

For external use only in concentrations of 1:100-1:10,000. The monohydrate of cetyl pyridinium chloride. $C_{21}H_{38}Cl$ N.H_2O. Mol. wt. 357.99. M.p. 77-83°. S: vs. A, C, W. A white powder with a slight odour. Available as concentrated solution, Ceepryn Chloride 10% which also contains in each 100 cc., 8 Gm. of monobasic sodium phosphate. Also available as Isotonic Solution Ceepryn Chloride 1:1000 which contains sodium phosphates.

⟪ For pre-operative sterilization of skin 1:100 solution may be used. For ordinary cuts, fungal infections, and other household uses, the usual strength is 1:1000. Cetyl pyridinium chloride is a cationic detergent.

Activated Charcoal U.S.P. XIII. *Carbo Activatus.* (Carbo Medicinalis C.F.)

DOSES: C.F. 1-10 Gm. (15-150 gr.).   A fine black tasteless powder free from gritty matter.   1 Gm. in 50 cc. water adsorbs 0.1
Gm. strychnine sulphate in 5 min.

⊄ The adsorptive power of Activated Charcoal makes it a useful
antidote for a variety of poisons such as $HgCl_2$ or alkaloids.   It
should be followed by a purge.   It may be given to relieve diarrhoea.

Oil of Chenopodium B.P.   *Oleum Chenopodii.*   (Oil of American Wormseed)

DOSES: 0.2-1 cc. (3-15 min.).   Gm./cc. 0.956-0.977.   S at 15.5°:
3-10 A 70%.   A pale-yellow or colourless liquid having a characteristic odour and bitter, burning taste.   Obtained from the fresh
flowering and fruiting plants, excluding the roots, of *Chenopodium
ambrosioides*, var. *anthelminticum*, by steam distillation.   Contains
not less than 65% w/w of ascaridole.

⊄ Oil of Chenopodium is used for the treatment of roundworms
and hookworms.

Cherry Juice U.S.P., C.F.   *Succus Cerasi*

The juice expressed from the fresh ripe fruit of *Prunus Cerasus*.
Sp. gr. 1.045-1.075.

Cherry Syrup U.S.P., C.F.   *Syrupus Cerasi*

Cherry Juice 475, Sucrose 800, Alcohol 20, Water to make 1000 cc.

Chiniofon.   *Chiniofonum.*   (Chiniofon Powder.   T.N. Yatren, Quinoxyl)

DOSES: B.P. oral, 60-500 mg. (1-8 gr.); by rectal injection, 1-5
Gm. (15-75 gr.); U.S.P. 1 Gm. (15 gr.).   S: 25 W (with effervescence);
ins. A, E, C.   A canary-yellow powder with a slight odour; taste
bitter at first but followed by a sweetish after taste.   A mixture of
iodohydroxyquinoline sulphonic acid, its sodium salt and sodium
bicarbonate, hence the effervescence on solution.   Contains about
28% of iodine.

⊄ Chiniofon is given by mouth or by enema for the treatment of
amoebic dysentery.   It should not be given when the liver is
diseased or to persons sensitive to iodine.

Chiniofon Tablets U.S.P.   *Tabellae Chiniofoni*

Size, 0.25 Gm. (4 gr.).

Chloral Hydrate. *Chloralis Hydras.* (Chloral)

DOSES: B.P. 0.3-2 Gm. (5-30 gr.); U.S.P. 0.6 Gm. (10 gr.). $CCl_3CH(OH)_2$. Mol.wt. 165.42. S: 0.25 W, 1.3 A, 2 C, 1.5 E, fs. in olive oil and in oil of turpentine. Colourless crystals; odour pungent, aromatic, penetrating; taste slightly bitter and burning.

⟨ In the recommended doses by mouth chloral hydrate is absorbed rapidly and may produce sleepiness in a few minutes. Such doses induce sleep of a natural character, lasting 6 or 8 hours. The patient can be aroused without much trouble at any time. The drug has no analgesic action so that severe pain will prevent the induction of sleep. Chloral hydrate is very irritating and must be taken well diluted; 1 Gm. in 6 cc. of Syrup and 2 cc. of Compound Syrup of Sassafras is a suitable mixture. It should be diluted with 3-4 times its volume of water before swallowing and then quickly washed down with water to remove the burning after taste.

Chloral and camphor when triturated in equal parts form a liquid known as Camphorated Chloral B.P.C. which may be applied to the skin to allay itching.

Chloramine B.P. *Chloramina.* (Chloramine T.)

$CH_3.C_6H_4.SO_2Na.NCl.3H_2O$. Mol.wt. 281.7. S: 7 W; 2 W at 100°; ins. C, E; sol. A but decomposes. White or faintly yellow crystalline powder; odour faintly of chlorine; taste unpleasant and bitter; contains about 12% active chlorine.

⟨ Solutions of Chloramine are germicidal by the liberation of free chlorine. They are more stable than Dakin's Solution. For irrigating the bladder or for a mouth wash, a 0.5% solution is suitable. Chloramine solutions do not possess the property of dissolving dead tissues which is characteristic of Dakin's Solution. A 1% solution in water may be used as a mouth wash to overcome foul odours in the mouth of local origin.

Chloramphenicol U.S.P. *Chloramphenicol.* (T.N. Chloromycetin)

DOSES: Initial, oral, 0.5-1 Gm. every hour for 3 hours, followed by 0.25-0.5 Gm. four times a day. $C_{11}H_{12}N_2O_5Cl_2$. Mol.wt. 323.14. S: 400 W, 7 propylene glycol; fs. A, acetone and ethyl acetate. A white crystalline substance with a bitter taste; stable at pH's from 2-9 and for several hours in boiling water. Available in capsules each containing 0.25 Gm.

⟨ Originally isolated from cultures of *Streptomyces Venezuelae*, chloramphenicol may be prepared now either by fermentation or

by chemical synthesis.   Clinical experience with this compound
dates from early 1948, when it was shown to be an effective treatment for typhus.   Since that time its effectiveness has been demonstrated in scrub typhus, typhoid fever and other salmonella infections, E. coli infections, whooping cough, rickettsial infections, and
certain cases of atypical pneumonia, also perhaps in measles and
herpes zoster.

Intramuscular or subcutaneous injection of chloramphenicol
causes pain, inflammation and necrosis.   Intravenous injection is
feasible but not recommended.

No toxic effects have been reported following oral doses, except
for nausea which may make it necessary to administer the drug by
duodenal tube.

Most of the drug is excreted in the urine as inactive nitro-com-
pounds; only 4%-8% is excreted in the active form.

Chloroazodin U.S.P.   *Chloroazodinum*

No Dose. $C_2H_4Cl_2N_6$.   Mol.wt. 183.01.   S: ss. W, A, G; less
sol. C.   Bright yellow needles or flakes; odour faintly of chlorine;
taste slightly burning.   Contains 37.5-39.5% of active chlorine.

Chloroazodin Solution U.S.P.   *Liquor Chloroazodini*

Chloroazodin 2.6, Glyceryl Triacetate to make 1000.   A clear
yellow, oily liquid.

℃ Chloroazodin is an antiseptic which has claims to superiority
over chloramine and hypochlorite solutions in stability and
efficiency.   Solutions of 1:6000 to 1:3000 are non-irritant and
actively disinfectant.   It is suggested for use in the sterilization of
dental pulp canals and periapical abscesses.   It may be used for the
treatment of fistulas and as a wet dressing for infected wounds.

Chlorbutol B.P.   *Chlorbutol.*   Chlorobutanol U.S.P.   *Chlorobutanol.*
(Acetone Chloroform, T.N. Chloretone)

Doses: B.P. 0.3-1.2 Gm. (5-20 gr.); U.S.P. 0.6 Gm. (10 gr.).
$Cl_3C.C(CH_3)_2OH$.   Mol.wt. 177.47.   M.p. not below 76°.   S: 125 W,
1 A, 10 G; readily sol. E, C and in volatile oils.   Colourless crystals
with a characteristic, musty, camphoraceous odour and taste.

℃ Chloretone has a long history of widely varied uses but its
most common use at present is to preserve various solutions, e.g.
of epinephrine or pituitary extract, for which it is used at concentrations of 0.1-0.5%.

It is also a hypnotic with dosage and action practically identical with chloral hydrate. In somewhat smaller doses it has been used to alleviate seasickness or post-operative vomiting, and to alleviate spasm of the bladder in cystitis. It has been used externally for itching and sprayed in the nose for colds.

Chloroguanide Hydrochloride U.S.P. Proguanil Hydrochloride B.P. (T.N. Paludrine, Guanatol, Chlorguanide)

Doses: oral, prophylactic, 0.1 Gm. twice a week; suppressive, 0.3 Gm. weekly; curative, 0.1 Gm. three times daily or 0.3 Gm. daily. $C_{11}H_{16}N_5Cl.HCl$. N^1-(p-chlorophenyl)-N^5-isopropylbiguanide hydrochloride. Mol.wt. 290.2. M.p. 248-252°. S: Sol. A; ss. W; ins. C,E. A colourless, odourless, fine, crystalline powder; taste bitter. Available as tablets, sizes, 25, 50, 100 and 300 mg.

℄ Chlorguanide is particularly effective against malignant tertian malaria (*P. falciparum*) but is less effective than mepacrine or chloroquine against *P. vivax*. Toxic effects are rare with the usual doses of chlorguanide but large doses (1 Gm.) may produce vomiting, abdominal pain and diarrhoea. Still larger doses may produce haematuria and casts in the urine. Chlorguanide is rapidly eliminated from the body after usual doses and is seldom detectable in body fluids after 48 hours. About half of the drug is excreted in the urine.

Chlorocresol B.P *Chlorocresol*. (Parachlorometacresol)

$CH_3.C_6H_3(Cl)OH-1:6:3$. Mol.wt. 142.58. M.p. 64-66°. S: 250 W 15.5°; more sol. in hot W; sol. A, E, terpenes, fixed oils and in sodium hydroxide; volatile in steam. Colourless crystals; odour characteristic.

℄ In a concentration of 0.1% chlorocresol is used as a bacteriostatic agent to preserve solutions for injection.

Chloroform. *Chloroformum*. (Trichloromethane)

Doses: B.P. 0.06-0.3 cc. (1-5 min.). No dose U.S.P. $CHCl_3$. Mol.wt. 119.4. B.p. 61°. Sp.gr. 1.474-1.478. S: 210 W; misc. A, E, B, petroleum benzin, fixed and volatile oils. A clear, colourless, mobile liquid having a characteristic ethereal odour and a burning sweet taste; non-inflammable.

℄ One per cent of chloroform vapour in air v/v is sufficient to induce general anaesthesia. In spite of many favourable characteristics, chloroform is not regarded on this continent as a safe anaesthetic. The favourable characteristics are fast and fairly pleasant induction, small volume required, and excellence of relaxation obtained. The unfavourable characteristics are ease of overdosage, with depression of heart and circulation, danger of sudden death by ventricular fibrillation in the early stages of anaesthesia, and danger of liver damage post-operatively.

Externally, Chloroform is a rubefacient and is often included in liniments. Chloroform Water is sweet and is used as a carminative flavour. The Spirit of Chloroform is frequently used as a source of alcohol in place of Rectified Spirit.

Emulsion of Chloroform B.P. *Emulsio Chloroformi*
DOSES: 0.3-2 cc. (5-30 min.). Chloroform 5, with Liquid Extract of Quillaia, Mucilage of Tragacanth, and Distilled Water to make 100. Chloroform content is equal to that of Spirit of Chloroform.

Spirit of Chloroform B.P. *Spiritus Chloroformi*
DOSES: 0.3-2 cc. (5-30 min.). Chloroform 5% v/v in 84-87% v/v C_2H_5OH.

Chloroform Water B.P. *Aqua Chloroformi*
DOSES: 15-30 cc. ($\frac{1}{2}$-1 fl.oz.). Chloroform 0.25% v/v in Distilled Water.

Chloroquine Phosphate U.S.P. *Chloroquinae Phosphas.* (Chloroquine Diphosphate, T.N. Aralen Diphosphate)
DOSES: oral, suppressive 0.5 Gm. at exactly seven-day intervals; curative, initial 1 Gm. to be followed by 0.5 Gm. after 6-8 hours and 0.5 Gm. on each of two consecutive days (total of 2.5 Gm. in 3 days). $C_{18}H_{32}ClN_3O_8P_2$. 7-chloro-4-(4-diethylamino-1-methylbutylamino) quinoline diphosphate. Mol.wt. 515.88. M.p. of one form 193-195° and of a second form 215-218°. S: fs. W; almost ins. A, B, C, E. A white crystalline powder; taste bitter. Available as tablets, size, 0.25 Gm.

℃ Chloroquine diphosphate is particularly useful for the treatment, suppression, and prevention of malignant tertian malaria (*P. falciparum*). It is less effective in preventing or suppressing benign tertian malaria (*P. vivax*). It will, however, terminate acute attacks of *vivax* malaria. The drug remains in the body in detectable amounts for a week or more after usual doses. Toxic manifestations are rarely serious but may include headache, blurring of vision, and pruritus.

Chloroxylenol B.P. *Chloroxylenol.* (Parachlorometaxylenol)

C_8H_9OCl. Mol.wt. 156.6. M.p. 114-115.5°. S: 3000 W at 15.5°; sol. A, E, B, terpenes, fixed oils and in solutions of alkali hydroxides. White to creamy crystals; odour characteristic.

Solution of Chloroxylenol B.P. *Liquor Chloroxylenolis.* (Roxenol. T.N. Dettol, Det)

Chloroxylenol 5, Terpineol 10, with Alcohol, Ricinoleic Acid, Solution of Potassium Hydroxide, and Distilled Water to make 100. Contains 17%-22% v/v of C_2H_5OH. When diluted with 19 vols. of water it forms a stable emulsion.

℣ Roxenol is widely used under the trade name Dettol (or Det in the U.S.A.) as an antiseptic for cuts and abrasions, and for cleansing the perineum in obstetrics. It is relatively non-irritant but active when diluted 1:20. Large quantities can be swallowed without serious harm.

Cholesterol U.S.P. *Cholesterol.* (Cholesterin)

$C_{27}H_{46}O$. Mol.wt. 386.64. M.p. 147-150°. S: ins. W; sps. A; sol. hot A, C, E, ethyl acetate, petroleum benzin and in vegetable oil. White or faintly yellow, almost odourless, pearly leaflets or granules; becomes darker on exposure to air.

Chrysarobin U.S.P. *Chrysarobinum*

S: ss. W, 400 A, 15 C, 160 E. A mixture of anthranols from Goa Powder, a substance deposited in the wood of *Andira Araroba*. A brown to orange-yellow crystalline powder; odourless and tasteless; irritating to the mucous membranes. See Dithranol.

Chrysarobin Ointment U.S.P. *Unguentum Chrysarobini*

Chrysarobin 6, Chloroform 7, Yellow Ointment 87.

Cinchophen B.P. *Cinchophenum.* (Quinophan. T.N. Atophan)

DOSES: 0.3-0.6 Gm. (5-10 gr.). $C_6H_5C_9H_5N.COOH$. Mol.wt. 249.3. S: ins. W, 120 A, 100 E, 400 C; sol. in alkali hydroxides, carbonates, and bicarbonates. A white or yellowish powder or crystals; almost odourless; taste slightly bitter.

℣Cinchophen is an antipyretic and analgesic. It increases the excretion of uric acid by the kidneys and was once thought to be a specific for gout. The beneficial effects are now attributed to the analgesic action. Hepatitis and jaundice sometimes follow its use.

Cinnamon. *Cinnamomum.* (Cinnamon Bark, Saigon Cinnamon U.S.P., Ceylon Cinnamon)
The dried inner bark from *Cinnamomum zeylanicum* (B.P.) or from *Cinnamomum Loureirii* (Nees). Contains a volatile oil; with tannin and mucilage; odour characteristic and aromatic; taste warm, sweet, aromatic, and pungent.

Powdered Cinnamon B.P. *Cinnamomi Pulvis*
A dull yellowish-brown powder.

Cinnamon Oil U.S.P. Oil of Cinnamon B.P. *Oleum Cinnamomi.* (Cassia Oil U.S.P., Can. Gaz.)
DOSES: B.P. 0.06-0.2 cc. (1-3 min.); U.S.P. 0.1 cc. (1½ min.). Gm./cc. 0.994-1.034. Sp. gr. 1.045-1.063. A pale-yellow oily liquid, darkening with age; contains between 50 and 65% cinnamic aldehyde; odour and taste that of cinnamon. *Can. Gaz. and U.S.P.* specify not less than 80% by vol. of the total aldehydes of oil of cinnamon.

Cinnamon Spirit C.F. *Spiritus Cinnamomi*
DOSE: 1 cc. (15 min.). Oil of Cinnamon 10, Alcohol to make 100.
⟪Cinnamon is a carminative flavour with a persistent taste which makes it useful for covering the taste of unpleasant medicines.

Concentrated Cinnamon Water B.P. *Aqua Cinnamomi Concentrata*
DOSES: 0.3-1 cc. (5-15 min.). Oil of Cinnamon 2% v/v, in 52-56% v/v of C_2H_5OH. Contains 80-87% v/v of C_2H_5OH.

Cinnamon Water U.S.P. *Aqua Cinnamomi*
A clear saturated solution of cinnamon oil in water.

Citric Acid. *Acidum Citricum*
DOSES: B.P. 0.3-2 Gm. (5-30 gr.) No dose U.S.P.
$OH.C_3H_4(COOH)_3.H_2O$. Mol.wt. 210.14. S: 0.5 W, 2 A, 30 E.
Large, colourless, translucent crystals or a white crystalline powder; odourless; taste acid; efflorescent in dry air.
⟪The main use of citric acid is in effervescent powders of various kinds and in syrups to improve their keeping qualities.

Citric Acid Syrup U.S.P. *Syrupus Acidi Citrici*
Lemon Tincture U.S.P. 10, Citric Acid 10, Distilled Water and Syrup to make 1000 cc.

Syrup of Citric Acid C.F.
Tincture of Lemon B.P. 30, Citric Acid 30, Syrup to 1000 cc.

℄ The Syrup of Citric Acid C.F. is a useful substitute for Syrup of Lemon because it keeps better.

Clove B.P. *Caryophyllum*
The dried flower buds of *Eugenia caryophyllata*; odour and taste spicy, pungent, and characteristic; produces a slight numbness of the tongue.

Powdered Clove B.P. *Caryophylli Pulvis*
A brown powder.

Concentrated Infusion of Clove B.P. *Infusum Caryophylli Concentratum*
DOSES: 2-4 cc. (30-60 min.). Clove 20 with 110 cc. of 25% Alcohol, by maceration. Contains 23-25% v/v of C_2H_5OH.

Infusion of Clove B.P.
DOSES: 15-30 cc. ($\frac{1}{2}$-1 fl.oz.). The Concentrated Infusion diluted to 8 times its volume with water.

Clove Oil U.S.P. **Oil of Clove B.P.** *Oleum Caryophylli.* (Oil of Cloves)
DOSES: B.P. 0.06-0.2 cc. (1-3 min.). No dose U.S.P. Gm./cc. 1.041-1.054. Sp.gr. 1.038-1.060. S: 2 A 70%. A colourless or pale-yellow liquid; odour and taste those of cloves; darkens on exposure to air. Contains, (B.P.) 85-90%, (U.S.P.) not less than 82% v/v of eugenol.

℄ The main constituent of Clove Oil is eugenol, a methoxy phenol, with germicidal and rubefacient actions. Either clove oil or eugenol is used in dentistry for a variety of purposes, as an obtundent and antiseptic dressing, and in periodontal packs.

Cochineal. *Coccus.* (Coccus Cacti)
The dried female insect *Dactylopius coccus*. Contains the red dye carmine, which turns yellow in acid solution.

Tincture of Cochineal B.P. *Tinctura Cocci*
Cochineal 10 Gm. to make 100 cc. by maceration. Contains 42-45% v/v of C_2H_5OH.

Coconut Oil Can. Gaz. *Oleum Cocois*

M.p. 23-26°. S: 2 A at 60°; readily sol. E, C, and carbon disulphide. The fat expressed from the kernels of the fruit of the coconut tree, *Cocos nucifera* and *butyracea*. A solid, pearly white fat; odour slightly of coconut; taste bland and agreeable.

℄ Coconut Oil is used in bases for ointments and to make marine soap which will lather in sea water.

Colchicine. *Colchicina*

DOSES: B.P. 0.5-1 mg. ($\frac{1}{120}$-$\frac{1}{60}$ gr.), total dose 2-8 mg. ($\frac{1}{30}$-$\frac{1}{8}$ gr.); U.S.P. 0.5 mg. ($\frac{1}{120}$ gr.). $C_{22}H_{25}NO_6$. Mol.wt. 399.43. M.p. 153-157°. S: 25 W, 220 E; fs. A, C. An alkaloid from the corm and seeds of *Colchicum autumnale*. Pale-yellow amorphous scales or powder; odourless; taste bitter; darkens on exposure to light. *Colchicine is extremely poisonous.*

Colchicine Tablets U.S.P.

Size, 0.5 mg. ($\frac{1}{120}$ gr.).

Colchicum Corm B.P. *Colchici Cormus*

The corm of *Colchicum autumnale*; taste bitter; contains not less than 0.25% of Colchicine.

Powdered Colchicum Corm B.P. *Colchici Cormi Pulvis*

A light-grey powder.

Dry Extract of Colchicum B.P. *Extractum Colchici Siccum*

DOSES: 10-30 mg. ($\frac{1}{6}$-$\frac{1}{2}$ gr.). A dried alcoholic extract of Colchicum Corm adjusted with lactose to contain about 1% of colchicine. The maximum dose contains 0.3 mg. ($\frac{1}{200}$ gr.) of colchicine.

Colchicum Seed B.P. *Colchici Semen*

The seeds of *Colchicum autumnale*; taste acrid and bitter. Contains not less than 0.3% of colchicine.

Powdered Colchicum Seed B.P. *Colchici Seminis Pulvis*

A brown powder.

Liquid Extract of Colchicum B.P. *Extractum Colchici Liquidum*

Colchicum Seed and Alcohol, by percolation. Contains 0.27-0.33% w/v of colchicine and 50-60% v/v C_2H_5OH.

Tincture of Colchicum B.P. *Tinctura Colchici*

DOSES: 0.3-1 cc. (5-15 min.). Liquid Extract of Colchicum

diluted to contain 0.027-0.033% w/v of colchicine and 58-60% v/v of C_2H_5OH. Maximum dose contains 0.3 mg. ($\frac{1}{200}$ gr.) colchicine.

℄ The preparations of Colchicum are used only in the treatment of acute gout. The relief obtained is attributed to colchicine but the mode of action is unknown. Colchicine in toxic doses has the remarkable property of arresting cell division in the metaphase. Whether this action has anything to do with the relief of gout is unknown.

Collodion U.S.P. *Collodium*
Pyroxylin 4, with Ethyl Oxide and Alcohol to make 100 cc. A clear, slightly opalescent, syrupy liquid; odour that of ether; highly inflammable.

Flexible Collodion B.P. *Collodium Flexile*
Pyroxylin 2, Colophony 3, Castor Oil 2, with Alcohol and Ether to make 100 cc. Contains 20-23% v/v of C_2H_5OH.

Flexible Collodion U.S.P. *Collodium Flexile*
Camphor 2, Castor Oil 3, Collodion to make 100.

℄ The various collodions are used mainly to attach dressings to the skin or sometimes as vehicles for drugs to be applied to the skin, e.g. corns and callouses.

Colocynth B.P. *Colocynthis*. (Colocynth Pulp)
The dried pulp of the fruit of *Citrullus Colocynthis*; odourless; taste intensely bitter.

Powdered Colocynth B.P. *Colocynthidis Pulvis*
A yellowish-white powder.

Compound Extract of Colocynth B.P. *Extractum Colocynthidis Compositum*
DOSES: 0.12-0.5 Gm. (2-8 gr.). Dried alcoholic extract of 27 Gm. of Colocynth, with Aloes 56 Gm., Ipomoea Resin 18.5 Gm. with Curd Soap and Cardamom Seed to make about 100 Gm.

Pill of Colocynth and Hyoscyamus B.P. *Pilula Colocynthidis et Hyoscyami*
DOSES: 0.25-0.5 Gm. (4-8 gr.). Colocynth 12.5, Aloes 25, Ipomoea Resin 25, Dry Extract of Hyoscyamus 12.5, with Curd Soap, Oil of Clove, and Syrup of Liquid Glucose to make about 100 Gm.

⟪ Colocynth is described as a drastic, hydrogogue cathartic, meaning that it produces copious watery stools with much griping. The hyoscyamus is added to the pill to reduce the griping. Colocynth should not be given to nursing mothers as the active principle passes into the milk.   Nor should it be given in pregnancy for fear of inducing uterine contractions.   The active principle or principles have not been identified.

Colophony B.P.   *Colophonium.*   (Resin, Rosin, *Resina*)

S: ins. W; sol. A 90%, B, E, CS₂; partially sol. in light petroleum. The residue left after distillation of the volatile oil from the oleoresin obtained from various species of Pinus.   Translucent pale-yellow or brownish, brittle, readily fusible glassy masses. Odour and taste faintly like turpentine.

Congo Red U.S.P.   *Rubrum Congo*

$C_{32}H_{22}N_6Na_2O_6S_2$. Mol.wt. 696.67. S: 25 W; ss. A. A dark red or reddish brown powder; odourless.   The pH of its solution is 8-9.5.

Congo Red Injection U.S.P.

Each 10 cc. contains 100 mg. (1½ gr.).

⟪ Congo red injected intravenously disappears more rapidly from the blood stream of patients with amyloid disease than it does from the blood of normal subjects.   The congo red is taken up by the organs which contain deposits of amyloid.   Congo red is thus used as a diagnostic agent for the detection of amyloid disease.

Copper Sulphate B.P.   Cupric Sulphate U.S.P.   *Cupri Sulphas*

DOSES: B.P. 16-120 mg. (¼-2 gr.); emetic, 0.3-0.6 Gm. (5-10 gr.). No dose. U.S.P. $CuSO_4.5H_2O$. Mol.wt. 249.71. S: 3 W, 500 A, 3 G, 0.5W at 100°.   Deep-blue triclinic crystals or a blue powder; odourless; taste astringent and nauseous.

⟪ Crystals of copper sulphate or sticks fused with alum are used to touch unhealthy granulation tissues, cuts and ulcers in the mouth, and the eyelids in trachoma.

Copper sulphate is an antidote for phosphorus poisoning. It is a prompt and effective emetic but if it does not act it should be washed out of the stomach for fear of poisoning by the absorption of the copper salt.

Coriander B.P. *Coriandrum.* (Coriander Fruit)

The dried ripe fruits of *Coriandrum sativum*. Odour aromatic; taste spicy and characteristic.

Powdered Coriander B.P. *Coriandri Pulvis*

A fawn to brown powder.

Coriander Oil U.S.P. Oil of Coriander B.P. *Oleum Coriandri*

DOSES: B.P. 0.06-0.2 cc. (1-3 min.). No dose U.S.P. Gm./cc. 0.865-0.879. Sp.gr. 0.863-0.875. S: 3 A 70%. The volatile oil distilled from the dried ripe fruit of *Coriandrum sativum*. A pale-yellow liquid; odour and taste characteristic of coriander.

℃ Because of its agreeable flavour and alleged carminative action, Oil of Coriander is added to laxative medicines to decrease griping.

Corn Oil U.S.P. *Oleum Maydis.* (Maize Oil)

DOSES: Can. Gaz. 15-30 cc. (½-1 fl.oz.). Sp.gr. 0.918-0.924 (U.S.P). S: ss. A; misc. E, C, B, and petroleum benzin. The refined fixed oil expressed from the embryo of *Zea Mays*; a clear, light-yellow, oily liquid with a faint characteristic odour and taste.

℃ Corn Oil has uses similar to those of Cotton Seed Oil.

Cottonseed Oil. *Oleum Gossypii Seminis*

Sp.gr. 0.915-0.921. S: ss. A; misc. E, C, petroleum benzin and with carbon disulphide. The refined fixed oil obtained from the seed of cultivated plants of various varieties of *Gossypium hirsutum* or other species of *Gossypium;* a pale yellow, oily, liquid; odourless or nearly so; taste bland.

℃ Cottonseed Oil may be used instead of Olive Oil for rubbing on the skin. It has no particular medicinal properties but is used as salad oil, for making soap, liniments, and as a vehicle for oily injections.

Creosote B.P. *Creosotum.* (Creasote)

DOSES: 0.12-0.6 cc. (2-10.min.). S: ss. W; misc. A 90%, E, fixed and volatile oils. A colourless or pale-yellow liquid; odour penetrating and smoky; taste burning; obtained by distillation of wood tars. Protect from light.

℀ Creosote consists largely of guaiacol, which is antipyretic and expectorant in action. At one time it was used in the treatment of pulmonary tuberculosis but without impressive effect.

Cresol. *Cresol*

$CH_3.C_6H_4.OH$. Mol.wt. 108.13. B.p. 195-205°. Gm./cc. 1.029-1.044. Sp.gr. 1.030-1.038. S: 50 W (cloudy); misc. A, E, G; sol. in fixed alkali hydroxide solutions. A mixture of isomeric cresols with other phenols. A colourless or yellowish or pinkish highly refractive liquid; odour phenol-like or tarry; taste pungent.

Solution of Cresol with Soap B.P. *Liquor Cresolis Saponatis.* (T.N. Lysol)

Cresol 50, Linseed Oil 18, with Potassium Hydroxide and Distilled Water to make 100. An amber-coloured to reddish-brown liquid; odour that of cresol; soapy to touch. S: 10 W; misc. A.

℀ The saponated cresols are effective antiseptics in proper dilution and may be used effectively to sterilize instruments or bed-pans. Cresols are more powerful antiseptics than phenol, but being only slightly soluble in water, must be dissolved with the aid of soap. They confer an odour of sanitation at dilutions which are virtually inactive, but are effective germicidally if diluted with not more than 100 volumes of water.

Crystal Violet B.P. *Viola Crystallina.* **Methylrosaniline Chloride.** *Methylrosanilinae Chloridum.* (Gentian Violet, Methyl Violet, Crystal Violet)

$C_{25}H_{30}N_3Cl$. Mol.wt. 408.0. S: 30-40 W, 10 A, 15 G; sol. C; ins. E. Greenish-bronze crystals or powder, having a metallic lustre; odourless or nearly so. Hexamethylpararosaniline chloride usually with some pentamethyl and tetramethyl compounds.

℀ According to Sollmann, crystal violet means more or less pure hexamethyl-compound; methylviolet means more or less pure pentamethyl-compound; while gentian violet means a mixture. All three substances are selectively toxic to gram positive microorganisms.

A triple dye solution of 1% gentian violet, 1% brilliant green and 0.1% acriflavine has been used to treat burns. It forms an eschar, like tannic acid. The principal objection to this treatment is the fear that islands of epithelium, which might survive under milder therapy, may be killed.

Enteric coated capsules of gentian violet are prescribed for pinworms. For this purpose an average dose for children is 30 mg. three times a day.

Cumidine Red Can. Gaz. *Rubrum Cumidinum.* (Ponceau-3R) $C_{19}H_{16}N_2O_7S_2Na_2$. Mol.wt. 494.3. S: W; sparingly sol. A. A dark-red powder, used for colouring medicines (1:10.000).

CURARE

The name Curare was given to a crude drug (or more correctly to a family of drugs) prepared from various plants by several tribes of South American Indians. The outstanding property of the curare drugs is their ability to paralyze skeletal muscle by preventing the transmission of impulses from motor nerves to muscles. Plants of several genera (*Chondodendron, Strychnos, Erythrina*) produce a number of alkaloids with "curare-like" action. In addition, many synthetic drugs, notably quaternary ammonium bases, have a similar action. For therapeutic purposes the curare-like action should be as pure as possible, i.e. side effects such as bronchiolar constriction, elevation or depression of the blood pressure, should be minimal.

One of the first natural alkaloids to be fully identified chemically was d-tubocurarine, a very complex organic molecule containing two quaternary ammonium groups. Relatively pure preparations of this alkaloid have been available for several years. More recently, a more potent derivative, the dimethyl-ether of d-tubocurarine, has been prepared by chemical modification of natural alkaloids. At about the same time, two synthetic curare-like drugs, Decamethonium and Flaxedil, which are very different in structure from the natural alkaloids, were made available.

The main use for the curare-like drugs is to produce muscular relaxation during light anaesthesia, thus permitting surgical operations with much less anaesthetic. Another application is to reduce the violence of convulsions during electro-shock therapy, as used in psychiatry. Some experimentation is proceeding on the use of long-lasting curare-like preparations for the treatment of a number of states characterized by spasm of skeletal muscles such as lumbago and sciatica. They have been used, with claims of success, for reducing spasm in spastic paralytic states, thus permitting more effective re-education in the use of paralyzed muscles. They have been used also to alleviate the spastic manifestations of Parkinsonism.

The action of d-tubocurarine and its dimethyl ether, is thought to consist in blocking the action of acetylcholine on skeletal muscle. Why it has so little effect on other structures which are stimulated by acetylcholine is not clear. With very large doses some blocking of cholinergic transmission in autonomic ganglia and at parasympathetic endings, can be demonstrated. In large doses, it interferes with central nervous functions producing changes in the electroencephalogram, and even anaesthesia. These effects can be shown only with doses which completely paralyze the muscles of respiration in animals (or patients) kept alive by artificial respiration.

A curious action which can be demonstrated with ordinary doses is the release of histamine in peripheral tissues. This may explain the spasm of bronchioles which may occur with ordinary doses and cause serious interference with pulmonary ventilation in spite of artificial respiration. Laryngeal spasm may also occur. The mechanism of this effect is not known.

The anticholinesterase drugs, particularly neostigmine, will antagonize the paralytic effects of d-tubocurarine on skeletal muscles. However, it is important to realize that the most effective measure for dealing with overdosage is to institute artificial respiration. This requires intubation of the larynx and inflation of the lungs with oxygen under intermittent positive pressure.

The more obvious effects of an intravenous injection of d-tubocurarine pass off in 15-30 minutes. A certain amount of the drug is excreted in the urine. The remainder probably diffuses into the body fluids, accounting for the rapid disappearance of its more obvious effects. Actual destruction of the drug seems to be slow, which accounts for the fact that some weakness and fatigability may last for several hours.

Frequently d-tubocurarine is given with sodium thiopentone. If too high a proportion of the curare solution is added, precipitation will occur. This is partly due to the acidity of the solution causing precipitation of the thiobarbituric acid. It is also partly due to alkaloidal impurities. The purer preparations of d-tubocurarine can be added in greater amounts without precipitation of thiopentone.

Tubocurarine Chloride U.S.P.   *Tubocurarinae Chloridum.* (Curare, d-Tubocurarine Chloride Pentahydrate)

Doses: 1-3 cc. intravenously, given slowly over a period of 1-2 minutes. *With ether anaesthesia give 1/3 the usual dose.* Each cc. contains 3 mg. of $C_{38}H_{44}Cl_2N_2O_6.5H_2O$, which is a white or slightly yellowish, odourless crystalline powder, obtained from the bark and stems of *Chondodendron tomentosum* and related species. Mol.wt. 785.74. M.p. 265-278°. S: sol. w; ss. A; ins. C, E. Specific optical rotation at 25° is 208-218°. Solutions are assayed biologically against a standard, using the rabbit "head drop" method. Available in vials containing 10 or 20 cc., each cc. contains the equivalent of 3 mg. of standard preparation, or 20 "units"; and also as the so-called "high potency" injection in 1 cc. ampuls as shown below.

Tubocurarine Chloride Injection U.S.P.
15 mg. ($\frac{1}{4}$ gr.) in 1 cc.; 30 mg. ($\frac{1}{2}$ gr.) in 10 cc.

Dimethyl Tubocurarine Iodide Solution N.N.R. (T.N. Metubine Iodide Solution)
Doses: 1-3 cc. intravenously, injected slowly over a period of 1-2 minutes. *With ether anaesthesia give 1/3 the usual dose.* Each cc. contains 1.0 mg. of dimethyl d-tubocurarine iodide, $C_{40}H_{48}O_6N_2I_2$. Mol.wt. 906.56. Decomposes at 257°. A white or pale yellow crystalline powder, odourless. S: ss. W, dil. HCl, dil. NaOH; vss. A; ins. B, C, E. Specific optical rotation at 25°+ 159° to + 160°. Available in vials containing 10 cc. (1.0 mg. per cc.).

℟ Dimethyl-tubocurarine is about three times as potent in humans as d-tubocurarine. It acts more rapidly and lasts a little longer than d-tubocurarine. The same precautions must be taken with the dimethyl compound as with d-tubocurarine. Provision must be made for laryngeal intubation and controlled artificial respiration, and a suitable antidote, neostigmine methylsulphate (1:2000) must be at hand.

Decamethonium Bromide N. (C 10, T.N. Syncurine)
Doses: 1-2 cc. intravenously over a period of 1-2 minutes; may be repeated several times during an operation as required to secure adequate relaxation. Each cc. contains 1 mg. of C 10, which is

decamethylene-1, 10-bistrimethylammonium dibromide. $C_{16}H_{38}Br_2$.
Mol.wt. 550.84. A white crystalline powder. S: sol. W, A. Aqueous
solutions are not irritating to tissues, are stable, and may be sterilized by heat. They are compatible with procaine and with thiopentone sodium.

℃ Like d-tubocurarine, decamethonium bromide blocks the transmission of impulses from motor nerves to skeletal muscles. Relaxation produced in this way is almost immediate in onset after
intravenous injection, and is much shorter in duration than that
produced by curare. Many injections may be required during a
long operation. The same dose may be used with any of the
common anaesthetics. Ether has no synergistic action with C 10
as it has with curare, thus smaller doses of C 10 are not required
when ether is the anaesthetic.

Decamethonium differs from tubocurarine in three other important respects. (1) It is not antagonized by neostigmine or eserine.
(2) Second and third injections produce less effect than the first—
a phenomenon known as tachyphylaxis. (3) Relaxation of muscles
may be preceded by twitching. All four differences suggest that
C 10 has a different mechanism of action from tubocurarine. It has
been postulated that C 10 on reaching the motor nerve ending first
acts like acetylcholine and causes depolarization of the muscle,
hence the twitches. It then persists near the nerve ending, blocking
the action on the muscle of acetylcholine liberated by nerve impulses. Tubocurarine blocks acetylcholine without causing depolarization of the muscle.

Cyclopropane. *Cyclopropanum*

C_3H_6. Mol.wt. 42.08. B.p. −34.5° at 760 mm.Hg. S: 1 vol.
in 2.7 W at 15°; fs. A, E, C, and in fixed oils. A colourless gas;
odour characteristic, resembling petroleum benzin. Contains not
less than 99% of C_3H_6 v/v.

℃ Cyclopropane is an anaesthetic gas with only a slight odour and
taste. It is usually administered in a "rebreather" type of gas
machine with oxygen. In concentrations of 20% v/v, anaesthesia
is produced very rapidly. Relaxation is not so complete as with
ether but subsequent nausea, vomiting, and pulmonary complications are less frequent. It is sometimes fortified with ether to
improve relaxation. Cardiac irregularities are sometimes produced
with higher concentrations and—very rarely—an abrupt cardiac
death occurs, presumably from ventricular fibrillation.

Deoxycortone Acetate B.P. *Deoxycortoni Acetas.* **Desoxycortico-sterone Acetate U.S.P.** *Desoxycorticosteroni Acetas*

DOSES: B.P. intramuscular, 2-10 mg. ($\frac{1}{30}$-$\frac{1}{6}$ gr.); implantation, 0.2-0.4 Gm. (3-6 gr.); U.S.P. intramuscular and implantation as prescribed. $C_{23}H_{32}O_4$. Mol.wt. 372.49. M.p. 154-160°. S: ins. W; sol. A, acetone, propylene glycol, and in fixed oils. Colourless crystals or crystalline powder; odourless.

Injection of Deoxycortone Acetate B.P.

DOSES: intramuscular, 2-10 mg. ($\frac{1}{30}$-$\frac{1}{6}$ gr.). Strength, 5 mg. per cc. ($\frac{1}{12}$ gr. in 15 min.).

℘ Deoxycortone acetate is a synthetic substance which partly corrects the adrenal insufficiency of Addison's disease. Because it is cheaper than adrenal cortical extracts, it is used to eke them out. Overdosage must be avoided, as excessive retention of sodium chloride may occur, with oedema and dilatation of the heart.

Desoxycorticosterone Acetate Pellets U.S.P.

Pellets contain 75 and 125 mg. (1$\frac{1}{4}$ and 2 gr.) of Desoxycortico-sterone Acetate, for subcutaneous implantation for prolonged therapy.

Dextrose B.P. *Dextrosum.* (Anhydrous Dextrose)

$C_6H_{12}O_6$. Mol.wt. 180.2. S: less than 1 W, 50 cold A 90%, 5 boiling A 90%. A white crystalline or granular powder; odourless; taste sweet.

Dextrose Monohydrate B.P. *Dextrosum Hydratum.* **Dextrose U.S.P.** *Dextrosum.* (Medicinal Glucose, Purified Glucose, d-Glucose)

$C_6H_{12}O_6.H_2O$. Mol.wt. 198 .17. S: 1 W, 60 A; more sol. W 100°, A 78°. Colourless crystals or a cream-coloured crystalline granular powder; odourless; taste sweet.

℘ The word dextrose is now used in both U.S.P. and B.P. to designate highly purified preparations of the sugar suitable for incorporation in solutions for injection. Note that in the B.P. Dextrose means anhydrous dextrose but in the U.S.P. it means the monohydrate.

Dextrose and Sodium Chloride Injection U.S.P.

Solutions having this title are available in various strengths for various purposes.   They range in strength from $2\frac{1}{2}\%$ to 25% in isotonic sodium chloride solution.

Dextrose Injections U.S.P.
Solutions having this title are available in various strengths for various purposes.   They range in strength from 5% to 50%.

Injection of Dextrose B.P.
Strength, when not otherwise stated, is 5% w/v (sterile).

❨ A 5% solution of Dextrose is approximately isotonic with erythrocytes and may be injected intravenously alone or with physiological salt solution to treat dehydration, or to supply nourishment to the tissues.

A 50% solution may be injected intravenously to draw fluid from the tissues into the blood stream, e.g. for the treatment of cerebral oedema.   The effects are temporary but often striking.   Diuresis with glycosuria follows.   Strong solutions may also be used for sclerosing varicose veins (dextrose 25% with NaCl 15%.)

DIGITALIS AND ITS DERIVATIVES

Digitalis Leaf B.P.   *Digitalis Folium*.   Digitalis U.S.P.   *Digitalis*.
(Foxglove)
The dried leaf of *Digitalis purpurea* (Foxglove).   In the leaf are contained the glycosides digitoxin, gitoxin and gitalin, and other glycosides in varying proportions.   Saponins are also present.

Powdered Digitalis Leaf B.P.   *Digitalis Folii Pulvis*.
A greenish powder.

Powdered Digitalis U.S.P.   *Digitalis Pulverata*.   Prepared Digitalis B.P.   *Digitalis Praeparata*
Doses: B.P. 30-100 mg. ($\frac{1}{2}$-$1\frac{1}{2}$ gr.) repeated; U.S.P. 0.1 Gm. ($1\frac{1}{2}$ gr.).   A powdered leaf standardized biologically and adjusted so that each gramme contains 10 International or U.S.P. Units. U.S.P. assay is by lethal effect on intravenous injection into pigeons.   The B.P. permits assay on cats, guinea pigs, or frogs. Whichever animal is used the potency of the unknown is compared with that of a preparation from a standard powder.

Digitalis Capsules U.S.P.
Sizes, 50 and 100 mg. ($\frac{3}{4}$ and $1\frac{1}{2}$ gr.).

Digitalis Injection U.S.P.

Sizes, 1 unit per cc. or 1 unit in 2 cc. for intravenous injection.

Digitalis Tablets U.S.P.

Sizes, 50 and 100 mg. ($\frac{3}{4}$ and $1\frac{1}{2}$ gr.).

Tablets of Prepared Digitalis B.P.

Size, 60 mg. (1 gr.).

Digitalis Tincture U.S.P.   Tincture of Digitalis B.P.   *Tinctura Digitalis*

DOSES: B.P. 0.3-1 cc. (5-15 min.); U.S.P. 1 cc. (15 min.). A tincture prepared from Digitalis Leaf or Prepared Digitalis adjusted so that 1 cc. is equivalent to 1 International Unit of potency (B.P.) or 1 U.S.P. Digitalis Unit, which is approximately the same.

Digitoxin U.S.P.   *Digitoxinum*

DOSE: oral, 0.1 mg. ($\frac{1}{600}$ gr.); intravenous as prescribed. S: ins. W; ss. E, 40 C, 60 A. Either pure digitoxin ($C_{41}H_{64}O_{13}$) or a mixture of cardiac glycosides obtained from *Digitalis purpurea*, consisting chiefly of digitoxin. A white or pale buff powder; odourless; taste bitter. *Digitoxin is extremely poisonous.* Biologically standardized against U.S.P. Digitoxin Reference Standard.

Digitoxin Injection U.S.P.

Sizes, 0.2 mg. ($\frac{1}{300}$ gr.) in 1 cc. or 0.4 mg. ($\frac{1}{150}$ gr.) in 2 cc. of 40-50% alcohol.

Digitoxin Tablets U.S.P.

Sizes, 0.1 and 0.2 mg. ($\frac{1}{600}$ and $\frac{1}{300}$ gr.).

Digoxin.   *Digoxinum*

DOSES: B.P. 1-1.5 mg. ($\frac{1}{60}$-$\frac{1}{40}$ gr.) oral initial; 0.25 mg. ($\frac{1}{240}$ gr.) once or twice daily (maintenance); 0.5-1 mg. ($\frac{1}{120}$-$\frac{1}{60}$ gr.) intravenously; U.S.P. oral, 0.5 mg. ($\frac{1}{120}$ gr.); intravenous as prescribed. $C_{41}H_{64}O_{14}$. Mol.wt. 780.92. M.p. 265°. S: ins. W, C, E; fs. in pyridine and dil. A. A crystalline glycoside obtained from leaves of *Digitalis lanata*; colourless four- or five-sided tabular crystals; odourless; taste (in dilute alcohol solution) bitter. *Digoxin is extremely poisonous.*

Digoxin Injection U.S.P.

Size, 0.5 mg. ($\frac{1}{120}$ gr.) in 1 cc. of 70% alcohol. Bioassay against U.S.P. Digoxin Reference Standard is required.

Injection of Digoxin B.P.

DOSES: intravenous, 10-20 cc. (150-300 min.). Supplied in ampoules of 50 mg. in 100 cc. of 70% alcohol. To be diluted 1 cc. with 9 cc. of Injection of Sodium Chloride.

Digoxin Tablets U.S.P.

Size, 0.25 mg. ($\frac{1}{250}$ gr.).

Tablets of Digoxin B.P.

Size, 0.25 mg. ($\frac{1}{240}$ gr.).

❰ The active principles of Digitalis and its preparations are known as cardiac glycosides. A number of these are available in pure form for administration orally or by intravenous injection, but not by hypodermic injection because they are very irritating. Digitoxin is probably the most important active principle of *Digitalis purpurea*. The pure glycosides which have been studied most thoroughly are Digitoxin, Digoxin, the Lanatosides, and Strophanthin. They differ in rate and completeness of absorption when taken by mouth and also in rate of excretion, consequently they differ in the dosage required. No other important differences in pharmacological action have been demonstrated as yet but they may exist.

The cardiac glycosides have a number of actions which are particularly beneficial in the treatment of congestive heart failure with oedema. The circulation is improved, the symptoms are relieved, and diuresis is produced as a result of the improved circulation. Relief is particularly dramatic in auricular fibrillation with congestive heart failure. Venous pressure is reduced, the pulse rate and pulse deficit are decreased, the cardiac output is increased, but the fibrillation usually persists.

Cardiac glycosides can be shown to increase the contractility of failing heart muscle. This in itself could explain all the beneficial effects of these drugs. Other actions, however, probably make very important contributions to the overall favourable effect. Oxygen consumption of all muscular tissue is reduced. The reduction in venous pressure may be due in part to an independent action which is not understood. Under full doses, the contraction period and refractory period of cardiac muscles is prolonged. This is particularly favourable in auricular fibrillation because it prevents the ventricle from responding to many of the impulses from the auricle. Directly, or indirectly, (i.e. through circulatory reflexes), vagal activity is increased and helps to slow the ventricular rate.

The toxic effects of the cardiac glycosides are nausea and vomiting, extra systoles in the previously regular heart, and, occasionally, diarrhoea. If any of these occur, the dosage should be decreased. The purified glycosides, when taken orally in large doses, produce much less nausea and vomiting of the type due to direct irritation of the gastrointestinal tract than do the galenical preparations. Nausea and vomiting due to central effects after absorption occur with about equal frequency with both types of preparation. Cumulation is characteristic of digitalis and digitoxin due to slow elimination or inactivation or the active glycosides. Digoxin and lanatoside are less persistent in action and the strophanthins have the least persistence of all. Effects of a single large dose of digitoxin do not disappear for nearly two weeks, while the effects of strophanthin last only a day or so.

Cardiac glycosides are said to sensitize the heart to epinephrine and calcium, increasing the tendency of these substances to produce ventricular fibrillation. They should be withheld from digitalized patients or used with caution.

Lantoside C U.S.P. *Lanatosidum C*

DOSE: oral 0.5 mg. ($\frac{1}{120}$ gr.); parenteral dosage as prescribed. $C_{49}H_{76}O_{20}$. Mol.wt. 984.58. S: 20,000 W, 45 A, 20 methanol, 2000 C; readily sol. pyridine and dioxane; ins. E and petroleum benzin. A glycoside obtained from the leaves of *Digitalis lanata*. Colourless or white crystals or a white crystalline powder; odourless; taste bitter. *Extremely poisonous.*

Lanatoside C Injection U.S.P.

Sizes, 0.4 mg. ($\frac{1}{150}$ gr.) in 2 cc. or 0.8 mg. ($\frac{1}{80}$ gr.) in 4 cc. of 10% alcohol.

Lanatoside C Tablets

Size, 0.5 mg. ($\frac{1}{120}$ gr.).

⟪ Some experimental evidence suggested that Lanatoside C has a more beneficial effect on cardiac muscle than other cardiac glycosides at doses which are not likely to produce cardiac irregularities. Clinical investigation has not substantiated this claim. Lanatoside C is not as well absorbed from the gastrointestinal tract as digitoxin or digoxin.

Ouabain. *Ouabainum.* (G-Strophanthin, Strophanthin-G)

DOSES: B.P. intravenous, 0.12-0.25 mg. ($\frac{1}{500}$-$\frac{1}{240}$ gr.); U.S.P. intravenous, 0.25 mg. ($\frac{1}{250}$ gr.). $C_{29}H_{44}O_{12}.8H_2O$. Mol.wt. 728.8. M.p. about 190°. S: 75 W, 100 A; more sol. in hot A; almost insol. E, C. Small colourless crystals or a white crystalline powder; odourless; taste bitter. Obtained from the seeds of *Strophanthus gratus*; the B.P. also recognizes the wood of *Acokanthera Schimperi* as a source. A very poisonous glycoside and should not be tasted except in very dilute solution.

❡ The purity and potency of Ouabain can be verified by chemical means, so that it is used as an International Standard for determination of potency of other preparations of strophanthus by bioassay. The absorption of the strophanthins from the alimentary tract is somewhat uncertain so that many authorities feel that the oral preparations are of little use. By intravenous injection the effects are prompt but relatively transient.

Injection of Ouabain B.P.

A sterile solution for injection, containing 0.25 mg. in 1 cc. ($\frac{1}{240}$ gr. in 15 min.).

Ouabain Injection U.S.P.

Sizes, 0.25 mg. ($\frac{1}{250}$ gr.) in 1 cc. and 0.5 mg. ($\frac{1}{120}$ gr.) in 1 cc. Must be bioassayed against U.S.P. Ouabain Reference Standard.

Strophanthin Can. Gaz. *Strophanthinum*

DOSE: 0.5 mg. ($\frac{1}{120}$ gr.) intravenously. S: sol. W, A 60%, but less sol. in dehydrated A; almost ins. C, E, B. A glycoside or a mixture of glycosides obtained from the seeds of *Strophanthus kombé*. It shall possess in each mg. a potency corresponding to 0.5 mg. of International Standard Ouabain. A white or yellowish powder containing varying amounts of water; taste bitter. *Strophanthin is very poisonous* and should not be tasted except in very dilute solution.

Strophanthus B.P. *Strophanthus.* (Strophanthus Seeds)

The dried ripe seed of *Strophantus kombé*. *Strophanthus hispidus* may also be used in Canada.

Powdered Strophanthus B.P. *Strophanthi Pulvis*

Greenish-yellow powder with brown specks.

Tincture of Strophanthus B.P.   *Tinctura Strophanthi*

DOSES: 0.12-0.3 cc. (2-5 min.).   Strophanthus extracted by percolation.   Contains 67-70% v/v of C_2H_5OH.   The tincture must be assayed biologically and adjusted until equal in potency to the standard tincture of strophanthus.

Dihydrostreptomycin U.S.P.   *Dihydrostreptomycinum*

DOSES: Intramuscular 1-4 Gm. daily. $C_{21}H_{41}N_7O_{12}$.   Mol.wt. 583.59.   S: vs. W; almost ins. C, A, E.   White or faintly yellow powder; odourless; taste slightly bitter.   Produced by hydrogenation of Streptomycin.   Not available as the base, but as hydrochloride or sulfate.   *Dihydrostreptomycin must not be injected intravenously.*

Dihydrostreptomycin is said to cause damage to the auditory nerve less frequently than does Streptomycin.

Streptomycin U.S.P.   *Streptomycinum*

DOSES: Intramuscular, 1-4 Gm. daily. $C_{21}H_{39}N_7O_{12}$.   Mol. wt. 581.58.   S: vs. W; almost ins. A, C, E.   Available as the hydrochloride, sulfate, phosphate, or double salt with calcium chloride. Although a formula is given for Streptomycin base, the product is not regarded as a pure substance but may contain more than one substance derived from certain strains of *Streptomyces griseus*.

The various preparations of Streptomycin and Dihydrostreptomycin are supplied as dry sterile powders in vials containing the equivalent of 1 or 5 Gm. of the base, to be dissolved immediately before use in water, isotonic sodium chloride or 5% dextrose solution (with 1% of procaine hydrochloride or other suitable local anaesthetic if desired).

To minimize painful local reactions the strength of solutions should not exceed 0.5 Gm. per cc.   Injections are commonly given at intervals of 12 hours, although therapeutic concentrations are seldom maintained in the blood for more than 6 hours after a single injection.

℄ Streptomycin is an antibiotic agent of particular interest because it is effective against tuberculous infections, and infections by a number of gram negative organisms, such as *Pasteurella tularense* and *B. proteus*.   Streptomycin is poorly absorbed from the gastro-intestinal tract.   Oral dosage is thus ineffective against systemic infections but may be useful in treatment of infections in the alimentary tract.   Streptomycin is usually given intramuscularly.

One injection every 12 hours suffices to maintain adequate levels
in the blood.   With doses of 1 Gm. per day toxic effects are rare.
With larger doses of 3-4 Gm. per day, which are sometimes given,
toxic reactions are fairly frequent and include fever, rash, dizziness,
pain in joints, and pain at the site of injection.   After a few weeks
of heavy dosage tinnitus and deafness are common.   The dosage
should be reduced at the first occurrence of tinnitus, to avoid the
possibility of permanent damage to the eighth nerve.   One serious
disadvantage of streptomycin is the rapidity with which many
organisms, including *M. tuberculosis*, can develop resistance to its
action.   For this reason it is not considered advisable to treat
tuberculous infections with streptomycin if good results can be
expected with other treatment.   It would seem wise to save the
streptomycin in case a serious emergency such as tuberculous
meningitis develops later. . The immediate effects of streptomycin on
various kinds of tuberculous infections are often dramatic but the
later effects are often disappointing.   Combination with other
chemotherapeutic agents is being actively investigated.

Diiodohydroxyquinoline U.S.P.   *Diiodohydroxyquinolinum.*
  (T.N. Diodoquin, Yodoxin)
  DAILY DOSE: 1.5 Gm. (22 gr.). $C_9H_5I_2NO$. Mol.wt. 396.98.
S: almost ins. W; ss. A, E.   Colourless to light brown crystalline
powder; may have a faint odour; melts with decomposition.

Diiodohydroxyquinoline Tablets U.S.P.
  Size, 200 mg. (3 gr.).
  ⓒ Diiodohydroxyquinoline is usually given three times a day for
the treatment or prevention of amoebic dysentry.

Dill B.P.   *Anethum.*   (Dill Fruit, Anethi Fructus)
  The dried ripe fruit of *Anethum graveolens* Linn.

Powdered Dill B.P.   *Anethi Pulvis*
  A pale-brown powder.

Oil of Dill B.P.   *Oleum Anethi*
  DOSES: 0.06-0.2 cc. (1-3 min.). Gm./cc. 0.895-0.910. S: 1 A 90%.
A colourless or pale-yellow liquid with a characteristic odour; taste
at first sweet and aromatic, subsequently pungent.

Concentrated Dill Water B.P. *Aqua Anethi Concentrata*
DOSES: 0.3-1 cc. (5-15 min.). Oil of Dill 2% in 52-56% v/v C$_2$H$_5$OH.

A stock solution for making Dill Water, which is used as a mild carminative flavour, and which is made by diluting the concentrated water to 40 times its volume.

Dimercaprol U.S.P. *Dimercaprol.* (Bal, 2-3 dimercaptopropanol)
DOSE: 0.2 Gm. (3 gr.) intramuscularly. C$_3$S$_2$H$_7$OH. Mol.wt. 124.23 Sp.gr. 1.238-1.240. S: 13 W; sol. A, methanol, benzyl benzoate. A clear colourless liquid with a strong sulphurous or offensive mercaptan odour; can be autoclaved without destruction.

Dimercaprol Injection U.S.P.
4.5 cc. contains 450 mg. (7 gr.) of Dimercaprol, in oil.

℃ The action of Bal is based on the high affinity of the SH groups for arsenic and other heavy metals such as mercury, antimony, and gold. These substances combine with Bal and are excreted with it in the urine and are thus prevented from exerting their toxic effects in the body. Bal is usually administered by intramuscular injection as a 10% solution in peanut oil. The dose of 2.5 mg. per kg. body weight may be given every 4 hours. Bal is absorbed through the skin. The pure liquid may be given by inunction or an aqueous solution may be given by mouth. In large doses Bal is toxic, producing nausea, and in larger doses convulsions and death. The convulsions can be ameliorated by sodium pentobarbitone.

Dimethylphthalate U.S.P. *Dimethylis Phthalas*
C$_{10}$H$_{10}$O$_4$. Mol.wt. 194.18. Sp.gr. 1.188-1.192. S: ins. W; misc. A, E, C. A clear colourless oily liquid having an aromatic odour. Used as an insect repellent either alone or in the following solution. It may be applied freely to the skin but should be kept away from the eyes and lips.

Compound Dimethylphthalate Solution U.S.P. *Liquor Dimethylis Phthalatis Compositus*
Dimethylphthalate 600, Ethohexadiol 200, Butopyronoxyl to make 1000 Gm. This preparation is effective against a larger number of insect species than is Dimethylphthalate.

Injection of Diodone B.P. *Injectio Diodoni.* (Solution of Diodone, Solution of diethanolamine salt of 3:5-diiodo-4-pyridone-N-acetic acid)

DOSE: intravenous, adult, 20 cc. (300 min.), child, 8-10 cc. (120-150 min.), infant, 2-3 cc. (30-45 min.). Strength, 17.3-17.7% w/v of iodine corresponding to 34.7-35.5% w/v of the diethanolamine salt. Clear, almost colourless liquid. Protect from light. See Iodopyracet Injection U.S.P.

Diphenan B.P. *Diphenanum.* (T.N. Butolan)
DOSES: 0.5-1 Gm. (8-15 gr.). $C_{14}H_{13}O_2N$. Mol.wt. 227.3. M.p. 147-150°. S: almost ins. W; ss. A 90%; sol. A abs., C, E. A white or very pale cream crystalline powder; odourless; tasteless.

℀ Diphenan is an anthelmintic which is said to be particularly effective against thread-worms. It may be given 3 times daily for a week and then followed by a purge. The treatment may be repeated after an interval of a week. The worms are usually killed or rendered incapable of depositing eggs in the anal region so that re-infestation is not likely to occur.

Diphenylhydantoin Sodium U.S.P. *Diphenylhydantoinum Sodicum.*
Phenytoin Sodium B.P. *Phenytoinum Sodium.* (Soluble Diphenyl Hydantoin. T.N. Dilantin Sodium, Epanutin, Eptoin, Solantoin)
DOSES: B.P. 50-100 mg. ($\frac{3}{4}$-1$\frac{1}{2}$ gr.); U.S.P. 0.1 Gm. (1$\frac{1}{2}$ gr.). $C_{15}H_{11}N_2O_2Na$. Mol.wt. 274.3. S: fs. W (solution somewhat turbid); sol. A; almost insol. E, C. A white micro-crystalline powder; odourless; taste slightly bitter; somewhat hygroscopic.

Diphenylhydantoin Sodium Capsules U.S.P.
Sizes, 30 and 100 mg. ($\frac{1}{2}$ and 1$\frac{1}{2}$ gr.).

℀ Diphenylhydantoin sodium controls or suppresses the convulsions of epilepsy in doses which have relatively little hypnotic or stupefying action. It is more effective against *grand mal* than *petit mal* seizures and will control many cases which are not controlled by phenobarbitone or bromides. Toxic reactions to phenytoin are numerous and may be serious. Sometimes reducing the dosage for a few days may cause the less serious one to disappear. These include nausea, dizziness, and skin rashes. They often do not reappear when the dose is raised to its previous level. More serious reactions, which may force discontinuation of the treatment, are fever, mental confusion, exfoliative dermatitis, and tenderness and hypertrophy of the gums. The doses shown above are often given 3 times a day and may be increased if necessary.

Dithranol B.P. *Dithranol.* (Dioxyanthranol)
$C_{14}H_{10}O_3$. Mol.wt. 226.2. M.p. 174-178°. S: ins. W; ss. A, E; sol. C, B, acetone, and in fixed oils. A yellow odourless and tasteless powder.

Ointment of Dithranol B.P. *Unguentum Dithranolis*
Dithranol 0.1 Gm., Soft Yellow Paraffin to make 100.

℄ Dithranol and Chrysarobin have the same actions and uses. They are antiseptic and irritant to the skin. In low concentrations they are keratoplastic, i.e. they increase proliferation of cornified epithelium. In higher concentrations they produce inflammation and itching. Absorption may occur when large areas are treated. The urine is coloured red and renal irritation may occur. The main use of dithranol is in the treatment of psoriasis and other chronic skin ailments. Great care should be taken to keep these materials away from the eyes, and the genitalia.

Emetine and Bismuth Iodide B.P. *Emetinae et Bismuthi Iodidum*
Doses: 60-200 mg. (1-3 gr.) daily. A reddish-orange powder; odourless; taste bitter and acrid. S: ins. W, A; sol. acetone.

℄ Emetine and Bismuth Iodide is intensely irritant and when taken by mouth usually causes nausea and vomiting. It may be given in enteric coated pills or capsules for the treatment of amoebic dysentery.

Emetine Hydrochloride. *Emetinae Hydrochloridum*
Doses: B.P. daily by subcutaneous or intramuscular injection, 30-60 mg. ($\frac{1}{2}$-1 gr.); U.S.P. average daily intramuscular, 60 mg. (1 gr.). $C_{29}H_{40}N_2O_4.2HCl$ (U.S.P.); $+7H_2O$ (B.P.). Mol.wt. 553.56 (U.S.P.); 679.7 (B.P.). S: sol. W, A. Hydrochloride of an alkaloid obtained from ipecacuanha root or prepared synthetically. It is a white or faintly yellowish crystalline powder; odourless; taste bitter. Protect from light.

Emetine Hydrochloride Injection U.S.P.
Sizes, 1 cc. contains 20 mg. ($\frac{1}{3}$ gr.) or 30 mg. ($\frac{1}{2}$ gr.) or 60 mg. (1 gr.).

Injection of Emetine Hydrochloride B.P.
DOSES: by subcutaneous or intramuscular injection, 30-60 mg. ($\frac{1}{2}$-1 gr.) daily. Strength, 60 mg. per cc. (1 gr. in 15 min.).

《 Emetine is the main active principle of Ipecacuanha. It has a very irritant action on mucous membranes. As little as 6 mg. by mouth will cause vomiting, presumably by irritating nerve endings in the stomach, since larger doses (60 mg.) by injection are usually not emetic. The drug is given by intramuscular injection for the treatment of amoebic dysentery once a day for 10 days, usually in conjunction with other drugs by mouth, such as Carbarsone or Emetine and Bismuth Iodide.

Anhydrous Ephedrine Can. Gaz. *Ephedrina Sicca.* **Ephedrine U.S.P.** *Ephedrina*
DOSES: Can. Gaz. 15-100 mg. ($\frac{1}{4}$-1$\frac{1}{2}$ gr.). U.S.P. no dose. $C_{10}H_{15}NO$. Mol.wt. 165.23. M.p. 33-40°. S: sol. W, A, C, E; 20 G, 25 olive oil, 100 liquid paraffin, giving a turbid solution if ephedrine contains more than 1% H_2O. An alkaloid from *Ephedra equisetina*, *Ephedra sinica* and other species of *Ephedra*, or produced synthetically. An unctuous, almost colourless, hygroscopic solid or white crystals or granules; odour unpleasant.

Ephedrine B.P. *Ephedrina.*
$(C_{10}H_{15}ON)_2.H_2O$. Mol.wt. 348.5. M.p. 40-41°. S: sol. W, A, E, C; the chloroform solution is turbid owing to the separation of water; 20 G, 25 olive oil, 100 liquid paraffin (with turbidity). An alkaloid obtained from *Ephedra sinica*, *Ephedra equisetina* or other species of *Ephedra* or by synthesis. Colourless crystals; odourless or with a slight unpleasant smell.

Ephedrine Hydrochloride. *Ephedrinae Hydrochloridum*
DOSES: B.P. 16-60 mg. ($\frac{1}{4}$-1 gr.); U.S.P. 25 mg. ($\frac{3}{8}$ gr.). $C_{10}H_{15}NOHCl$. Mol.wt. 201.7. M.p. 217-220°. S: 3W, 14 A; ins. E. Fine white odourless crystals or powder; affected by light; taste bitter. Contains between 80.4 and 82.5% of anhydrous ephedrine (U.S.P.).

Ephedrine Hydrochloride Capsules U.S.P.
Sizes, 25 and 50 mg. ($\frac{3}{8}$ and $\frac{3}{4}$ gr.).

Ephedrine Hydrochloride Tablets U.S.P.
Sizes, 15, 25 and 30 mg. ($\frac{1}{4}$, $\frac{3}{8}$ and $\frac{1}{2}$ gr.).

Tablets of Ephedrine Hydrochloride B.P.
Size, 30 mg. ($\frac{1}{2}$ gr.).

Ephedrine Sulfate U.S.P. *Ephedrinae Sulfas*
DOSE: 25 mg. ($\frac{3}{8}$ gr.). $(C_{10}H_{15}NO)_2H_2SO_4$. Mol.wt. 428.53.
S: fs. W and hot A; less sol. in cold A. Colourless crystals; odourless;
taste bitter; affected by light. Contains 75.5-77.3% of anhydrous
ephedrine.

Ephedrine Sulfate Capsules U.S.P.
Sizes, 25 and 50 mg. ($\frac{3}{8}$ and $\frac{3}{4}$ gr.).

Ephedrine Sulfate Injection U.S.P.
1 cc. contains 25 mg. ($\frac{3}{8}$ gr.) or 50 mg. ($\frac{3}{4}$ gr.).

Ephedrine Sulfate Tablets U.S.P.
Size, 25, 30, mg. ($\frac{3}{8}$, $\frac{1}{2}$, gr.).

❡ The effects of ephedrine and its salts closely resemble those of
epinephrine, with the important differences that they last longer
(1-2 hours), and that they can be produced by oral administration.
The most important actions are vasoconstriction, bronchiolar
dilatation, pupillary dilatation, and analepsis. The last-named
action may be used to combat poisoning by morphine or barbiturates.
Ephedrine in ordinary dosage may produce certain unpleasant side
effects, viz. anxiety, tremor, and palpitation.

The main uses are shrinking of nasal mucous membranes by the
local application of 0.5 to 1% aqueous solutions, prevention or
abortion of asthmatic attacks by oral administration, and maintenance of blood pressure by injection during spinal anaesthesia.
Successive injections of ephedrine produce decreasing effect, a
phenomenon known as tachyphylaxis.

Adrenaline B.P. *Adrenalina.* **Epinephrine U.S.P.** *Epinephrina.*
Adrenalinum. (T.N. Adrenalin). (N.B. in Canada Adrenaline
is regarded as a trade name)

Doses: Subcutaneous, 0.1-0.5 mg. ($\frac{1}{600}$-$\frac{1}{120}$ gr.). $C_9H_{13}O_3N$. Mol.wt. 183.2. M.p. 205-212°. S: ss. W; ins. A, E, C, fixed and volatile oils; sol. in dilute acids. A colourless or pale-buff powder; an active principle extracted from the suprarenal medulla; may be prepared synthetically; affected by light.

Injection of Adrenaline B.P. (Injection of Adrenaline Tartrate)

Doses: subcutaneous, 0.12-0.5 cc. (2-8 min.). Adrenaline 0.1 with Tartaric Acid, Sodium Metabisulphite, Sodium Chloride 0.8, and Water for Injection to make 100 cc.

℃ A subcutaneous injection of 0.5 cc. of 1:1000 aqueous solution of epinephrine produces first a vasoconstriction locally. Absorption is thus slightly delayed but in 5-10 minutes systemic effects are noticeable. These may include a tremor and a sensation of pounding of the heart. In asthma, relaxation of bronchiolar muscles is produced, with easing of respiratory effort. With urticaria (hives), the itching and swelling are relieved. If the blood pressure is low, e.g. in spinal anaesthesia, it will be raised. In normal persons the blood pressure may not rise much because of regulatory reflexes. The pulse rate usually increases slightly. The pulse pressure is usually increased, indicating an increased cardiac output per beat. The blood sugar increases, an effect which may be used to counteract severe insulin hypoglycaemia.

If epinephrine is given intramuscularly (1 cc. of 1:500) in oil, the absorption is slower and the systemic effects are less intense but more prolonged, which is desirable in the treatment of asthma or hives.

Given intravenously, 0.2-0.4 mg., epinephrine raises the blood pressure by constricting the arterioles of the splanchnic region and the skin. The coronary arteries are, however, dilated, as are those of the voluntary muscles. The spleen is contracted, increasing the volume of circulating blood. The contractility of the heart muscle is increased. The net effect is an increase in cardiac output per minute, although the pulse rate may be decreased by the carotid sinus and depressor reflexes. An injection of epinephrine into the left ventricle of a heart which has apparently stopped, as in deep anaesthesia, may restore its activity, but this should not be tried except as a last resort. The injection should be made in a large volume; at least 50 cc. of isotonic saline.

The effects of epinephrine on uterine muscle are mixed but during parturition the net effect is to inhibit temporarily the expulsive contractions. This action has been used together with deep ether anaesthesia to relax uterine muscle in the spastic state known as Bandl's Ring.

Large doses of epinephrine may produce pulmonary oedema as a result of left ventricular failure consequent on hypertension. In patients under chloroform anaesthesia or cyclopropane anaesthesia, or under the influence of digitalis, much smaller doses of epinephrine may produce ventricular fibrillation.

Epinephrine may be applied locally to produce vasoconstriction and arrest of haemorrhage in the nose, throat, gums. It may also be used in nasal packs to shrink the mucous membranes. Small amounts may be used in eye-drops and in solutions of local anaesthetics to prolong the action of the anaesthetic by means of vascular constriction.

Epinephrine Inhalation U.S.P.   *Inhalatio Epinephrinae*
An aqueous solution containing 1% of epinephrine hydrochloride.

℃ The 1% solution is meant to be administered by inhalation, *not* by injection. A special nebulizer is required to make a very fine suspension (aerosol) which will pass well down into the bronchioles. Particle sizes must be about 10 microns or less to penetrate deeply into the lungs.

Epinephrine Injection U.S.P.
A sterile aqeous solution of epinephrine as hydrochloride, for injection. The potency shall be stated on the label. Usual strength is 1:1000, supplied in ampules or vials of dark glass of 1 cc., 10cc.

Epinephrine in Oil Injection U.S.P.
1 cc. contains 2 mg. (1/30 gr.) Epinephrine.

Epinephrine Bitartrate U.S.P.   *Epinephrinae Bitartras*
$C_9H_{13}NO_3.C_4H_6O_6$. Mol.wt. 333.29. M.p. 147-154°. S: 3 W; ss. A. A white, grayish white or brownish gray crystalline powder; odourless; decomposes on melting.

Epinephrine Bitartrate Ophthalmic Ointment U.S.P.   *Unguentum Epinephrinae Bitartratis Ophthalmicum*
Epinephrine Bitartrate 1, Water 10, Hydrophilic Petrolatum to make 100 Gm.

Epinephrine Solution U.S.P. *Liquor Epinephrinae*
A solution of epinephrine in distilled water, dissolved with the aid of HCl. Its potency is equivalent to 1 Gm. of standard epinephrine in 1000 cc. as determined by bioassay.

Solution of Adrenaline Hydrochloride B.P. *Liquor Adrenalinae Hydrochloridi.* (Epinephrine Solution)
Adrenaline 1 Gm., Sodium Chloride 9 Gm., with Chlorbutol, Sodium Metabisulphite, Dilute Hydrochloric Acid and Distilled Water to make 1000 cc. Used to make the Strong Injection of Procaine and Adrenaline.

Ergometrine Maleate B.P. *Ergometrinae Maleas.* **Ergonovine Maleate U.S.P.** *Ergonovinae Maleas*
DOSES: B.P. oral 0.5-1 mg. ($\frac{1}{120}$-$\frac{1}{60}$ gr.); intramuscular 0.25-0.5 mg. ($\frac{1}{240}$-$\frac{1}{120}$ gr.); intravenous, 0.125-0.25 mg. ($\frac{1}{480}$-$\frac{1}{240}$ gr.); U.S.P. oral 0.5 mg. ($\frac{1}{120}$ gr.); intramuscular or intravenous 0.2 mg. ($\frac{1}{300}$ gr.). $C_{19}H_{23}N_3O_2.C_4H_4O_4$. Mol.wt. 441.5. M.p. 195-197°. S: 36 W, 120 A, 100 A 90%; ins. E, C. A white or faintly yellow odourless micro-crystalline powder, affected by light.

Ergonovine Maleate Injection U.S.P.
Sizes, 0.2 mg. ($\frac{1}{300}$ gr.) or 0.5 mg. ($\frac{1}{120}$ gr.) in 1 cc.

Ergonovine Maleate Tablets U.S.P.
Sizes, 0.2 mg. ($\frac{1}{300}$ gr.) or 0.5 mg.($\frac{1}{120}$ gr.).

Injection of Ergometrine Maleate B.P.
Strength, 0.5 mg. ($\frac{1}{120}$ gr.) in 1 cc. (15 min.).

⟪ The galenical preparations of ergot have now been largely replaced by the purified alkaloids. These are derivatives of lysergic acid and the important ones are Ergometrine (Ergonovine), Ergotamine, and Ergotoxine. Crude ergot contains many other similar alkaloids in addition to histamine, choline, and tyramine. All three of the alkaloids mentioned above cause powerful contractions of the uterus but the one now used mostly for this effect is Ergometrine because it is active by mouth, while the others are not, and also because it acts more rapidly on injection. Ergometrine is mainly used after parturition to check bleeding and it is often given for several days to encourage involution of the uterus.

Ergotamine Tartrate is given, usually by injection, for migraine. It is thought to act by constriction of cerebral vessels. Pulsations of the temporal artery which are often visible during an attack decrease or disappear in a few minutes if symptomatic relief is obtained. Both Ergotamine and Ergotoxine may be given by injection to promote uterine contractions after parturition. They act more slowly than Ergometrine but last longer.

All three ergot alkaloids, if given over too long a period, may cause gangrene of extremities, but Ergometrine is much less likely to do so than the other two.

Ergot B.P. *Ergota.* (Secale Cornutum I.A.)

The dried sclerotium of the fungus *Claviceps purpurea* developed on rye plants. Contains about 0.2% of alkaloid; taste disagreeable; odour characteristic.

Prepared Ergot B.P. *Ergota Praeparata*

Doses: 0.15-0.5 Gm. ($2\frac{1}{2}$-8 gr.). A purplish-brown powder; odour and taste characteristic; Ergot defatted and standardized to contain 0.2% of total alkaloids calculated as ergotoxine; 0.5 Gm. contains 1 mg. (8 gr. contain $\frac{1}{60}$ gr.) of total alkaloids and 0.5 Gm. contains 0.015 mg. (8 gr. contain $\frac{1}{400}$ gr.) of water-soluble alkaloids calculated as ergometrine.

Tablets of Prepared Ergot B.P.

Size, 150 mg. ($2\frac{1}{2}$ gr.).

Liquid Extract of Ergot B.P. *Extractum Ergotae Liquidum*

Doses: 0.6-1.2 cc. (10-20 min.). Contains, after storage, not less than 0.04% of total alkaloids; 1.2 cc. contain 0.7 mg. (20 min. contain $\frac{1}{90}$ gr.) of total alkaloids.

Ergotamine Tartrate. *Ergotaminae Tartras*

Doses: B.P. single oral, 1-2 mg. ($\frac{1}{60}$-$\frac{1}{30}$ gr.); subcutaneous, 0.25-0.5 mg. ($\frac{1}{240}$-$\frac{1}{120}$ gr.); U.S.P. 0.5 mg. ($\frac{1}{120}$ gr.) intramuscular; 1 mg. ($\frac{1}{60}$ gr.) oral. $(C_{33}H_{35}N_5O_5)_2C_4H_6O_6$. Mol.wt. 1313.4. M.p. 177-184°. S: 500 W, 500 A. An alkaloid obtained from ergot; colourless crystals or a white crystalline powder usually containing solvent of crystallization.

Ergotamine Tartrate Injection U.S.P.

1 cc. contains 0.5 mg. (1/120 gr.).

Ergotamine Tartrate Tablets U.S.P.

Sizes, 0.5 and 1 mg. ($\frac{1}{120}$ and $\frac{1}{60}$ gr.).

Erythrityl Tetranitrate Tablets U.S.P. *Tabellae Erythritylis Tetranitratis.* (Erythrol Tetranitrate Tablets, Tetranitrol Tablets)

DOSE: 30 mg. ($\frac{1}{2}$ gr.). Contains $C_4H_6(NO_3)_4$. Sizes, 15 and 30 mg. ($\frac{1}{4}$ and $\frac{1}{2}$ gr.).

₡ Erythrityl tetranitrate slowly releases nitrite ions in the body. These depress smooth muscles generally, particularly those of arterioles. The effects of this drug are milder and more prolonged than those of amyl nitrite or nitroglycerine. Peak effects occur 2 to 3 hours after an oral dose. Headache may accompany its use. The drug has been tried in angina pectoris, asthma, and hypertension and may be useful in some cases.

Ethanolamine B.P. *Aethanolamina.* (Monoethanolamine)

C_2H_7ON. Mol.wt. 61.08. F.p. 9.5-10.5.° S: sol. W, A 90%; ss. E, B, light petroleum. A clear colourless or pale-yellow liquid; odourless; volatile in steam.

Injection of Ethanolamine Oleate B.P. *Injectio Aethanolaminae Oleatis*

DOSES: intravenous, 2-5 cc. (30-75 min.). Ethanolamine 0.91 Gm., Oleic Acid 4.23 Gm., Benzyl Alcohol and Water for Injection to make 100 cc.

₡ This injection is used as a sclerosing agent for varicose veins. It should be protected from light.

Anaesthetic Ether B.P. *Aether Anaestheticus.* **Ether U.S.P.** *Aether.* (Ether, Ethyl Ether, Diethyl Ether)

$C_2H_5.O.C_2H_5$. Mol.wt. 74.12. B.p. 34-35°. Gm./cc. 0.7135. Sp.gr. 0.713-0.716. S: 12 W; misc. A 90%, C and with fixed and volatile oils. A highly purified, colourless, transparent, very volatile liquid; odour characteristic; taste sweet and burning; inflammable; explosive in certain concentrations when mixed with air, oxygen or nitrous oxide; must be stored in a cool place, protected from light in dry containers.

₡ Ether vapour when inhaled irritates the mucous membrane of the respiratory tract and increases secretion of saliva and mucus. It stimulates breathing mostly by reflex action as a result of local irritation. Concentrations in the blood which produce deep anaesthesia depress the breathing. Death from overdosage is by respiratory failure. Ether is considered one of the safest and most effective of the general anaesthetics but it should not be used when the lungs are diseased. The anaesthetic concentration in the blood is 100-150 mg. per 100 cc., in air, about 5% by volume.

Ethohexadiol U.S.P.   *Ethohexadiol*

2-ethyl hexane-1, 3-diol. $C_8H_{18}O_2$. Mol.wt. 146.22 Sp.gr. 0.936-0.940. S: 50 W; misc. A, C, E. A clear colourless oily liquid; odourless; used as an insect repellent.

Ethyl Chloride.   *Aethylis Chloridum*

C_2H_5Cl. Mol.wt. 64.50. B.p. 12-13°. Gm./cc. 0.919. Sp.gr. 0.921 at 0°. S: ss. W; fs. A, E. A clear colourless very mobile liquid; odour characteristic, ethereal; taste burning; gaseous at ordinary temperatures; *very inflammable.*

℃ Sprayed on the skin, ethyl chloride evaporates so rapidly that local freezing results. It thus produces a very transient local anaesthesia which may be employed for incising a superficial abscess.

Inhalation of the vapour produces anaesthesia very rapidly. Great caution must be used to avoid overdosage. It is used for brief operations or for anaesthetic induction. The anaesthetic concentration in air is about 4% by volume. It is sometimes used in dentistry.

Ethyl Oleate B.P.   *Aethylis Oleas*

$C_{20}H_{38}O_2$. Mol.wt. 310.5. Gm./cc. 0.869-0.870. S: ins. W; misc. vegetable oils. A pale-yellow oil with a strong disagreeable odour and taste. Contains not less than 98% of ethyl oleate w/w. Used as a vehicle for injections of substances soluble in oil or dispersible in it.

Ethyl Oxide U.S.P.   *Aethylis Oxidum.*   Solvent Ether B.P.   *Aether Solvens*

$C_4H_{10}O$. Mol.wt. 74.12. B.p. 34-36°. Gm/.cc. 0.714-0.718. S: as for anaesthetic ether. *Caution—not to be used for anaesthesia.* Used in the preparation of collodions.

Spirit of Ether B.P.   *Spiritus Aetheris.*   (Hoffmann's Drops)

DOSES: 1-4 cc. (15-60 min.). Anaesthetic Ether 33% v/v in 59-65% v/v C_2H_5OH.

℃ Hoffmann's Drops were once a favourite remedy for asthma and hysteria.

Ethylene. *Aethylenum*

$CH_2:CH_2$. Mol.wt. 28.05. S: 1 vol. in 9.2 W, 0.5 A, 0.05 E at 15.5°. A colourless, inflammable gas; odour and taste slightly sweet; explosive in certain concentrations when mixed with air or oxygen; contains not less than 99% by volume C_2H_4, (U.S.P.) or 98% (B.P.)

℃ Inhalation of ethylene produces anaesthesia very rapidly with no irritation. Muscular relaxation is poor. Anaesthetic concentration in blood is about 140 mg. per 100 cc., in air, about 85% by volume.

Ethylenediamine Solution U.S.P. *Liquor Aethylenediaminae*

S: misc. W, A. A clear colourless, or slightly yellow oily liquid having an ammonia-like odour and a strong alkaline reaction. Contains 67-71% of (H_2N-CH_2-CH_2-NH_2).

℃ Ethylenediamine is used in Aminophylline to increase the solubility of the theophylline. In doses which are given in that preparation the ethylenediamine cannot be said to have any definite pharmacological action.

Eucalyptol. *Eucalyptol.* (Cineole)

DOSES: B.P. 0.06-0.2 cc. (1-3 min.). $C_{10}H_{18}O$. Mol.wt. 154.2. Gm./cc. 0.922-0.924. Sp.gr. 0.921-0.924. S: ins. W; sol. 5 vols. A 60%; misc. A, C, E, glacial acetic acid and with fixed and volatile oils. A colourless liquid having a characteristic aromatic, distinctly camphoraceous, odour with a pungent, cooling, spicy taste.

Oil of Eucalyptus B.P. *Oleum Eucalypti*

DOSES: B.P. 0.06-0.2 cc. (1-3 min.). Sp.gr. 0.905-0.925. S: 5 A 70%. Volatile oil from fresh leaves of *Eucalyptus Globulus* and other species. It contains not less than 70% of cineole.

℃ Eucalyptol and Oil of Eucalyptus are traditionally associated with the treatment of colds, by inhalation of the vapour or by nasal sprays containing about 1% of either. Their use declined when it was reported that they depressed the activity of cilia of the nasal mucosa.

Eucatropine Hydrochloride U.S.P. *Eucatropinae Hydrochloridum*
(Euphthalmine Hydrochloride N.N.R.)
$C_{17}H_{25}O_3N.HCl$. Mol.wt. 327.84. M.p. 183°. S: vs. W; fs. A,
C; ins. E. A white granular odourless powder.

℃ Eucatropine Hydrochloride is instilled in the eye in 5-10%
solution to produce dilatation of the pupil. It produces little or no
paralysis of accommodation and its effects wear off more rapidly
than those of Homatropine.

Eugenol U.S.P. *Eugenol*
$C_{10}H_{12}O_2$. Mol.wt. 164.20. Sp.gr. 1.064-1.070 at 25°. S: ss. W;
misc. A, C, E and fixed oils, 2 A 70%. A colourless or pale-yellow
liquid having a strong aromatic odour of clove; taste spicy and
pungent. See Clove.

Fennel B.P. *Foeniculum*. (Fennel Fruit)
The dried ripe fruit of *Foeniculum vulgare*; taste sweet, aromatic,
and agreeable.

Powdered Fennel B.P. *Foeniculi Pulvis*
A greenish-yellow to yellowish-brown powder.

Fennel Oil U.S.P. *Oleum Foeniculi*
Sp.gr. 0.953-0.973. S: 8 A 80%, 1 A 90%. The volatile oil
steam-distilled from the dried ripe fruit of *Foeniculum vulgare*; a
colourless or pale-yellow liquid having the characteristic odour and
taste of Fennel.

℃ Fennel Oil has a reputation as a carminative. It is sometimes
included in cathartic pills to diminish griping.

Fluorescein Sodium. *Fluoresceinum Sodicum U.S.P. Fluores-*
ceinum Sodium B.P. (Disodium Fluorescein, Resorcinolphthalein
Sodium)
$C_{20}H_{10}O_5Na_2$. Mol.wt. 376.3. S: 1 W, 5 A 90% at 15.5°. An
orange-red powder; odourless; almost tasteless; hygroscopic.

℃ A 2% solution of disodium fluorescein is used to show small
ulcers or foreign bodies in the cornea. The dye tends to accumulate
in the injured spots, which thus appear green when illuminated.
Fluorescein is relatively non-toxic and may be given orally for
kidney function tests and tests of permeability of ocular blood
vessels.

Folic Acid U.S.P. *Acidum Folicum.* (Pteroylglutamic Acid)

DAILY DOSE: 10 mg. (1/6 gr.). $C_{19}H_{19}N_7O_6$. Mol.wt. 441.40. S: ins. W, A, B, C; sol. in alkalis. A yellowish orange crystalline powder; odourless.

Folic Acid Capsules U.S.P.

Size 5 mg. (1/12 gr.).

Folic Acid Tablets U.S.P.

Size 5 mg. (1/12 gr.).

⟨ In the course of its investigation Folic Acid has been referred to as *L. casei* factor, Vitamin B_c and Vitamin M. It is particularly effective in treating the diarrhoea and the anaemia of sprue. It also produces improvement in the blood picture in nutritional macrocytic anaemia and pernicious anaemia. It does not prevent spinal cord lesions in pernicious anaemia and hence will not replace liver extracts in the treatment of pernicious anaemia. Certain cases of coeliac disease respond favourably to treatment by folic acid.

Solution of Formaldehyde B.P. *Liquor Formaldehydi.* (Formalin)

A clear colourless or nearly colourless liquid having a pungent irritating odour; contains 37-41% w/v CH_2O. S: misc. W, A. Gm./cc. 1.076-1.091. Contains variable amounts of ethanol or methanol or both to prevent polymerization.

⟨ Formalin diluted 1:200 of water is a powerful antiseptic but is seldom used externally or internally on account of its irritant properties. A 2% solution is used as a preservative for pathological specimens, and a 4% solution as a hardening agent for tissues for microscopic examination. Dilute solutions of formaldehyde, e.g. 2%, usually mean per cent of formalin by volume, not per cent of CH_2O. Gelatin capsules may be hardened and rendered resistant to pepsin and hydrochloric acid by dipping for 2 minutes in a 10% solution of formalin and drying. The capsules will dissolve in the small intestine.

In the practice of dentistry formalin is used in the treatment of pulp gangrene but with great caution because necrosis of the periapical tissues may occur. It may be used in suitable dilution for the sterilization of some instruments.

Gelatin. *Gelatinum*
Dried protein material, extracted with boiling water from skin, tendons, ligaments, and bones of animals. It occurs in sheets, flakes, shreds, or as a coarse or fine powder. S: ins. A, E, C; sol. hot W. Forms a gel on cooling.

⟪ Gelatin is used for making capsules and pastilles.

Glycerinated Gelatin U.S.P. *Gelatinum Glycerinatum*
Gelatin 100 Gm., Glycerin 100 Gm., Distilled Water to make 200 Gm.

⟪ Glycerinated Gelatin is solid at room temperature but melts at body temperature . It may be used as a base for suppositories.

Gelatin of Zinc B.P. *Gelatinum Zinci.* (Unna's Paste)
Zinc Oxide 15 Gm. with Gelatin, Glycerin, and Distilled Water to make 100 Gm.

Zinc Gelatin U.S.P. *Gelatinum Zinci.* (Zinc Gelatin Boot)
Zinc Oxide 100, Gelatin 150, Glycerin 400, Distilled Water to make about 1000 Gm.

⟪ Unna's Paste is used to provide a protective cover for chronic skin lesions caused or aggravated by scratching or even exposure to dry air. The paste is melted and applied warm. It hardens as it cools.

Gentian. *Gentiana.* (Gentian Root)
The dried rhizome and roots of *Gentiana lutea*; taste sweetish at first, then persistently bitter.

Powdered Gentian B.P. *Gentianae Pulvis*
A light-brown or yellowish-brown powder.

Concentrated Compound Infusion of Gentian B.P. *Infusum Gentianae Compositum Concentratum*
DOSES: 2-4 cc. (30-60 min.). Gentian 10 Gm., Dried Bitter Orange Peel, Lemon Peel, Alcohol, and Water to make about 120 cc. by maceration. Contains 20-24% v/v C_2H_5OH.

Compound Infusion of Gentian B.P. *Infusum Gentianae Compositum*
DOSES: 15-30 cc. ($\frac{1}{2}$-1 fl.oz.). Concentrated Infusion of Gentian 12.5, Distilled Water to make 100 cc.

Compound Gentian Tincture U.S.P. Compound Tincture of Gentian B.P. *Tinctura Gentianae Composita*
DOSES: B.P. 2-4 cc. (30-60 min.); U.S.P. 4 cc. (1 fl.dr.). B.P.—Gentian 10 Gm., with Dried Bitter Orange Peel, Cardamom, and Alcohol 45% to make 100 cc. by maceration. Contains 41-45% v/v of C_2H_5OH. U.S.P.—Gentian 10 Gm., Bitter Orange Peel, Cardamom Seed, Glycerin, with Alcohol and Water to make 100 cc. by percolation. Contains 43-47% v/v of C_2H_5OH.

❡ Preparations of gentian are now used only as bitter flavours. They contain tannic acid.

Ginger B.P. *Zinigiber*
The dried rhizome of *Zingiber officinale* Roscoe scraped to remove the dark outer skin. It is known in commerce as unbleached Jamaica ginger. Odour agreeable and aromatic; taste pungent and burning.

Powdered Ginger B.P. *Zingiberis Pulvis*
DOSES: 0.3-1 Gm. (5-15 gr.). A light yellow powder.

Strong Tincture of Ginger B.P. *Tinctura Zingiberis Fortis* (Essence of Ginger)
DOSES: 0.3-0.6 cc. (5-10 min.). Ginger 50 Gm. to make 100 cc. by percolation. Contains 80-88% v/v of C_2H_5OH.

Weak Tincture of Ginger B.P. *Tinctura Zingiberis Mitis*
DOSES: 2-4 cc. (30-60 min.). Strong Tincture of Ginger 20 cc. to make 100 cc. Contains 88-90% v/v of C_2H_5OH.

Syrup of Ginger B.P. *Syrupus Zingiberis*
DOSES: 2-8 cc. (30-120 min.). Strong Tincture of Ginger 5, Syrup to make 100.

Antihemophilic Globulin U.S.P. *Globulinum Antihemophilicum*
DOSE: intravenous, 200 mg. protein (the contents of 1 container). A dry sterile preparation containing a fraction of normal human plasma of unknown composition which shortens the clotting time of hemophilic blood when it is shed; to be dissolved in 15-20 cc. of sterile saline immediately before administration.

Human Immune Globulin U.S.P. *Globulinum Immune Humanum.*
(Measles Prophylactic, Placental Extract)

Doses: intramuscular for modification, 2-5 cc. (30-75 min.); for prevention, 2-10 cc. (30-150 min.). A sterile solution of antibodies obtained from the placenta and placental blood expelled by healthy women.

Liquid Glucose. *Glucosum Liquidum*
S: misc. W; ss. A. A colourless or almost colourless, very viscous syrup; odourless; taste sweet. Consists chiefly of dextrose with dextrins, maltose, and water.

℃ Liquid glucose is given orally or rectally but not by injection. It is used as a sweetening agent, as an excipient in pills, as a diagnostic agent (glucose tolerance), and for infant feeding. See Dextrosum.

Syrup of Liquid Glucose B.P. *Syrupus Glucosi Liquidi.* (Syrup of Glucose)
Liquid Glucose 33.3 Gm. with Syrup 66.7 Gm.

Glycerin. *Glycerinum*
CH₂OH.CHOH. CH₂OH. Mol.wt. 92.09. Gm./cc. 1.255-1.260. Sp.gr. not less than 1.249 at 25°. S: misc. W, A; ins .E, C, fixed and volatile oils. A clear, colourless, syrupy liquid; odourless; taste sweet; hygroscopic.

Glycerin Suppositories U.S.P. Suppositories of Glycerin B.P. *Suppositoria Glycerini*
U.S.P.—Glycerin with Sodium Stearate and Distilled Water. Contains about 92% w/w of Glycerin. B.P.—Glycerin with Distilled Water and Gelatin. Contains about 70% w/w of Glycerin.

℃ A glycerin suppository initiates defaecation usually within half an hour. It may be used to establish regular habits in infants or to produce soft stools when haemorrhoids are troublesome.

Glyceryl Triacetate U.S.P. *Glycerylis Triacetas.* (Triacetin)
C₉H₁₄O₆. Mol.wt. 218.2. S: sol. W; misc. A, C, E; ins. CS₂. A colourless somewhat oily liquid with a slight fatty odour.

℃ Triacetin is not used as a medicine but as a solvent for cosmetics and also to dissolve the disinfectant, azochloramide.

Glyceryl Trinitrate Tablets U.S.P. *Tabellae Glycerylis Trinitratis.* (Nitroglycerin Tablets, Trinitrin Tablets)

Dose: 0.4 mg. ($\frac{1}{150}$ gr.). Sizes, 0.3, 0.4, 0.6 and 1.2 mg. ($\frac{1}{200}$, $\frac{1}{150}$, $\frac{1}{100}$ and $\frac{1}{50}$ gr.).

Tablets of Glyceryl Trinitrate B.P. (Nitroglycerin Tablets)
Doses: 0.5-1 mg. ($\frac{1}{130}$-$\frac{1}{60}$ gr.).
Size, 0.5 mg. ($\frac{1}{130}$ gr.). To be chewed up before swallowing. See Amyl Nitrite.

Glycyrrhiza U.S.P. Liquorice B.P. *Glycyrrhiza.* (Liquorice Root, Licorice Root)
The peeled root and subterranean stem of *Glycyrrhiza glabra* and other species; odour characteristic; taste sweetish.

Powdered Liquorice B.P. *Glycyrrhizae Pulvis*
A buff or yellow powder of the peeled drug.

Extract of Liquorice B.P. Glycyrrhiza Extract U.S.P. *Extractum Glycyrrhizae.* (Liquorice Root Extract, Licorice)
Doses: B.P. 0.6-2 Gm. (10-30 gr.). B.P.—a percolate of liquorice root with chloroform water evaporated to a soft consistency. U.S.P.—A brown powder or in flattened cylindrical rolls or in masses. Both are evaporated aqueous extracts.

Pure Glycyrrhiza Extract U.S.P. *Extractum Glycyrrhizae Purum.* (Pure Licorice Root Extract)
Powdered Glycyrrhiza is percolated with boiling water. The percolate is made ammoniacal and evaporated until a soft mass is obtained of a consistency suitable for making pills.

Glycyrrhiza Fluidextract U.S.P. *Fluidextractum Glycyrrhizae.*
Liquid Extract of Liquorice B.P. *Extractum Glycyrrhizae Liquidum*
Doses: B.P. 2-4 cc. (30-60 min.); U.S.P. 2 cc. (30 min.). B.P.— Liquorice unpeeled in coarse powder extracted with chloroform water by percolation. Alcohol is added later. The final product contains 16-20% v/v of C_2H_5OH. U.S.P.—Glycyrrhiza in very coarse powder is extracted with boiling water. Ammonia and alcohol are added later. The final product contains 20-24% v/v of C_2H_5OH.

Glycyrrhiza Syrup U.S.P. *Syrupus Glycyrrhizae.* (Licorice Syrup)
Glycyrrhiza Fluidextract 25 cc., Fennel Oil, Anise Oil, and Syrup to make 100 cc. Contains 5-6% v/v of C_2H_5OH.

℟ Liquorice has a persistent flavour which is useful for covering unpleasant drugs such as ammonium chloride or bromides. The taste is due to a glycoside, glycyrrhizin, which precipitates if dispensed in acid solution.

Compound Powder of Liquorice B.P.   *Pulvis Glycyrrhizae Compositus*
DOSES: 4-8 Gm. (60-120 gr.). Senna Leaf 16 Gm., Powdered Liquorice 16 Gm., Sulphur 8 Gm., Sucrose, and Fennel to make 100 Gm.

℟ The action of this laxative powder is due to the senna and the sulphur.

Hamamelis B.P.   *Hamamelis.*   (Witch Hazel Leaves)
Leaves of *Hamamelis virginiana* (Witch Hazel); taste bitter and astringent.

Powdered Hamamelis B.P.   *Hamamelidis Pulvis*
A dull-green powder.

Dry Extract of Hamamelis B.P.   *Extractum Hamamelidis Siccum*
(Extract of Witch Hazel)
A dried alcoholic extract of Hamamelis.

Liquid Extract of Hamamelis B.P.   *Extractum Hamamelidis Liquidum*
A dilute alcoholic extract of 100 Gm. of Hamamelis adjusted to 100 cc. Contains 32-40% v/v of C_2H_5OH.

Ointment of Hamamelis B.P.   *Unguentum Hamamelidis*
An ointment containing about 10% of Liquid Extract of Hamamelis in Wool Fat and Yellow Soft Paraffin.

℟ The preparations of witch hazel contain tannic acid and hence exert some astringent action. They have a popular reputation for possessing healing properties and are used in a variety of preparations for local application.

Suppositories of Hamamelis B.P.
Dry extract of Hamamelis 0.2 Gm. (3 gr.) in a suitable base.

Suppositories of Hamamelis and Zinc Oxide B.P.
Dry extract of Hamamelis 0.2 Gm. and Zinc Oxide 0.6 Gm. in a suitable base.

Helium U.S.P. *Helium*

He. At.wt. 4.003. S: ss. W. A colourless, odourless, tasteless gas which does not burn or support combustion; contains not less than 95% by volume of He, the remainder consisting of nitrogen.

℃ The very low viscosity of helium makes it useful for treating asthma. By breathing a mixture of 20-30% oxygen in helium, nitrogen can be removed from the lungs and ventilation through the constricted bronchioles can be accomplished with less effort.

Heparin B.P. *Heparinum.* **Heparin Sodium U.S.P.** *Heparinum Sodicum*

DOSES: B.P. intravenous, 6000-12,000 units. S: sol. in water or saline solution. Pale amorphous powder; odourless; hygroscopic. The sodium salt is a complex organic acid present in mammalian tissues (lung or liver is used commercially as the source) having the characteristic property of delaying the clotting of shed blood. Each mg. contains not less than 75 units (B.P.) or 100 units (U.S.P.).

Heparin Sodium Injection U.S.P.

10 cc. contain 10,000 units.

Injection of Heparin B.P. *Injectio Heparini*

DOSES: intravenous, 6,000-12,000 Units. A clear, colourless, or straw-coloured sterile solution in Water for Injection, free from turbidity and matter which deposits on standing.

℃ Heparin given intravenously has no notable effect other than prolongation of the clotting time of the blood. Indications for its administration are not generally agreed upon. It should be of value to prevent the spread of an embolus by preventing deposition of a fresh clot. It has also been used with apparent success with penicillin and sulphonamide in the treatment of subacute bacterial endocarditis. It allows these drugs to act on the bacteria by preventing fibrinous deposits around them.

Hexamine. See Methenamine.

Hexylresorcinol U.S.P. *Hexylresorcinol*

DOSE: 1 Gm. (15 gr.). $C_{12}H_{18}O_2$. Mol.wt. 194.26. M.p. 62-67°. S: 2000 W 25°; fs. A, G, E, C, B, and vegetable oils. White needle-shaped crystals; odour faintly fatty; taste astringent followed by a sensation of numbness.

℃ Hexylresorcinol is a powerful antiseptic and germicide. It is used externally as a general-purpose antiseptic in a solution of 1:1000 in 30% glycerin in water. For administration internally for pinworms or roundworms, it is available in enteric coated pills of 0.1 or 0.2 Gm. It may also be given dissolved in corn oil in capsules.

Hexylresorcinol Pills U.S.P.

DOSE: 1 Gm. (15 gr.) anthelmintic. Sizes, 0.1 and 0.2 Gm. (1½ and 3 gr.).

Histamine Acid Phosphate B.P.   *Histaminae Phosphas Acidus.*
Histamine Phosphate U.S.P.   *Histaminae Phosphas*

DOSES: B.P. subcutaneous, 0.5-1 mg. ($\frac{1}{120}-\frac{1}{60}$ gr.); U.S.P. intramuscular, 0.3 mg. ($\frac{1}{200}$ gr.). $C_5H_9N_3.2H_3PO_4$. Mol.wt. 307.2. M.p. 130-133°. S: 4 W; ss. A. Clear, colourless, odourless crystals.

Histamine Phosphate Injection U.S.P.

Sizes, 0.1 mg. or 1.0 mg. in 1 cc.; 0.2 mg. in 5cc.

Injection of Histamine Acid Phosphate B.P.

DOSES: subcutaneous, 0.5-1 mg. ($\frac{1}{120}-\frac{1}{60}$ gr.). Strength, 1 mg. per cc. ($\frac{1}{60}$ gr. in 15 min.).

℃ Histamine on injection causes increased secretion by salivary and gastric glands. On the latter the effect is particularly to increase the secretion of hydrochloric acid. For this reason it is used diagnostically to determine whether the stomach is capable of secreting any hydrochloric acid. A headache of short duration usually follows the injection. An overdose will cause prostration by vasodilation. Histamine may also be used to produce local vasodilation, when administered by iontophoresis. This is done sometimes in peripheral vascular disease or for rheumatoid arthritis.

Homatropine Hydrobromide.   *Homatropinae Hydrobromidum*

$C_{16}H_{21}O_3NHBr$. Mol.wt. 356.26. S: 6 W, 40 A, 420 C; ins. E. White crystals or a white crystalline powder; odourless; taste bitter.

Lamellae of Homatropine B.P.

Each gelatin disc contains 0.65 mg. ($\frac{1}{100}$ gr.) of homatropine hydrobromide.

₡ Homatropine like atropine may block, depending on concentration, the action of acetylcholine at certain cholinergic nerve endings. It is given mainly by local application to the eye to produce dilatation of the pupil. Its effects subside more quickly than those of atropine and are usually over in 24 hours. Partial paralysis of accommodation is also produced but it is seldom complete.

Homatropine Methyl Bromide U.S.P. *Homatropinae Methylbromidum*

DOSE: 2.5 mg. (1/25 gr.). $C_{17}H_{24}BrNO_3$. Mol.wt. 370.29. M.p. 190-198°. S: vs. W; fs. A; almost ins. E, acetone. A white odourless powder; taste bitter; darkens on exposure to light.

Homatropine Methyl Bromide Tablets U.S.P.

Size, 2.5 mg. (1/25 gr.).

₡ Homatropine Methyl Bromide is advocated as a substitute for atropine for the treatment of gastro-intestinal spasm and hyperchlorhydria.

Purified Honey B.P. *Mel Depuratum*

Honey melted, strained, and adjusted to a density of 1.355 Gm./cc. A thick syrupy, translucent, pale-yellow or yellowish-brown liquid, having a characteristic odour and a sweet characteristic taste. See Oxymel.

Diluted Hydriodic Acid U.S.P. *Acidum Hydriodicum Dilutum*

Sp.gr. 1.1. A colourless or pale-yellow liquid; odourless; contains 9.5-10.5 Gm. of HI in 100 cc.

Hydriodic Acid Syrup U.S.P. *Syrupus Acidi Hydriodici*

DOSE: 4 cc. (1fl.dr.). Diluted Hydriodic Acid 14, Sucrose 45, Distilled Water to make 100 cc.

₡ The syrup of hydriodic acid is used chiefly as an expectorant, and also as a palatable way of giving iodides internally.

Hydrochloric Acid. *Acidum Hydrochloricum.* (Muriatic Acid)

HCl. Mol.wt. 36.47. Sp.gr. about 1.18. A colourless, fuming liquid; odour pungent; contains between 35 and 38% HCl. When distilled it gives a constant boiling point mixture (110°) containing approximately 20% w/w HCl.

Dilute Hydrochloric Acid B.P. Diluted Hydrochloric Acid U.S.P.
Acidum Hydrochloricum Dilutum
DOSES: B.P. 0.6-8 cc. (10-120 min.); U.S.P. 4 cc. (1 fl.dr.).
Gm./cc. 1.042-1.049. Sp.gr. 1.05. A colourless, odourless liquid;
taste sharply acid. Contains 9.5-10.5 Gm. HCl in 100 cc.

℃ Taken well diluted (4 cc. in 150 cc.) and suitably flavoured,
Dilute Hydrochloric Acid may be used to produce systemic acidosis
for such purposes as the treatment of lead poisoning. It may also
be used to relieve gastro-intestinal symptoms associated with
achlorhydria. In dentistry it may be applied locally to remove
spicules of bone from tooth sockets.

Hydnocarpus Oil B.P. *Oleum Hydnocarpi*
DOSES: oral, 0.3-1 cc. (5-15 min.) gradually increasing to 4 cc.
(60 min.). Gm./cc. 0.946-0.956. S: almost completely sol. in hot
A 90%; less sol. in cold A 90%; misc. E, C, and carbon disulphide.
The fatty oil obtained by cold expression from the fresh ripe seeds
of *Hydnocarpus Wightiana*; a yellowish or brownish-yellow oil or
soft, creamy fat; odour slight and characteristic; taste somewhat
acrid.

Injection of Hydnocarpus Oil B.P.
DOSES: subcutaneous or intramuscular, 2 cc., increasing gradually
to 5 cc. (30-75 min.). Unmodified oil sterilized by heating.

℃ In the U.S.P. XII the name Chaulmoogra Oil was applied to
oil from three species of plants, including that from which the
Hydnocarpus Oil B.P. is derived. These oils have been used since
1900 for the treatment of leprosy. The nature of their beneficial
action is not well understood but is presumably due to some
bacteriostatic effect on the infecting organism. Some irritation is
commonly observed at the site of injection of the oil and also signs
of systemic toxicity, including headache, abdominal pain, and
albuminuria.

Ethyl Esters of Hydnocarpus Oil B.P. *Oleum Hydnocarpi Aethyli-
cum*
DOSES: see Hydnocarpus Oil. Consists mainly of the ethyl esters
of chaulmoogric and hydnocarpic acids; colourless or faintly yellow
limpid oil; odour characteristic; taste acrid. S: 6 A 90%; misc. E,
C, CS₂. Gm./cc. 0.900-0.905.

Injection of Ethyl Esters of Hydnocarpus Oil B.P.

DOSES: subcutaneous or intramuscular, 2 cc., increasing gradually to 5 cc. (30-75 min.). Unmodified liquid esters, sterilized by heating.

℀ The ethyl esters of hydnocarpus oil are said to be less irritating than the oil and as they are less viscous, they are more easily injected.

Hydrogen Peroxide Solution U.S.P.   Solution of Hydrogen Peroxide

B.P. *Liquor Hydrogenii Peroxidi.* (Hydrogen Dioxide Solution) Sp.gr. about 1.01. A colourless liquid having no odour or an odour resembling that of ozone; slightly acid; contains about 2.5-3.5% w/v of H_2O_2 (U.S.P.) or 5.0-7.0% w/v (B.P.).

℀ Hydrogen peroxide is an oxidizing antiseptic agent. Its action is brief and unreliable as a germicide.

Hyoscine Hydrobromide B.P.   *Hyoscinae Hydrobromidum.*

Scopolamine Hydrobromide U.S.P. *Scopolaminae Hydrobromidum*

DOSES: B.P. 0.3-0.6 mg. ($\frac{1}{200}$-$\frac{1}{100}$ gr.); U.S.P. 0.6 mg. ($\frac{1}{100}$ gr.). $C_{17}H_{21}NO_4 \cdot HBr \cdot 3H_2O$. Mol.wt. 438.3. M.p. of anhydrous salt 194-197°. S: 1.5 W, 20 A; ss. C; ins. E. Colourless or white crystals or a white granular powder; odourless; taste bitter; efflorescent in dry air. The hydrobromide of the laevo-rotatory alkaloid, 1-hyoscine, obtained from various plants of the family *Solanaceae.*

Injection of Hyoscine Hydrobromide B.P.

DOSES: subcutaneous, 0.3-0.6 mg. ($\frac{1}{200}$-$\frac{1}{100}$ gr.). Strength, 0.4 mg. per cc. ($\frac{1}{160}$ gr. in 15 min.).

℀ Hyoscine hydrobromide has many of the actions of atropine. It may block, depending on concentration, the action of acetylcholine liberated at the endings of cholinergic autonomic nerves. In a therapeutic dose by mouth the effects are hardly distinguishable from those of atropine. The same dose injected hypodermically produces drowsiness and some stupor. Larger doses may cause delirium. A 0.5% solution dropped in the eye produces dilatation of the pupil and paralysis of accommodation about as well as a 1% solution of atropine sulphate, but the effects do not last so long.

Hyoscine hydrobromide is frequently given by injection with morphine as a pre-operative sedative, or to produce obstetrical analgesia. The hyoscine often produces complete amnesia regarding the labour, but may induce delirium and excitement which is hard to control.

Therapeutic doses of hyoscine by mouth are often helpful in preventing seasickness, airsickness, and carsickness. Taken this way undesirable side effects are negligible except for some dryness of the mouth. Somewhat larger doses by mouth are used to treat post-encephalitic Parkinsonism.

Hyoscine Hydrobromide Ointment for the Eye B.P. *Oculentum Hyoscinae*
Contains 0.125% hyoscine hydrobromide.

Scopolamine Hydrobromide Tablets U.S.P.
Sizes 0.3 and 0.6 mg. (1/200 and 1/100 gr.).

Hyoscyamus B.P. *Hyoscyamus.* (Hyoscyamus Leaves, Henbane)
The dried leaves, with or without the tops of *Hyoscyamus niger*; contains not less than 0.05% (B.P.) or 0.04% (N.F.) of the alkaloids calculated as hyoscyamine.

Powdered Hyoscyamus B.P. *Hyoscyami Pulvis*
Green or grayish-green powder; odour strong and characteristic; taste bitter and somewhat acrid.

Dry Extract of Hyoscyamus B.P. *Extractum Hyoscyami Siccum*
DOSES: 16-60 mg. ($\frac{1}{4}$-1 gr.). Dry Extract of Hyoscyamus contains 0.27-0.33% of the alkaloids of hyoscyamus calculated as hyoscyamine; 60 mg. (1 gr.) of Dry Extract of Hyoscyamus contain 0.18 mg. ($\frac{1}{350}$ gr.) of alkaloids calculated as hyoscyamine.

Liquid Extract of Hyoscyamus B.P. *Extractum Hyoscyami Liquidum*
DOSES: 0.2-0.4 cc. (3-6 min.). An alcoholic extract standardized to contain 0.045-0.055% of alkaloids; contains 50-60% v/v of C_2H_5OH; 0.4 cc. contains 0.2 mg. of alkaloid calculated as hyoscyamine (6 min., $\frac{1}{320}$ gr.).

Tincture of Hyoscyamus B.P. *Tinctura Hyoscyami*
DOSES: B.P. 2-4 cc. (30-60 min.). Alkaloidal content calculated as hyoscyamine; 4.5-5.5 mg. per 100 cc. Alcoholic content, 66-71% v/v C_2H_5OH.

℄ The galenical preparations of hyoscyamus contain l-hyoscyamine and some atropine and hyoscine. Atropine is racemic (dl) hyoscyamine. The actions are consequently those of atropine (q.v.). The tincture and liquid extract are often used in diuretic mixtures to decrease bladder spasm in cystitis. They may also be used to treat Parkinson's syndrome.

Hypophosphorous Acid U.S.P.   *Acidum Hypophosphorosum*
HPH_2O_2. Mol.wt. 66.0. Sp.gr. 1.13. A colourless or slightly yellow odourless liquid. Contains 30-32% HPH_2O_2.

Dilute Hypophosphorous Acid B.P.   *Acidum Hypophosphorosum Dilutum*
DOSES: 0.3-1 cc. (5-15 min.). A clear, colourless liquid; odourless; taste strongly acid; contains 9.8-10.2% w/w H_3PO_2. Gm./cc. 1.037-1.039.

℃ Hypophosphorous acid is used as a reducing agent in Syrup of Ferrous Chloride C.F. and other preparations of ferrous iron, to keep the iron in the ferrous form.

Ichthammol B.P.   *Ichthammol.*   (Ammonium Ichthosulphonate, T.N. Ichthyol)
S: sol. in W; partly sol. in A 90% and in E; misc. with glycerin and with fixed oils. Soluble ammonium salts prepared from sulphonated, sulphur containing distillate of a bituminous schist which contains the fossil remains of fish; black and viscid; odour strong and characteristic.

℃ Ichthammol contains a number of organic sulphonates which have considerable antiseptic potency. Applied undiluted to the skin, ichthammol is rubefacient and irritant. About 5% in an ointment allays itching and is said to stimulate the skin. It is used mostly in chronic skin diseases.

Injection of Insulin B.P.   Insulin Injection U.S.P.   *Injectio Insulini.* (Insulin)
A clear, colourless or almost colourless sterile liquid, free from turbidity and from insoluble matter. Insulin Injection is supplied in Canada in strengths of 40, 80, or 100 insulin units per cc. The B.P. specifies that a strength of 20 units per cc. is to be supplied unless another strength is stated. Insulin is usually given by subcutaneous injection but in diabetic coma a part of the total dose may be given intravenously.

❡ Insulin is a protein and destroyed when taken by mouth. After injection it lowers the blood sugar by decreasing the production of glucose by the liver and increasing the storage and utilization of sugar by the tissues. Overdosage results in hypoglycaemia with faintness, sweating, incoordination, coma, convulsions, and death, if treatment is not given. In the early stages treatment is simple and consists of giving sugar by mouth. In later stages glucose may have to be given intravenously, with or without epinephrine, which mobilizes sugar from the liver.

Unmodified insulin is available as solutions of amorphous (regular) and zinc crystalline insulin. The latter may be preferred for patients who show signs of sensitivity to foreign protein in the amorphous insulin.

Modified insulins are those treated to give a prolonged action. The longest acting is protamine zinc insulin which may take 12-24 hours to exert its peak effect. Globin and histone insulins have actions of intermediate duration.

Insulin may be used for shock therapy of psychiatric patients, or in small doses to stimulate appetite and improve nutrition.

Globin Zinc Insulin Injection U.S.P. *Injectio Zinco Insulini Globini*

DOSE: By subcutaneous injection as prescribed. Strength, 40 or 80 units per cc. A sterile preparation in a hydrochloric acid medium containing insulin modified by the addition of Zinc Chloride and Globin (derived from the haemoglobin of beef blood). *Not to be injected intravenously.*

❡ Globin insulin exerts its peak effect 8-16 hours after administration. A dose given early in the morning is not likely to cause hypoglycaemia during the following night. It may be sufficient to supply the patient's insulin requirement for 24 hours.

Injection of Protamine Zinc Insulin B.P. *Injectio Insulini Protaminati cum Zinco.* **Protamine Zinc Insulin Injection U.S.P.** *Injectio Zinco-Insulini Protaminati.* (Protamine Zinc Insulin)

DOSES: by injection, as prescribed. Strengths, 40 or 80 units per cc. An almost colourless, turbid liquid. *Shake well before use.* The unit is the same as that of unmodified insulin. The zinc and protamine are added after the assay, together with some suitable preservative and buffers. *Not to be injected intravenously.*

N.P.H. Insulin N.

A suspension of *micro-crystals* of protamine with zinc insulin having a shorter duration of action than suspensions of amorphous Protamine Zinc Insulin. Available in vials of 10 cc. containing 40 or 80 units per cc.

Iodine. *Iodum*

I. At.wt. 126.92.   S: 2950 W, 13 A, 80 G, 4 CS_2; fs. E, CCl_4, C and aqueous solutions of iodides. Heavy bluish-black or grayish-black plates with a metallic lustre; odour characteristic. Sublimes at room temperatures, forming a purple vapour.

⟨ Iodine is required by the body for the manufacture of thyroid hormone. After administration a large amount of the circulating iodide is collected in the thyroid gland. The solutions of iodine are used largely as external antiseptics but Lugol's Solution is frequently given for temporary alleviation of the symptoms of hyperthyroidism.

As an antiseptic for preparing healthy skin for operation, Iodine has not been surpassed in spite of certain disadvantages. The main disadvantage is the tendency for free I and HI to blister sensitive skin. This can be avoided usually by care in its application, the use of milder solutions, and removal of most of the stain in a few minutes by swabbing with alcohol. A few people react to application of iodine by fever and general rash.

In wounds, solution of iodine, if used freely and early, will rapidly kill most pathogens, including spores, and if further infection is excluded, rapid healing occurs. For treating established infections in wounds or tissues, iodine is not so satisfactory because it combines with tissue proteins and is inactivated.

The Weak Solution of Iodine B.P. or Mild Tincture of Iodine U.S.P. are most suitable for general external use.

About 3 Gm. of iodine is usually fatal. The antidotes for iodine poisoning are starch, boiled flour, and 5% sodium thiosulphate (photographic hypo). In dentistry iodine is employed as a local antiseptic and as a disclosing stain in order to reveal carbohydrate plaques.

Aqueous Solution of Iodine B.P. *Liquor Iodi Aquosus.* **Strong Iodine Solution U.S.P.** *Liquor Iodi Fortis.* (Lugol's Solution, Compound Iodine Solution)

DOSES: B.P. 0.3-1 cc. (5-15 min.); U.S.P. 0.3 cc. (5 min.). Iodine 5, Potassium Iodide 10, Distilled Water to 100. An aqueous solution containing about 5% of Iodine. The aqueous solution contains in 1 cc. about 50 mg. of free iodine and about 130 mg. of total iodine (15 min. about $\frac{4}{5}$ gr. of iodine and about 2 gr. of total iodine free and combined).

Strong Solution of Iodine B.P. *Liquor Iodi Fortis.* (Strong Tincture of Iodine)
9.8-10.2% of iodine in 76-79% v/v of C_2H_5OH with Potassium Iodide, 5.8-6.2%.

Weak Solution of Iodine B.P. *Liquor Iodi Mitis.* (Weak Tincture of Iodine, Tincture of Iodine)
DOSES: 0.3-2 cc. (5-30 min.).
A solution of iodine containing about 2.5% of iodine and 85-88% v/v of C_2H_5OH with potassium iodide 2.5%. Two cc. contain about 50 mg. of free iodine and 88 mg. of total iodine (30 min. about $\frac{4}{5}$ gr. of iodine and $1\frac{1}{3}$ gr. of total iodine).

Iodine Tincture U.S.P. *Tinctura Iodi.* Mild Tincture of Iodine
Iodine 2, Sodium Iodide 2.4, Diluted Alcohol to make 100. Contains 44-50% v/v of C_2H_5OH.

Iodized Oil. *Oleum Iodisatum B.P. Oleum Iodatum U.S.P.*
S: ins. W; sol. C, E; 1 cc. in 10 cc. petroleum benzin gives a clear solution. Gm./cc. 1.34-1.37. An iodine addition product of poppy-seed oil containing 39-41% of organically combined iodine (B.P.). The U.S.P. allows the use of other vegetable oils iodinated to the extent of 38-42%. A colourless or pale-yellow, clear, viscous, oily liquid having an odour of garlic; taste bland and oily.

℀ Iodized oil is used for diagnostic purposes to produce opacity to x-rays in the lungs and thus show up the dilatations characteristic of bronchiectasis.

Iodoalphionic Acid U.S.P. *Acidum Iodoalphionicum.* (Pheniodol, T.N. Priodax)
DOSE: 3 Gm. (45 gr.). $C_{15}H_{12}I_2O_3$. Mol.wt. 494.09. M.p. 160-164°. S: ins. W; sol. A, E; ss. B, C. White crystals or a white to faintly yellow powder; taste and odour faint and characteristic.

Iodoalphionic Acid Tablets U.S.P.

Size, 0.5 gm. (7½ gr.).

℃ Iodoalphionic Acid is given orally for radiographic examination of the gall bladder. The average dose is taken late in the afternoon with several glasses of water and nothing is eaten until after the radiological examination on the following morning.

Iodochlorhydroxyquin U.S.P. *Iodochlorhydroxyquinum*

(Iodochlorohydroxyquinoline.   T.N. Vioform)

Daily DOSE: 0.75 Gm. (12 gr.). $C_9H_5ClI.N.O.$ Mol.wt. 305.52. M.p. about 172° with decomposition. S: ins. W, A; sol. hot ethyl acetate and hot glacial acetic acid. A voluminous spongy brownish yellow powder; taste slight and characteristic; affected by light. Available in tablets for the prevention or treatment of amoebic or bacillary dysentery, and in ointments (2-3%) for infections of the skin.

Compound Iodochlorhydroxyquin Powder U.S.P. *Pulvis Iodochlor-hydroxyquini Compositus*

Iodochlorhydroxyquin 250, Boric Acid 100, Lactic Acid 25, Zinc Stearate 200, Lactose to make 1000 Gm.; for vaginal insufflation, for the treatment of trichomonas vaginitis.

Iodoform B.P. *Iodoformum*

CHI_3. Mol.wt. 393.8. M.p. 120-122°. S: at 15.5°, 100 A 90%, 8 E, 10 C, 3 CS_2; sol. volatile oils and fixed oils; vss. W. Lemon-yellow crystals having a characteristic, strong, persistent disagreeable odour and taste.

Suppositories of Iodoform B.P. *Suppositoria Iodoformi*

In each—0.2 Gm. (3 gr.) in a suitable base.

℃ Iodoform has been used as a dusting powder or on dressings for infected wounds. Iodine is liberated slowly, and probably exerts a prolonged antiseptic action in infected wounds. Poisoning has occurred from absorption of iodoform from closed cavities such as empyema cavities. Symptoms may be due to the iodine or to iodoform itself, which may act like chloroform to produce stupor. Some patients show sensitivity to iodoform, manifested as skin rashes.

In dentistry it is employed to some extent in the form of iodoform gauze (containing 5 or 10% w/w of CHI_3), for packing infected sockets, or cystic cavities. Some root canal fillings contain it as an ingredient but its use is limited.

Iodophthalein B.P. *Iodophthaleinum.* **Iodophthalein Sodium U.S.P.** *Iodophthaleinum Sodicum.* (Tetraiodophthalein Sodium Tetiothalein Sodium, Soluble Iodophthalein, Tetraiodophenol-phthalein Sodium)

DOSES: B.P. 40-60 mg. per kg. body weight, up to 5 Gm. ($\frac{1}{3}$-$\frac{1}{2}$ gr. per lb.); U.S.P; doses per 10 kg. body weight; oral, 0.5 Gm. ($7\frac{1}{2}$ gr.), intravenous 0.3 Gm. (5 gr.). $C_{20}H_8O_4I_4Na_2.3H_2O$. Mol.wt. 919.99. S: 7 W; ss. A. A pale blue-violet crystalline powder; odourless; taste saline and astringent.

⚓ Iodophthalein may be given intravenously or orally for diagnostic radiography of the gall bladder. The substance is excreted by the liver and concentrated in the gall bladder. It should not be given in serious heart disease or liver disease.

Iodopyracet Injection U.S.P. *Injectio Iodopyraceti* (T.N. Diodrast) $C_5H_2I_2ONCH_2COONH_2(CH_2CH_2OH)_2$. A clear and nearly colour-less sterile solution of the diethanolamine salt of 3, 5-diiodo-4-pyridone-N-acetic acid in a concentration of 34-36% w/v. The salt contains 61.5-63.5% of iodine. See Injection of Diodone B.P.

⚓ Iodopyracet injection is used for intravenous urography. An average dose is 20 cc. injected slowly. Stronger solutions of this material are available for particular purposes. See N.N.R. Liver disease and severe renal insufficiency are contra-indications for urography by excretion.

Iodoxyl B.P. *Iodoxylum.* **Sodium Iodomethamate U.S.P.** *Sodii Iodomethamas* (T.N. Neo-Iopax)

DOSES: intravenous, 10-15 Gm. (150-225 gr.) (B.P.) or 10 Gm. ($2\frac{1}{2}$ dr.) U.S.P. $C_8H_3NI_2O_5Na_2$. Mol.wt. 492.9. S: 1.2 W, 100 A 90% 15.5°; ins. E, C. A white odourless powder, the disodium salt of N-methyl-3:5-diiodo-4-pyridone-2:6-dicarboxylic acid.

Injection of Iodoxyl B.P.
Strength, 0.75 Gm. per cc. (12gr. in 15 min.).

Sodium Iodomethamate Injection U.S.P.
5 Gm. (75 gr.) in 10 cc.; 7.5 Gm. (2 dr.) in 10 cc.; 10 Gm. ($2\frac{1}{2}$ dr.) in 20 cc.; 15 Gm. (4 dr.) in 20 cc.; 15 Gm. (4 dr.) in 30 cc.

℃ Iodoxyl is a diagnostic agent used in radiographic examination of the kidneys and urinary tract. It may be used for intravenous urography or retrograde pyelography. Irritation and pain at site of injection sometimes occurs. The drug appears in the urinary tract 5-30 minutes after injection. Liver disease and severe renal insufficiency are contra-indications.

Ipecac U.S.P. Ipecacuanha B.P. *Ipecacuanha.* (Ipecacuanha Root)
The dried root of *Cephaelis Ipecacuanha* or of *Cephaelis acuminata*; odour slight; taste bitter.

Powdered Ipecacuanha B.P. *Ipecacuanhae Pulvis*
A light-grey to yellowish-brown powder.

℃ The actions of Ipecacuanha are due mostly to the alkaloids, emetine (q.v.) and cephaeline. They are very irritant to mucous membranes, and reflexly stimulate salivary secretion and bronchial secretion, and in larger doses produce nausea and vomiting. Sweating also occurs but the mechanism of its production is not clear.

The galenical preparations are used mostly as expectorants but occasionally as emetics. The Powder of Ipecac and Opium (Dover's Powder) is used for the symptomatic treatment of febrile coughs and colds.

Prepared Ipecacuanha B.P. *Ipecacuanha Praeparata*
Doses: expectorant, 30-120 mg. ($\frac{1}{2}$-2 gr.); emetic, 1-2 Gm. (15-30 gr.). Contains 1.9-2.1% of alkaloids calculated as emetine. A light-grey to yellow-brown powder; odour slight; taste bitter.

Ipecac Fluidextract U.S.P. *Fluidextractum Ipecacuanhae.* **Liquid Extract of Ipecacuanha B.P.** *Extractum Ipecacuanhae Liquidum*
Doses: B.P. expectorant, 0.03-0.12 cc. ($\frac{1}{2}$-2 min.); emetic, 0.6-2 cc. (10-30 min.); U.S.P. emetic, 0.5 cc. (8 min.). An alcoholic extract standardized to contain about 2% of alkaloids w/v calculated as emetine. Contains 63-69% v/v C_2H_5OH (B.P.) or 28-33% v/v C_2H_5OH (U.S.P.).

Powder of Ipecacuanha and Opium B.P. *Pulvis Ipecacuanhae et Opii.* (Compound Powder of Ipecacuanha, Dover's Powder)
Doses: 0.3-0.6 Gm. (5-10 gr.). Ipecacuanha 10 Gm., Opium 10 Gm., Lactose 80 Gm. Each 0.6 Gm. (10 gr.) contains 6 mg. ($\frac{1}{10}$ gr.) of anhydrous morphine.

℄ Dover's Powder, by virtue of its content of morphine, acts as a cough sedative by depressing the cough reflex. It also stimulates bronchial secretion by the reflex initiated by the irritating action of the ipecac on the mucosa of the stomach. Opium and ipecac, acting together by mechanisms not well understood, have an antipyretic effect by causing vasodilation and sweating. Large doses of Dover's Powder, e.g. about three times the ordinary dose, will sometimes cause vomiting.

Tablets of Acetylsalicylic Acid with Ipecacuanha and Opium B.P.
(Tablets of Aspirin and Dover's Powder)
DOSES: 1 or 2 tablets. Acetylsalicylic Acid and Powder of Ipecacuanha and Opium in equal parts. Size, 0.32 Gm. (5 gr.).

Tablets of Ipecacuanha and Opium B.P. (Tablets of Powder of Ipecacuanha and Opium, Tablets of Compound Powder of Ipecacuanha, Dover's Powder Tablets)
Size, 0.3 Gm. (5 gr.).

Lozenges of Morphine and Ipecacuanha B.P. *Trochisci Morphinae et Ipecacuanhae*
Each lozenge contains about 2 mg. ($\frac{1}{32}$ gr.) of Morphine Hydrochloride and about 6 mg. ($\frac{1}{10}$ gr.) of Prepared Ipecacuanha.

Ipecac Syrup U.S.P. *Syrupus Ipecacuanhae*
DOSE: emetic 8 cc. (2 fl.dr.). Fluidextract of Ipecac 7 cc., with Glycerin and Syrup to make 100 cc.

Tincture of Ipecacuanha B.P. *Tinctura Ipecacuanhae*
DOSES: expectorant 0.6-2 cc. (10-30 min.); emetic 15-30 cc. ($\frac{1}{2}$-1 fl.oz.). Liquid Extract of Ipecacuanha 5 cc., with Dilute Acetic Acid, Alcohol, Glycerin and Distilled Water to make 100 cc. Contains 20-24% v/v of C_2H_5OH; 2 cc. contain 2 mg. (30 min. $\frac{1}{30}$ gr.) of total alkaloids. This tincture replaces the Wine of Ipecacuanha B.P. 1914.

Ipomoea B.P. *Ipomoea.* (Orizaba Jalap Root, Mexican Scammony Root)
The dried root of *Ipomoea orizabensis* Ledanois.

Powdered Ipomoea B.P. *Ipomoeae Pulvis*
A light-grey to greyish-brown powder.

Ipomoea Resin B.P. *Ipomoea Resina.* (Scammony Resin)
¶ Doses: 30-200 mg. ($\frac{1}{2}$-3 gr.). S: ins. W; sol. A 90%. Brownish, translucent, brittle fragments; odour characteristic and agreeable; taste acrid.

¶ Ipomoea resin is a drastic purgative. It irritates the intestinal tract throughout its length and produces copious watery stools.

Iron B.P. *Ferrum*
Fe. Mol.wt. 55.85. Fine bright iron wire.

¶ Many preparations of iron are available and most are used for the treatment of hypochromic anaemia. The normal dietary requirement of absorbable iron is about 4-10 mg. Hypochromic anaemia may be caused by inadequate intake of iron, excessive loss of blood (acute or chronic) or failure to assimilate dietary iron for reasons which may not be clear. It is thought that iron is absorbed only in the form of simple ferrous salts in that portion of the intestine where the contents are acidic. It is agreed that soluble ferrous salts are effective in smaller doses than are ferric salts. For best results, however, the doses must be far greater than the normal daily requirement. The iron content of the recommended daily dose of Ferrous Chloride or Ferrous Sulphate is 100-200 mg., of Iron and Ammonium Citrate 800-1600 mg., and of Reduced Iron 1.2-4.8 Gm.

Preparations of iron for oral use are best given during or after meals, to minimize gastric irritation. Stools may become very black during iron therapy and either diarrhoea or constipation may develop. The preparations of iron are usually considered to be almost without toxicity but ferrous sulphate tablets or soluble salts swallowed on an empty stomach have caused gastric perforation in children.

Ferric Ammonium Citrate U.S.P. *Ferri Ammonii Citras.* **Iron and Ammonium Citrate B.P.** *Ferri et Ammonii Citras*
Doses: B.P. 1-3 Gm. (15-45 gr.); U.S.P. 1 Gm. (15 gr.). S: 0.5 W; ins. A. Thin, dark-red, transparent scales or granules; deliquescent; taste slightly sweetish and astringent. Contains 16.5-18.5% Fe (U.S.P.) or 20.5-22.5% Fe (B.P.).

¶ Iron and Ammonium Citrate is relatively non-irritating and particularly suitable for prescribing in flavoured mixtures. It is often tolerated when other salts are not and its efficiency is well established. Large doses are necessary because the unionized salt must be split, presumably by the action of HCl in the stomach, and part of the iron must be reduced to the ferrous form before absorption can occur.

Ferric Ammonium Citrate Capsules U.S.P.

Size, 0.5 Gm. (7½ gr.).

Exsiccated Ferrous Sulphate. *Ferri Sulphas Exsiccatus*

DOSES: B.P. 60-200 mg. (1-3 gr.); U.S.P. 0.2 Gm. (3 gr.). S: dissolves slowly in W; ins. in A. A greyish-white powder; contains not less than 77% (B.P.) or 80% (U.S.P.) of FeSO₄. 0.2 Gm. contains about 60 mg. of Fe (3 gr., 1 gr. of Fe).

☾ The exsiccated sulphate is used only for making pills.

Ferrous Sulphate. *Ferri Sulphas*

DOSES: B.P. 0.2-0.3 Gm. (3-5 gr.); U.S.P. 0.3 Gm. (5 gr.). FeSO₄.7H₂O. Mol.wt. 278.02. S: 1.5 W; 0.5 W 100°; ins. A. Pale-green crystals with an astringent taste; 300 mg. contain about 60 mg. (or 5 gr., 1 gr.) of Iron.

Ferrous Sulfate Syrup U.S.P. *Syrupus Ferri Sulfatis*

DOSE: 8 cc. (2 fl. dr.). Ferrous Sulfate 40, Citric Acid 2.1, Peppermint Spirit 2, Sucrose 825, Water to make 1000 cc. Each 8 cc. dose contains 0.32 gm. (5 gr.) of ferrous sulfate.

Ferrous Sulfate Tablets U.S.P.

Size, 0.3 Gm. (5 gr.).

☾ Tablets of Ferrous Sulphate are a popular way of giving iron. They may be too irritating for some persons. Children swallowing a number of these tablets have developed gastric perforation. Ferrous sulphate is sometimes marketed as an enteric coated tablet; this coating may prevent the absorption of iron in the acidic portion of the intestine.

Saccharated Iron Carbonate B.P. *Ferri Carbonas Saccharatus*

DOSES: 0.6-2 Gm. (10-30 gr.). S: partly soluble in W. Ferrous Sulphate with Liquid Glucose, Sodium Carbonate, and Distilled Water q.s., dried to a powder. Two Gm. contain about 0.5 Gm. of Iron (or 30 gr. about 7½ gr.). An olive-brown powder with a slightly metallic taste.

℃ Saccharated Iron Carbonate may be administered in capsules, pills, or tablets, and is a satisfactory source of ferrous iron.

Pill of Iron Carbonate B.P. *Pilula Ferri Carbonatis.* (Blaud's Pill, Iron Pill, Blaud's Mass).

DOSES: 0.3-2 Gm. (5-30 gr.). Exsiccated Ferrous Sulphate 34%, Exsiccated Sodium Carbonate 21.6%, with Tragacanth, Acacia, Liquid Glucose, and Distilled Water. 2 Gm. contain about 0.2 Gm. (30 gr. contain 3 gr.) of iron.

℃ The usual recommended daily dose of Blaud's Pill is 3-4 Gm. (45-60 gr.); this contains about 0.3-0.4 Gm. (4½-6 gr.) of iron.

Solution of Ferric Chloride B.P. *Liquor Ferri Perchloridi*
DOSES: 0.3-1 cc. (5-15 min.). A very astringent aqueous solution containing 14.25-15.75 w/v of ferric chloride. One cc. contains about 50 mg. of iron. A strongly acid solution.

℃ The Solution of Ferric Chloride is seldom given internally but is more commonly applied locally to stop bleeding, e.g. after tonsillectomy. It is also used to prepare styptic gauze and styptic cotton.

Compound Syrup of Ferrous Phosphate B.P. *Syrupus Ferri Phosphatis Compositus.* (Parrish's Food, Parrish's Syrup, Chemical Food)
DOSES: 2-8 cc. (30-120 min.). A syrup containing ferrous phosphate and tricalcium phosphate, flavoured with orange and coloured with cochineal; 8 cc. contain about 34 mg. (½ gr.) of iron, and about 110 mg. (1¾ gr.) of tricalcium phosphate.

℃ Large doses of this preparation must be given if adequate iron therapy is to be achieved.

Heavy Kaolin B.P. *Kaolinum Ponderosum*
S: ins. W and in mineral acids. Native aluminium silicate powdered and freed from gritty particles by elutriation; odourless and tasteless. A soft, whitish powder which can be distinguished from light kaolin by the fact that it settles quite rapidly from aqueous suspensions.

Light Kaolin B.P. *Kaolinum Leve*
DOSES: 15-60 Gm. (½-2 oz.). S: ins. W, and in mineral acids.

Purified native aluminium silicate free from gritty particles. A light, white powder; odourless and tasteless.

℃ Kaolin has a number of medicinal uses both internal and external and some pharmaceutical uses. It is given by mouth to check diarrhoea by adsorbing irritants. It has also been given for peptic ulcer as a protective agent which coats the ulcer, and also for its rather feeble antacid effect (aluminium silicate + HCl →aluminium chloride + silicic acid). It is used externally in dusting powders and poultices (see Poultice of Kaolin). Pharmaceutically it is used to filter liquids and as an excipient in pills containing drugs which might react with organic excipients. Light kaolin is intended for internal use and in dusting powders and will be supplied on prescription, unless heavy kaolin is specified. Heavy kaolin is for poultices.

Poultice of Kaolin B.P. *Cataplasma Kaolini.* (T.N. Antiphlogistine)

A pasty mass containing Heavy Kaolin, Boric Acid, Methyl Salicylate, Oil of Peppermint, Thymol, and Glycerin.

℃ A rubefacient poultice.

Krameria B.P. *Krameria.* (Krameria Root, Rhatany Root)
DOSES: 0.6-2 Gm. (10-30 gr.). The dried root of *Krameria triandra*; taste bitter and astringent; odourless.

Powdered Krameria B.P. *Krameriae Pulvis*
A reddish-brown powder.

Dry Extract of Krameria B.P. *Extractum Krameriae Siccum*
DOSES: 0.3-1 Gm. (5-15 gr.). A dried aqueous extract.

Lozenges of Krameria B.P. *Trochisci Krameriae.* (Krameria Lozenge)
Each lozenge contains 60 mg. (1 gr.) of dry extract of krameria.

℃ Preparations of krameria are rich in tannins and consequently are astringent. The Dry Extract of Krameria may be used with or without opium in suppositories for the treatment of haemorrhoids. The lozenges are used to some extent for sore throats. Those with cocaine are presumably more effective in giving symptomatic relief by virtue of the local anaesthetic action of the cocaine.

Lozenges of Krameria and Cocaine B.P.   *Trochisci Krameriae et Cocainae.*   (Krameria and Cocaine Lozenges)

Each lozenge contains 60 mg. (1 gr.) of the dry Extract of Krameria and 3 mg. (1/20 gr.) of Cocaine Hydrochloride.

LOCAL ANAESTHETICS

Amethocaine Hydrochloride B.P.   *Amethocainae Hydrochloridum.*
Tetracaine Hydrochloride U.S.P.   *Tetracainae Hydrochloridum.*
(Pontocaine Hydrochloride N.N.R.)

$C_{15}H_{24}N_2O_2.HCl$.   Mol.wt. 300.82.   M.p. 147-150°.   S: vs. W; sol. A; ins, E, B.   A white crystalline powder; odourless; taste slightly bitter, followed by a sensation of numbness.

Injection of Amethocaine Hydrochloride B.P.

Provided as a solid drug in sealed containers to be dissolved in the required amount of Injection of Sodium Chloride.

⟪ Tetracaine (Pontocaine) is more potent and more toxic than cocaine.   It is effective as a surface anaesthetic.   A 0.5% solution may be used for corneal anaesthesia.   It is particularly useful for prolonged spinal anaesthesia.

Benzamine Hydrochloride B.P.C.   *Benzaminae Hydrochloridum.*
(Beta-Eucaine Hydrochloride, Eucaine Hydrochloride)

$C_{15}H_{21}O_2N.HCl$ Mol.wt. 283.79.   S: 30 W, 35 A, 30 C.   A white crystalline powder; odourless; taste slightly bitter followed by numbness when placed on the tongue.

⟪ In 2% solution Benzamine Hydrochloride is about as effective as a 1% solution of Cocaine Hydrochloride on the cornea.   It does not cause local vasoconstriction like cocaine.   By intravenous injection it is about as toxic as cocaine but is much less toxic by subcutaneous injection because it is destroyed fairly rapidly in the body.   It is included in the schedule of narcotic drugs in Canada.   Its use is declining.

Benzocaine B.P.   *Benzocaina.*   **Ethyl Aminobenzoate U.S.P.**
Aethylis Aminobenzoas.

$NH_2.C_6H_4.CO.OC_2H_5$.   Mol.wt. 165.2.   S: 2500 W, 5 A, 2 C, 4 E, 30-50 almond oil or olive oil.   Small white crystals or a white crystalline powder; odourless; taste slightly bitter followed by a sensation of numbness.

⟨ Benzocaine is almost insoluble in water and hence not used for injection. It may be applied in an ointment to relieve pruritus. In glycerin or propylene glycol it will penetrate mucous membranes to some extent and has been tried for topical anaesthesia around the gums.

Five to 10% of Benzocaine in dusting powders may be applied to ulcers, burns, or fissures to relieve discomfort.

Butethamine Hydrochloride N.N.R. (T.N. Monocaine Hydrochloride)

$C_{13}H_{20}N_2O_2HCl$. Mol.wt. 272.78. 2-Isobutylamino-ethyl-p-aminobenzoate hydrochloride. M.p. 192-196°. S: sps. W; ss. A, C. A 1% aqueous solution has a pH of about 4.7. A white, odourless, crystalline powder with a bitter taste.

⟨ Butethamine hydrochloride is a local anaesthetic with actions very similar to those of procaine hydrochloride. It is frequently used for nerve blocks in dentistry in a concentration of 1% with epinephrine 1:75,000. This strength is considered to be equivalent in potency and toxicity to a 1.3% solution of procaine hydrochloride. Preparations of *monocaine formate* are available and are suggested for spinal anaesthesia. Persons with allergic sensitivity to procaine will probably be sensitive also to monocaine.

Butacaine Sulphate. *Butacainae Sulphas.* (T.N. Butyn. γ-di-n-butyl-aminopropyl-paraminobenzoate)

$(C_{18}H_{30}O_2N_2)_2H_2SO_4$. Mol.wt. 710.95. M.p. 100-103°. S: less than 1 W, less than 1 A and 1 acetone; ss. C; ins. E. White crystalline powder; odourless; taste slightly bitter followed by numbness when placed upon the tongue.

⟨ Butacaine Sulphate is a local anaesthetic related chemically to Procaine but with a potency for surface anaesthesia resembling Cocaine. A 2% solution may be used in the eye and 2-5% solution in the nose and throat. It has no local vasoconstrictor action and does not dilate the pupil. Its intravenous toxicity roughly equals that of Cocaine. It is not recommended for injection anaesthesia. Solutions may be sterilized by boiling.

While not recommended for routine use in dentistry, Butacaine in solutions of 0.5-0.75% mixed with epinephrine may be employed for single extractions, using 1.5-2 cc. of a 0.75% solution. For multiple extractions at one sitting, not more than 8 cc. of a 0.75% solution should be injected. Stronger solutions may be used for topical application.

Butyl Aminobenzoate B.P. *Butylis Aminobenzoas.* (T.N. Butesin)
$NH_2.C_6H_4.CO.OC_4H_9$. Mol.wt. 193.24. M.p. 57-59°. S: 7000 W; sol. dilute acids, A, C, E, and in fatty oils. Slowly hydrolyzes when boiled with water.

⟪ Butyl Aminobenzoate is an ingredient of an ointment commonly used to treat small burns, Butesin Picrate Ointment.

Cinchocaine Hydrochloride B.P. *Cinchocainae Hydrochloridum.*
(Dibucaine Hydrochloride N.N.R., T.N. Nupercaine)
$C_{20}H_{29}O_2N_3.HCl$. Mol.wt. 379.9. S: at 15.5° 0.5 W; fs. A; sol. acetone and chloroform. Fine, white, hygroscopic, odourless crystals.

⟪ Cinchocaine Hydrochloride is a local anaesthetic with about five times the toxicity of Cocaine but it is at least 10 times as potent. A solution of 0.1% may be used on the cornea and for urethral instillations. An ointment containing 1% may be used for anal fissure or pruritus ani, or for sunburn. Solutions may be sterilized by autoclaving or boiling in hard glass containers. *Because of its great potency every precaution must be taken not to use this drug by mistake in the concentrations usual for Procaine. Many deaths have occurred from such errors.*

Cocaine. *Cocaina*
$C_{17}H_{21}O_4N$. Mol.wt. 303.35. M.p. 96-98°. S: 600 W, 7 A, 1 C, 3.5 E, 12 olive oil, 80-100 liquid petrolatum. An alkaloid obtained from *Erythroxylon Coca* or other species of *Erythroxylon*, or by synthesis from ecgonine. Colourless crystals; odourless; taste bitter, followed by a sensation of tingling and numbness.

Cocaine Hydrochloride. *Cocainae Hydrochloridum.* (*Cocaini Hydrochloridum I.A.*)

DOSES: B.P. 8-16 mg. ($\frac{1}{8}$-$\frac{1}{4}$ gr.). $C_{17}H_{21}O_4N.HCl$. Mol.wt. 339.81. M.p. not below 197°. S: 0.5 W, 3.5 A, 15 C; sol. G; ins. E and olive oil. Colourless transparent crystals; odourless; taste bitter with tingling and numbness.

Lamellae of Cocaine B.P. *Lamellae Cocainae*
Gelatin discs containing about 1.3 mg. (1/50 gr.) Cocaine Hydrochloride, for insertion in the eye.

Cocaine Ointment for the Eye B.P. *Oculentum Cocainae*
An ointment containing 0.25% of Cocaine Hydrochloride.

Cocaine Suppositories B.P. *Suppositoria Cocainae*
Cocaine Hydrochloride, 15 mg. ($\frac{1}{4}$ gr.) in each in a suitable base.

℄ Cocaine is particularly useful for its property of anaesthetizing intact mucous membranes. It was the first local anaesthetic to be used in medicine and its advantages and limitations are so well known that most others are described by reference to it. Cocaine was once an important drug of addiction and is still used by the underworld to lure novices into addiction. Its immediate effects of exhilaration are much more attractive to the beginner than the effects of the opiates. By decreasing the sensations of fatigue, it may give the individual a sensation of elation and physical vigour. Cocaine and all its derivatives are on the narcotic schedule. It is more likely than other drugs to produce in women hallucinations of a sexual nature.

A few people are very sensitive to Cocaine so that one or two drops of 1% solution in the eye, or injected subcutaneously, will cause fainting. A fatal dose to humans is considered to be about 1.2 Gm. but death has occurred from 20 mg. Cocaine is destroyed relatively slowly in the body. Half of it may be excreted unchanged in the urine.

Solutions of Cocaine Hydrochloride are used for surface anaesthesia, 2% solutions for superficial anaesthesia of the cornea, 4% solutions for operations. Constriction of blood vessels occurs, and dilatation of the pupil. Cocaine increases the sensitivity of some effector cells to circulating epinephrine. Solutions of cocaine hydrochloride may be sterilized by boiling for not more than 5 minutes.

Orthocaine B.P. *Orthocaina.* (T.N. Orthoform)
$OH.C_6H_3(NH_2)CO_2CH_3$. Mol.wt. 167.1. M.p. 141-143°. S: sps. W, 7 A 90%; sol. in solutions of sodium hydroxide. A white or faintly yellow crystalline powder; odourless; tasteless.

℄ Orthocaine is a local anaesthetic, but being almost insoluble it can be used only as a dusting powder or in ointments (10%). No great claims are made for its efficacy.

Piperocaine Hydrochloride U.S.P. *Piperocainae Hydrochloridum.*
(T.N. Metycaine)
$C_{16}H_{23}NO_2.HCl$. Mol.wt. 297.82. M.p. 172-175°. S: 1.5 W,
4.5 A; fs. C; almost ins. E and fixed oils. Small white crystals or
a crystalline powder; odourless; taste slightly bitter, followed by a
sensation of numbness.

Piperocaine Hydrochloride Injection U.S.P.
Sizes, 200 cc., 1.5% solution; 30 cc., 2% solution; 5 cc., 20%
solution.
Piperocaine has much the same uses as procaine, and in addition
may be used for topical effects, e.g. in the eye.

Procaine Hydrochloride. *Procainae Hydrochloridum.* (Ethocaine
Hydrochloride. T.N. Novocaine Hydrochloride)
$H_2N.C_6H_4CO_2C_2H_4N(C_2H_5)_2HCl$. Mol.wt. 272.77. M.p. 153-
156°. S: 1 W, 30 A; ss. C; almost ins. E. Small white crystals or a
white crystalline powder; odourless; taste bitter, producing a
transient numbness of the tongue.

Sterile Solution of Procaine Hydrochloride 2% B.P.
Procaine Hydrochloride 5, Sodium Chloride 2, with Chlorocresol
and Water for Injection to make 250 cc. For use in preparing the
Weak Injection of Procaine and Adrenaline.

Strong Injection of Procaine and Adrenaline B.P.
Procaine Hydrochloride 2, Sodium Chloride 0.5, Solution of
Adrenaline Hydrochloride 2 cc., with Chlorocresol, Sodium Metabi-
sulphite, and Water for Injection to make 100 cc.

Weak Injection of Procaine and Adrenaline B.P.
To be made up freshly from Sterile Solution of Procaine Hydro-
chloride 250, Injection of Sodium Chloride 750, Injection of
Adrenaline 2. Contains 0.5% of Procaine Hydrochloride with
Adrenaline 1:500,000.

Procaine Hydrochloride and Epinephrine Injection U.S.P.
Two percent Procaine Hydrochloride and 1:25,000 Epinephrine,
in 1 cc. and 30 cc. containers.

Procaine Hydrochloride Injection U.S.P.
1% in 1 cc.; 2% in 1, 2, and 5 cc. containers.

Sterile Procaine Hydrochloride U.S.P. *Procainae Hydrochloridum Sterile*

℀ Procaine Hydrochloride is considered to be the safest and most generally useful local anaesthetic. Its greatest disadvantage is its low potency in anaesthetizing intact mucous membranes and the cornea. On injection it tends to be carried away rapidly by the circulation, but its action can be prolonged by adding epinephrine to a concentration of 1:500,000, which, by causing vascular constriction locally, delays the removal of the procaine.

Recently Procaine Hydrochloride has been given intravenously to alleviate the itching of urticaria, the pain of severe burns, and even as an obstetrical analgesic. Anaesthetic doses are close to those producing convulsions but control is possible because procaine is rapidly destroyed by the liver.

Lactic Acid. *Acidum Lacticum*

$CH_3.CHOH.COOH$. Mol.wt. 90.08. Gm./cc. about 1.20. S: misc. W, A, E; ins. C. A colourless, syrupy, hygroscopic liquid containing the equivalent of about 87.5% w/w of $C_3H_6O_3$.

℀ Lactic Acid is used to make lactic acid milk for infant feeding, and is an ingredient of the Compound Injection of Sodium Lactate B.P.

Lactose. *Lactosum.* (Milk Sugar, *Saccharum Lactis*)

$C_{12}H_{22}O_{11}.H_2O$. Mol.wt. 360.31. S: 5 W, 2.6 W 100°; vss. A; ins. E, C. A white crystalline powder with a slightly sweet taste.

℀ Lactose is used in pharmacy as a diluent for powders and for making tablets. In artificial feedings for infants it is sometimes used when a laxative action is desired.

Laevulose B.P. *Laevulosum.* (Fructose, Fruit Sugar)

$C_6H_{12}O_6$. Mol.wt. 180.2. S: vs. W. A whitish crystalline powder with a sweet taste.

℀ Laevulose is used in a liver function test, the laevulose tolerance test.

Lard B.P. *Adeps*

M.p. 34-41°. S: ins. W; vss. A; sol. E, C. The purified abdominal fat of the hog (*Sus scrofa*).

Benzoinated Lard B.P.   *Adeps Benzoinatus*
Siam Benzoin 2, Lard 100.

¶ The main use of Lard is in the ointments of mercuric nitrate, and of phenol.

Lavender Oil U.S.P.   Oil of Lavender B.P.   *Oleum Lavandulae.*
(Lavender Flowers Oil)
Sp.gr. 0.875-0.888.   Gm./cc. (English oil) 0.879-0.897; (foreign oil) 0.880-0.892.   S: 4 A 70%.   The volatile oil distilled from the flowering tops of *Lavandula officinalis*.   A colourless or pale-yellow or yellowish-green liquid having the characteristic odour and taste of lavender flowers, slightly bitter.

¶ Lavender Oil is used only as a perfume or flavour, e.g. in the Ammoniated Liniment of Camphor B.P.

Lead Acetate B.P.   *Plumbi Acetas.*   (Sugar of Lead)
DOSES: B.P. 30-120 mg. ($\frac{1}{2}$-2 gr.).
$Pb(C_2H_3O_2)_2.3H_2O$.   Mol.wt. 379.35.   S: 1.6 W, 0.5 W 100°, 30 A; fs. G.   Colourless shining prisms or plates or heavy white crystalline masses; odour acetous; taste sweet and astringent; efflorescent and absorbs carbon dioxide from the air.

Dilute Solution of Lead Subacetate B.P.   *Liquor Plumbi Sub-acetatis Dilutus.*   (*Liquor Plumbi Subacetatis*, Goulard's Solution Goulard Water)
Strong Solution of Lead Subacetate 1.25, Distilled Water, recently boiled, to make 100.   Must be freshly prepared.

Strong Solution of Lead Subacetate B.P.   *Liquor Plumbi Subacetatis Fortis*
Lead Acetate 25, Lead Monoxide 17.5, Distilled Water to make 100.   A clear, colourless, alkaline liquid becoming turbid when exposed to air, owing to absorption of carbon dioxide.   Contains 19-21.5% w/w of total Pb.

¶ Lead Acetate is an effective astringent and less irritating than other astringents.   It has been used extensively for chronic inflammations and ulcerations of skin and mucous membranes.   Its use has declined on account of the possibility of absorption of lead from denuded surfaces and the production of lead poisoning.

Lead Monoxide B.P. *Plumbi Monoxidum.* (Lead Oxide, Litharge)
PbO.   Mol.wt. 223.2.   S: almost ins. W; ins. A 90%; sol. acetic
and dilute nitric acids and in warm solutions of alkali hydroxides.
Pale-orange or pale brick-red heavy scales or powder; odourless.

Fresh Lemon Peel B.P. *Limonis Cortex Recens.* **Lemon Peel U.S.P.**
Limonis Cortex
The fresh outer pericarp of *Citrus Limon.*

Dried Lemon Peel B.P. *Limonis Cortex Siccatus*
Dried outer pericarp of the ripe or nearly ripe fruit of *Citrus
Limon.*

Lemon Oil U.S.P.   Oil of Lemon B.P. *Oleum Limonis*
Gm./cc. 0.850-0.856.   Sp.gr. 0.849-0.855.   S: 3 A; misc. A abs.,
CS_2, glacial acetic acid.   A pale-yellow or greenish-yellow liquid
expressed from fresh lemon peel; odour that of lemons; taste warm
and slightly bitter.

Syrup of Lemon B.P. *Syrupus Limonis*
DOSES: 2-8 cc. (30-120 min.).   Fresh Lemon Peel 6.0 Gm.,
Alcohol q.s., Citric Acid 2.4 Gm., Syrup to produce 100 cc.   See
also Syrup of Citric Acid.

Lemon Tincture U.S.P.   Tincture of Lemon B.P. *Tinctura Limonis*
DOSES: 2-4 cc. ($\frac{1}{2}$-1 fl.dr.).   B.P.—Fresh Lemon Peel 25 Gm. to
make 100 cc. by maceration.   Contains 48-54% v/v of C_2H_5OH.
U.S.P.—Lemon Peel 50 Gm. to make 100 cc. by maceration.
Contains 70-75% v/v of C_2H_5OH.

Leptazol B.P.   Pentylenetetrazol U.S.P. (Metrazol, T.N. Cardiazol)
DOSES: 50-100 mg. ($\frac{3}{4}$-1$\frac{1}{2}$ gr.). $C_6H_{10}N_4$.   Mol.wt. 138.2.
M.p. 57-60°.   S: sol. A, E, C, W.   Colourless crystals or a white
crystalline powder; odourless; taste slightly pungent and bitter.
Available in tablets of 100 mg. or in sterile ampoules of 1 cc. and
3 cc. of 10% solution.

Pentylenetetrazol Injection U.S.P.
100 mg. (1$\frac{1}{2}$ gr.) in 1 cc.; 300 mg. (5 gr.) in 2 cc.

ℂ Metrazol is an analeptic and convulsant, i.e. it antagonizes the
action of anaesthetics and hypnotics on the central nervous system

and in larger doses produces convulsions of an epileptiform type. In smaller doses respiration is stimulated.

Metrazol is one of the most effective antidotes for barbiturate poisoning. It has also been used to produce convulsions for psychiatric therapy.

Injection of Leptazol B.P.

DOSES: subcutaneous, 0.5-1 cc. (8-15 min.). Strength, 10%.

Linseed Oil B.P. *Oleum Lini*

Gm./cc. 0.924-0.934. S: ss. A 90%; misc. E, C, light petroleum. A yellowish-brown oil with a characteristic odour and bland taste. Obtained from the ripe seeds of *Linum usitatissimum*. An ingredient of Saponated Cresol Solution.

Liquorice. See Glycyrrhiza

Liver Extract U.S.P. *Extractum Hepatis*. (Dry Liver Extract)

DOSE: 1 U.S.P. Unit. A dry, brownish, somewhat hygroscopic powder containing the soluble thermostable fraction of mammalian livers, which increases the number of red blood corpuscles in the blood of persons affected with pernicious anaemia.

Liquid Extract of Liver B.P. *Extractum Hepatis Liquidum*

DOSE: 30 cc. (1 fl.oz.). An alcoholic extract of ox or sheep liver, dissolved in a mixture of water, glycerin, and alcohol. Contains, in 30 cc., the equivalent of 240 Gm. of fresh liver.

℅ Liver extracts are used to treat pernicious anaemia. The active ingredient in the extract has not yet been identified. No test on animals is available to identify it, so assay must be done by clinical trial on untreated cases of pernicious anaemia. In the United States and also in Canada, evidence must be submitted to a special committee that the amount labelled as 1 Unit will produce a satisfactory reticulocyte response in an untreated patient when administered according to directions for the preparation. The unit for injections differs from the unit for preparations for oral use in the sense that the oral unit contains more of the active principle since absorption is incomplete.

Liver Injection U.S.P. *Injectio Hepatis*. (Liver Extract for Parenteral Use)

DOSE: intramuscular 1 U.S.P. Unit. Sizes, 10 and 15 U.S.P. Units (Injectable) per 1 cc. in 1cc. or 10 cc. ampoules.

Liver Solution U.S.P. *Liquor Hepatis.* Liquid Liver Extract

DOSE: 1 U.S.P. Unit (oral). A brownish liquid containing the factor obtained from liver which increases the number of red blood corpuscles in the blood of persons affected with pernicious anaemia.

Liver with Stomach U.S.P. *Hepar cum Stomacho*

DOSE: 1 U.S.P. Unit (oral). A brownish powder obtained by mixing a concentrated water solution of mammalian liver with minced fresh hog stomach tissue; the mixture after incubation is dried under reduced pressure and defatted. The hog stomach potentiates the action of the liver extract so that less of it is required to constitute one unit of oral activity. Not to be given in hot liquids as the activity of stomach preparation may be destroyed. Available in capsules or as a powder.

MAGNESIUM

The magnesium ion is poorly absorbed from the gastrointestinal tract and in consequence the soluble salts of magnesium retard by osmotic action the absorption of water and thus tend to produce liquid stools. The salts of magnesium with anions which are also poorly absorbed are the most effective purgatives, e.g. magnesium sulphate, but magnesium chloride also has considerable laxative power. Insoluble salts of magnesium, like the hydroxide and the carbonate, are partly converted by hydrochloric acid in the stomach into magnesium chloride, and in this form have a laxative action.

Magnesium sulphate injected intravenously (0.1 Gm. per kg. body weight) acts in some respects like a general anaesthetic. It is used to control convulsions in children due to cerebral oedema, and eclamptic convulsions. Calcium chloride or gluconate quickly reverses the anaesthetic effect of magnesium and should be at hand for intravenous injection after magnesium sulphate in case it is necessary to counteract excessive respiratory depression.

Saturated solutions of magnesium sulphate are sometimes applied to the skin in wet dressings to treat erysipelas or other infections. A paste of magnesium sulphate is sometimes applied to boils or carbuncles to relieve pressure and pain by osmotic action.

Magnesium oxide and magnesium carbonate are effective gastric antacids. The former neutralizes acid without the liberation of gas, which is an advantage in the treatment of poisoning by ingestion of a strong acid.

The light and heavy forms of magnesium carbonate and oxide differ only in particle size. The light powders act somewhat more rapidly as antacids because they are in a more finely divided state and they are commonly used in antacid mixtures.

Magnesia Magma U.S.P. *Magma Magnesiae.* **Mixture of Magnesium Hydroxide B.P.** *Mistura Magnesii Hydroxidi.* (Milk of Magnesia U.S.P., Cream of Magnesia B.P.)
DOSES: B.P. 4-16 cc. (1-4 fl.dr.); U.S.P. antacid, 4 cc. (1 fl.dr.); laxative, 15 cc. (4 fl.dr.). A thick suspension containing about 8% of $Mg(OH)_2$ w/v.

Solution of Magnesium Bicarbonate B.P. *Liquor Magnesii Bicarbonatis.* (Fluid Magnesia)
DOSES: 30-60 cc. (1-2 fl.oz.). A clear colourless liquid containing magnesium bicarbonate in a solution saturated with carbon dioxide. Contains about 2.5% w/v $Mg(HCO_3)_2$.

Heavy Magnesium Carbonate B.P. *Magnesii Carbonas Ponderosus.*
DOSES: 0.6-4 Gm. (10-60 gr.). $3MgCO_3.Mg(OH)_2.4H_2O$ (approximately). S: almost ins. W, A; sol. dilute acids. Hydrated basic magnesium carbonate; a white granular powder; odourless; almost tasteless.

Light Magnesium Carbonate B.P. *Magnesii Carbonas Levis.* **Magnesium Carbonate U.S.P.** *Magnesii Carbonas*
DOSES: B.P. 0.6-4 Gm. (10-60 gr.); U.S.P. antacid, 0.6 Gm. (10 gr.); laxative, 8 Gm. (120 gr.). $3MgCO_3.Mg(OH)_2.3H_2O$ (approximately). S: almost ins. W, A; sol. dilute acids. A light, fluffy, white powder; odourless; almost tasteless. Contains the equivalent of 40-43.5% MgO (U.S.P.).

Heavy Magnesium Oxide. *Magnesii Oxidum Ponderosum.* (Heavy Magnesia)
DOSES: B.P. 0.6-4 Gm. (10-60 gr.); U.S.P. antacid 0.25 Gm. (4 gr); laxative 4 Gm. (60 gr.). MgO. Mol.wt. 40.32. S: ins. W, A; sol. dilute acids. A relatively heavy white powder; odourless; taste slightly alkaline. Combines with CO_2 on exposure to air.

Light Magnesium Oxide B.P. *Magnesii Oxidum Leve.* **Magnesium Oxide U.S.P.** *Magnesii Oxidum.* (Magnesia, Light Magnesia)

DOSES: B.P. 0.6-4 Gm. (10-60 gr.). U.S.P. antacid, 0.25 Gm. (4 gr.); laxative, 4 Gm. (60 gr.). MgO. Mol.wt. 40.32. S: ins. W, A; sol. dilute acids. A light, bulky, white powder containing about 96% of MgO; odourless; taste slightly alkaline.

Exsiccated Magnesium Sulphate B.P. *Magnesii Sulphas Exsiccatus.* (Dried Epsom Salts)

DOSES: 2-12 Gm. (30-180 gr.). S: 2 W 15.5°. A white powder; odourless; taste saline and bitter. Contains between 62-70% $MgSO_4$; the remainder is mostly H_2O.

℃ Exsiccated Magnesium Sulphate is used in the preparation of Magnesium Sulphate Paste B.P.C. (Morison's Paste) which has been used to treat boils.

Magnesium Sulphate. *Magnesii Sulphas.* (Epsom Salt, Epsom Salts)

DOSES: B.P. 2-16 Gm. (30-240 gr.); U.S.P. 15 Gm. (½oz.). $MgSO_4.7H_2O$. Mol.wt. 246.49. S: 1 W, about 1 G, 0.2 W 100°; sps. A. Colourless crystals; odourless, with a cool, saline, bitter taste. Effloresces in warm dry air.

Magnesium Trisilicate. *Magnesii Trisilicas*

DOSES: B.P. 0.3-2 Gm. (5-30 gr.); U.S.P. 1 Gm. (15 gr.). $2MgO.3SiO_2.nH_2O$. S: almost ins. W, A; decomposed by mineral acids. A white or nearly white fine powder free from grittiness; odourless; tasteless; slightly hygroscopic.

℃ Magnesium trisilicate is favoured by some as an antacid for the treatment of peptic ulcer. It is said not to interfere with peptic digestion, which may or may not be an advantage.

Magnesium Trisilicate Tablets U.S.P.

Sizes, 0.3, 0.5 Gm. (5, 7½ gr.).

Mandelic Acid B.P. *Acidum Mandelicum.* (Phenylglycollic Acid)

DOSES: 2-4 Gm. (30-60 gr.). $C_6H_5CHOH.COOH$. Mol.wt. 152.1. M.p. 119-121°. S: 7W, 1 A. White crystals turning yellow when exposed to light; almost odourless; taste acid and saline.

Calcium Mandelate. *Calcii Mandelas*

DOSES: B.P. 2-4 Gm. (30-60 gr.); U.S.P. 4 Gm. (60 gr.).

$Ca(C_8H_7O_3)_2$.   Mol.wt. 342.35.   S: ss. cold W; 80 W at 100°; ins. A.   A white, almost odourless and tasteless powder.

Calcium Mandelate Tablets U.S.P.
Size, 500 mg. ($7\frac{1}{2}$ gr.).

⟪ Calcium Mandelate provides an easy way of taking Mandelic Acid by mouth, without gastric irritation.   It may not, however, make the urine sufficiently acid to enable the mandelic acid to act as a urinary antiseptic.   An acidifier should be given with it or Ammonium Mandelate used instead.

Mannitol N.N.R.
$C_6H_{14}O_6$.   1, 2, 3, 4, 5, 6-hexahydroxyhexane.   Mol.wt. 182.17. M.p. 166-168°.   S: fs. W; ss. A.   A white crystalline substance having a sweet taste.   Available in 50 cc. ampuls containing 12.5 Gm. Mannitol.

⟪ Mannitol is a hexahydric alcohol.   After intravenous injection it is rapidly and almost completely excreted by the kidneys.   None is reabsorbed by the renal tubules so that the rate of excretion may be used to measure the rate of glomerular filtration.   The number of milligrams excreted over a short period of time is measured and the average concentration in the plasma over the same period is also measured.   From these two measurements the number of cc. of plasma, filtered through the glomeruli per minute, may be calculated.   The assumption that no mannitol is reabsorbed through the walls of the renal tubules may not be valid in patients with renal tubular damage.

Mannitol Hexanitrate Tablets U.S.P.   *Tabellae Mannitolis Hexanitratis*
Sizes, 15 and 30 mg. ($\frac{1}{4}$ and $\frac{1}{2}$ gr.).   Contains $C_6H_8(NO_3)_6$, a slowly acting, persistent depressant of smooth muscles, which may be useful for temporary reduction of blood pressure.

Menthol.   *Menthol.*
$C_{10}H_{20}O$.   Mol.wt. 156.3.   S: ss. W; vs. A, E, C, petroleum benzin.   A saturated cyclic alcohol, laevo or racemic, obtained from various species of mint (*mentha*) or prepared synthetically. Colourless crystals; odour penetrating, resembling that of mint; taste warm and aromatic followed by a sensation of coolness.

⟪ Menthol imparts a sense of coolness to the skin and mucous membranes by some action on nerve endings which is not well understood. An ointment containing 1% of menthol applied to the nares during a cold is somewhat comforting.

In dentistry menthol has been combined with resins and phenols for the treatment of pulp canals.

Mepacrine Hydrochloride B.P. *Mepacrinae Hydrochloridum.*
Quinacrine Hydrochloride U.S.P. *Quinacrinae Hydrochloridum.*
(T.N. Atabrine, Chinacrine, Atebrine)

Doses: B.P. prophylactic, 0.1 Gm. ($1\frac{1}{2}$ gr.) daily; therapeutic, 0.2-0.5 Gm. (3-8 gr.) daily in divided doses; U.S.P. 0.1 Gm. ($1\frac{1}{2}$ gr.). $C_{23}H_{30}ON_3Cl.2HCl.2H_2O$. Mol.wt. 508.9. S: 35 W; sol. A. A bright yellow, crystalline powder; odourless; taste bitter.

Quinacrine Hydrochloride Tablets U.S.P.
Sizes, 50, 100 mg. ($\frac{3}{4}$, $1\frac{1}{2}$ gr.).

Tablets of Mepacrine Hydrochloride B.P.
Size, 0.1 Gm. ($1\frac{1}{2}$ gr.).

Mepacrine Methanesulphonate B.P. *Mepacrinae Methanosulphonas*
Doses: intramuscular, 0.1-0.3 Gm. ($1\frac{1}{2}$-5 gr.). $C_{23}H_{30}ON_3Cl.2(CH_3SO_3H).H_2O$. Mol.wt. 610.2. S: 3 W, 36 A 15.5°. A bright-yellow, crystalline solid without odour; taste bitter.

Injection of Mepacrine Methanesulphonate B.P.
Doses: intramuscular, 0.1-0.3 Gm. ($1\frac{1}{2}$-5 gr.). Supplied dry in sealed containers. Fresh solutions are to be made in Water for Injection immediately before use.

⟪ Mepacrine is a chemotherapeutic agent effective against malarial infections. It is as effective as quinine in benign tertian (P.*vivax*) and quartan (P.*malariae*) infections, and much more effective against malignant subtertian malaria (P. *falciparum*). Adequate dosage with mepacrine causes a yellow colouration of the skin which is harmless and disappears in a few weeks after stopping the treatment. The toxicity of the drug is low but with full doses some persons may experience nausea and vomiting; a very small number manifest a temporary toxic psychosis. For preventive (suppressive) therapy, 0.1 Gm. is given daily after the evening meal. For treatment of active infection, 0.2 Gm. is given every 6 hours for 5 days, followed by 0.1 Gm. thrice daily after meals for 6 to 10 days. With the larger doses it is recommended that plenty of water or sweetened drinks be given, together with 1 Gm. of sodium bicarbonate with each dose.

Mepacrine methanesulphonate is for intramuscular injection when oral medication is difficult or impossible.

Merbromin N.F. (T.N. Mercurochrome)

For external use only, usually as a 2% solution. Disodium salt of 2, 7 - dibrom-4-hydroxymercurifluorescein. $C_{20}H_8O_6Br_2Na_2Hg$. Mol.wt. 750.70. S: fs. W; ins. A, E, C, acetone. Iridescent, green scales or granules; odourless; stable in air. Available as 2% aqueous solution or 2% solution in alcohol 55, acetone 10, water 35, parts by volume.

ℂ Like other mercurial antiseptics, merbromin is not very reliable as a germicide but has excellent bacteriostatic properties. It also has prolonged fungistatic properties so that daily applications are often effective for the treatment of superficial fungal infections of the skin. One per cent solutions are sometimes used for irrigation of the bladder and of the renal pelvis.

Merbromin is incompatible with acids and with most local anaesthetics. If the red stain, which is produced on the skin by merbromin, is objectionable, it may be removed by washing with a solution of sodium hypochlorite.

Mercocresols N.N.R. (T.N. Mercresin)

For external use only, usually as a solution containing 0.1% w/v of secondary-amyltricresol and 0.1% w/v of orthohydroxyphenylmercuric chloride in 10% acetone and 50% alcohol in water.

ℂ Solution of mercocresols is germicidal and fungicidal. The undiluted solution may be applied to intact skin or superficial wounds. Diluted 1:10 or 1:20 it may be instilled into the urethra, the bladder, or the eye. Dilutions of 1:2 or 1:5 are often applied to the external auditory meatus on cotton pledgets for the treatment of external otitis.

Mercury B.P. *Hydrargyrum*

Hg. At.wt. 200.61. A shining silvery metal; liquid at ordinary temperatures. Gm./cc. 13.55.

❲ Mercury and its compounds are used in medicine for laxative, diuretic, and anti-infective action.   Mercury preparations presumably have some common fundamental action in intracellular processes but the various compounds of mercury differ strikingly in toxicity and other manifestations of action.   Factors of solubility, ionization, and penetration must determine these differences to a large extent.   Metallic mercury and the insoluble monovalent salts, such as calomel, are relatively non-toxic, while the soluble mercuric chloride is extremely poisonous.   Mild toxic reactions include salivation, diarrhoea, and gingivitis.   Severe poisoning by mercuric chloride results in violent gastro-enteritis and nephritis with suppression of urine, and death by uraemia.   Doses of 2 Gm. or more of mercuric chloride are usually fatal.   The most effective antidote is Bal (Dimercaprol).

Preparations of mercury should not be applied to the skin if preparations containing iodine or iodides are also on the skin. Mercuric iodide may be formed and cause blistering.   A similar effect may occur if a mercuric ointment is applied to the eye of a patient receiving iodide internally.

Ammoniated Mercury.   *Hydrargyrum Ammoniatum.*   (White Precipitate, Mercuric Aminochloride)

$HgNH_2Cl$.   Mol.wt. 252.09.   Sol: ins. W, E; sol. in warm hydrochloric, nitric and acetic acids.   A white powder; odourless; stable in air.   Contains about 80% of mercury. See Ammoniated Mercury Ointment.

Pill of Mercury B.P.   *Pilula Hydrargyri.*   (Mercury Pill, Blue Pill)

DOSES: 0.25-0.5 Gm. (4-8 gr.).   Mercury 33 Gm. with Syrup, Liquid Glucose, Glycerin, and Liquorice to make 100 Gm.

❲ A purgative pill now little used.   It must not be confused with tablets of Mercuric Chloride which are very poisonous.

Mercury with Chalk B.P.   *Hydrargyrum cum Creta.*   (Grey Powder)

DOSES: 60-300 mg. (1-5 gr.).   Mercury 33 Gm. with Chalk 66 Gm. and Dextrose to make 100 Gm.

Tablets of Mercury with Chalk B.P.   (Tablets of Grey Powder) Size, 60 mg. (1 gr.).

❲ Mercury with Chalk was once very popular as a laxative, particularly for children.   It is given at bedtime.

Mercuric Chloride. *Hydrargyri Perchloridum.* Corrosive Sublimate, Perchloride of Mercury, Mercury Bichloride)
DOSES: 2-4 mg. ($\frac{1}{32}$–$\frac{1}{16}$ gr.). $HgCl_2$. Mol.wt. 271.52. S: 13.5 W, 3.8 A, 12 G, 25 E, 2.1 W 100°, 1.6 A 78°. Heavy, colourless, odourless crystals or a white powder. *Perchloride of mercury is extremely poisonous.*

❡ Although a powerful antiseptic, mercuric chloride has little to recommend its use today. It is corrosive to instruments, irritant to skin, and quickly inactivated by pus or serum. Tablets of mercuric chloride are available. To decrease the chance of accidental ingestion, the tablets have a distinctive shape and are coloured with a blue dye.

Solution of Mercuric Chloride B.P. *Liquor Hydrargyri Perchloridi*
DOSES: 2-4 cc. (30-60 min.). An aqueous solution containing 0.1 Gm. of mercuric chloride in 100 cc. (0.1%); 4 cc. contain 4 mg. of mercuric chloride (60 min., $\frac{1}{16}$ gr.).

Oleated Mercury B.P. *Hydrargyrum Oleatum*
Yellow Mercuric Oxide with Liquid Paraffin and Oleic Acid (19-21% HgO).

❡ Oleated Mercury is used in an ointment for application to syphilitic lesions.

Yellow Mercuric Oxide. *Hydrargyri Oxidum Flavum*
HgO. Mol.wt. 216.6. S: ins. W, A; sol. dilute nitric and hydrochloric acids. An orange-yellow amorphous powder; odourless; becomes discoloured on exposure to light.

Mercuric Oxycyanide B.P. *Hydrargyri Oxycyanidum*
S: 18 W 15.5°. A white crystalline powder.

❡ A solution of 1:1000 of mercuric oxycyanide is an effective and non-irritant antiseptic suitable for disinfecting instruments or for application to mucous membranes. It has been largely supplanted by the complex organic mercurial antiseptics.

Mercurous Chloride B.P. *Hydrargyri Subchloridum* **Mild Mercurous Chloride N.F.** (Calomel, Subchloride of Mercury)
DOSES: B.P. oral, 30-200 mg. ($\frac{1}{2}$-3 gr.). HgCl. Mol.wt 236.1. S: ins. W, A. E and in cold dilute acids. A dull-white, heavy, odourless powder; almost tasteless.

Tablets of Mercurous Chloride B.P.
Size, 60 mg. (1 gr.). To be crushed before administration.

⟨ Calomel was once a favourite purgative but has little to recommend it today, when many safer cathartics are available. It is thought to act by forming small quantities of mercuric chloride which irritate the intestinal tract.

Ammoniated Mercury Ointment U.S.P. Ointment of Ammoniated Mercury B.P. *Unguentum Hydrargyri Ammoniati.* (White Precipitate Ointment)
B.P.—Ammoniated Mercury 2.5 Gm., Simple Ointment 97.5 Gm. U.S.P.—Ammoniated Mercury 5 Gm., Liquid Petrolatum 3 Gm., White Ointment 20 Gm. See also Ophthalmic Ointments.

⟨ Ammoniated mercury ointment is used for local antiseptic action, particularly in staphylococcal infections of the skin.

Dilute Ointment of Mercury B.P. *Unguentum Hydrargyri Dilutum.*
Mild Mercurial Ointment N.F. (Blue Ointment, Diluted Mercurial Ointment)
B.P.—Ointment of Mercury 33.3%, in Simple Ointment. N.F.—Strong Mercurial Ointment 20%, in White Ointment. *Both contain about 9-11% of Hg.*

Ointment of Mercury B.P. *Unguentum Hydrargyri*
Mercury 30, Oleated Mercury 1.5, with Wool Fat, White Beeswax, and Soft White Paraffin; contains about 30% of Hg. Unless it is very clearly indicated in a prescription that this strong ointment is to be supplied, the pharmacist will dispense the Dilute Ointment of Mercury.

⟨ The three preceding ointments are used principally in the treatment of syphilis. The ointments are rubbed into the skin (inunction). A certain amount of the mercury is absorbed and exerts a systemic action. Blue ointment has been used in the treatment of pediculosis pubis.

Not all of the following mercurial ointments seem essential but each has many advocates for one purpose or another.

Compound Ointment of Mercury B.P. *Unguentum Hydrargyri Compositum.* (Compound Mercury Ointment, Scott's Dressing)
Ointment of Mercury, Yellow Beeswax, Olive Oil, Camphor.

Arachis, Cottonseed, or Sesame Oil may be used in place of Olive Oil. Contains about 12% w/w of mercury and about 12% of camphor.

Strong Ointment of Mercuric Nitrate B.P. *Unguentum Hydrargyri Nitratis Forte.* (Mercuric Nitrate Ointment, Citrine Ointment)

Mercury 10 Gm., Nitric Acid 30 cc., with Lard and Olive Oil. Contains not less than 6.7% w/w of mercury.

Dilute Ointment of Mercuric Nitrate B.P. *Unguentum Hydrargyri Nitratis Dilutum.* (Dilute Mercuric Nitrate Ointment)

Strong Ointment of Mercuric Nitrate 20, Soft Yellow Paraffin 80. Contains about 1.3% w/w of mercury.

Ointment of Oleated Mercury B.P. *Unguentum Hydrargyri Oleati.* (Mercuric Oleate Ointment)

Oleated Mercury 25, Hydrous Ointment 75. Contains about 5% w/w of Yellow Mercuric Oxide. *Note*—this is 5 times as strong as Yellow Mercuric Oxide Ointment U.S.P.

Yellow Mercuric Oxide Ointment U.S.P. *Unguentum Hydrargyri Oxidi Flavi*

Yellow Mercuric Oxide 1% with Liquid Petrolatum, and White Ointment. Contains about 1% w/w of yellow mercuric oxide.

Yellow Mercuric Oxide Ointment for the Eye B.P. *Oculentum Hydrargyri Oxidi*

Contains 1% of yellow mercuric oxide.

The ointments containing 1% of yellow mercuric oxide are frequently used for the treatment of conjunctivitis.

Ointment of Mercurous Chloride B.P. *Unguentum Hydrargyri Subchloridi.* (Calomel Ointment)

Mercurous Chloride 20, Hydrous Ointment 80. Contains about 20% of mercurous chloride.

❨ Calomel ointment is used as a prophylactic against venereal disease.

MERCURIAL DIURETICS

Meralluride Injection U.S.P. (T.N. Mercuhydrin)

DOSES: 1-2 cc. by intramuscular or intravenous injection twice
weekly. A sterile aqueous solution containing in each cc. 119 mg.
of meralluride with an additional 13 mg. of theophylline adjusted
to a pH of about 7.5 with NaOH. Each cc. contains 39 mg. of Hg
and 48 mg. of theophylline. Meralluride is a combination of one
mol of methoxy-oxy-mercuri-propylamide with one mol theophylline.
The extra theophylline provides additional suppression of ionization
of the mercury and facilitates its absorption from the site of injection. Meralluride is $C_9H_{16}HgN_2O_6.C_7H_8N_4O_2.H_2O$. Available in
1 and 2 cc. ampuls.

℄ Meralluride Solution is a mercurial diuretic which causes somewhat less pain on intramuscular injection than do the older mercurial diuretics.

Mercaptomerin Sodium N.N.R. (T.N. Thiomerin)

DOSES: 0.2-2 cc. subcutaneously two or three times weekly. The
material is supplied dry in sterile vials. Water for Injection is
added shortly before use, to make a solution containing 39 mg. of
mercury per cc. Available in vials containing 1.4 Gm. of Mercaptomerin Sodium, to be dissolved in 10 cc. of water. Solutions are
stable for several hours or several days if kept in a cool place. They
should not be used after the appearance of turbidity.

℄ Mercaptomerin is a mixture or compound of mercurin (the
organic mercurial in Mercurophylline) and sodium thioglycollate.
The thioglycollate prevents the liberation of free mercuric ions by
forming an unionized compound R-Hg-S-R. The mercury is absorbed from the site of injection and transported by the blood
stream to the kidneys where it acts by depressing the reabsorption
of salt and water by the renal tubules. Mercaptomerin can be
injected subcutaneously. It does not as a rule cause pain or induration at the site of injection. The mercurial diuretics previously
available cause severe pain and necrosis when injected subcutaneously. Even deep intramuscular injection often causes pain and
induration, hence they are usually given intravenously.

Mercurophylline Injection U.S.P. *Injectio Mercurophyllinae.* (T.N.
Mercupurin)

Average dose by intramuscular injection—mercuri compound

100 mg. (1½ gr.), Theophylline 40 mg. (⅔ gr.). Mercuri compound is $C_{14}H_{24}NO_5HgNa$ (Mercurin N.N.R.). A clear, faintly yellow, odourless liquid (pH about 8 to 9). Sizes, mercuri compound 100 mg. (1½ gr.) and Theophylline 40 mg. (⅔ gr.) in 1 cc.; or mercuri compound 200 mg. (3 gr.) and Theophylline 80 mg. (1⅓ gr.) in 1 cc. See Mersalyl.

Mercurophylline Tablets U.S.P.

Size 80 mg. (1 1/3 gr.) of mercuri compound (which contains 31 mg. Hg), and 30 mg. (½ gr.) of theophylline. Usual dose: 1 tablet three times a day for 2 or 3 days a week.

Mersalyl. *Mersalylum.* (T.N. Salyrgan)

$C_{13}H_{16}NO_6HgNa$. Mol.wt. 505.87. S: 1 W, 2 A; ins. C, E. A white or almost white crystalline powder; odourless; taste bitter; deliquescent and slowly decomposed by light; contains 38.5-40.5% w/w of mercury.

❦ A number of related organic mercurial compounds are available for use as diuretics. They are usually given intravenously or intramuscularly. They are irritant to tissues and intramuscular injections may be very painful. If any is deposited outside the vein during an intravenous injection, severe pain occurs, sometimes followed by sloughing.

The mercurial diuretics are thought to act by inhibiting enzymes in the kidney tubules concerned with the reabsorption of water and salts. They are more powerful than any other type of diuretic but are contraindicated if the kidneys are diseased. Action is evident within a few hours and often causes a net loss of several litres of fluid. The main uses are to treat the oedema of congestive heart failure and the ascites of portal obstruction. Theophylline is added to increase the solubility and absorption of the mercury compound. Acidifying diuretics such as ammonium chloride are often given with the mercurials as they greatly enhance the action of the mercurial diuretics.

The full maximum dose of 2 cc. of the Injection of Mersalyl or Mercurophylline, when given intravenously, has on occasion caused, within a few minutes, sudden death by ventricular fibrillation.

Injection of Mersalyl B.P.

DOSES: intravenous or intramuscular 0.5-2 cc. (8-30 min.). Two cc. (30 min.) contain about 0.2 Gm. (3 gr.) of Mersalyl and 0.1 Gm. (1½ gr.) of Theophylline. Each cc. contains about 40 mg. of Hg.

Mersalyl and Theophylline Injection U.S.P. *Injectio Mersalylis et Theophyllinae*

DOSE: intramuscular, Mersalyl 200 mg. (3 gr.), Theophylline 100 mg. (1½ gr.). (Often given intravenously.) Composition same as preceding preparation.

Mersalyl and Theophylline Tablets U.S.P.

Size 80 mg. (1 1/3 gr.), of Mersalyl and 40 mg. (2/3 gr.) of Theophylline. Usual dose: 1 tablet three times daily for 2 or 3 days a week.

Merthiolate N.N.R. Thimerosal N.F.

For external use only, usually as 1:1000 solution. Sodium ethylthiomercurisalicylate. $C_9H_9HgNaO_2S$. Mol.wt. 404.83. S: 1 W, 8 A; ins. E, B. A light cream coloured crystalline powder with a slight odour; stable in air but unstable in light. A 1% aqueous solution has a pH of about 6.7. Available in solution, 1:1000 in water with sodium borate and sodium chloride to make an istonic solution, or 1:1000 in alcohol 50, acetone 10, water to make 100 cc. with 0.1 Gm. of monoethanolamine. Available also in a jelly, an ophthalmic ointment and in suppositories.

(Merthiolate, like other mercurial antiseptics, is not a very reliable germicide but it is fungistatic and bacteriostatic. Its action on the skin is not very persistent and it is said to be practically over in about thirty minutes when applied in solution.

Phenylmercuric Nitrate B.P. *Phenylhydrargyri Nitras*

$C_{12}H_{11}O_4NHg_2$. Mol.wt. 634.4. M.p. 185-190°. S: ss. W, 160 W 100°, 1000 A 15.5°; more sol. in G and in fixed vegetable oils. White lustrous plates or a white crystalline powder; odourless; taste weakly metallic and astringent.

(Phenylmercuric nitrate is an excellent antiseptic for external use. A concentration of 1:1500 is commonly used. It is non-corrosive to instruments and relatively non-irritant to tissues. Like other mercurial antiseptics it cannot be relied upon to kill spores.

Mesantoin N. (Phenantoin)

DOSES: oral, 0.1-0.5 Gm. (1½-7½ gr.) daily. 3-methyl-5, 5-phenylethylhydantoin. Available in tablets of 0.1 Gm. (1½ gr.).

(Mesantoin is an anticonvulsant drug related chemically to

phenytoin. It is effective in controlling *grand mal* seizures of epilepsy in smaller doses than those required with phenytoin sodium. It is said not to produce certain undesirable side effects of phenytoin, namely ataxia, diplopia, and hypertrophy of gum tissue; it may however cause skin rashes. Mesantoin has little or no hypnotic or sedative action and may be given advantageously together with small doses of phenobarbitone.

Methadon Hydrochloride N.N.R.   (T.N. Amidone, Dolophine, Adanon, Miadone, Physeptone)

DOSES: 2.5-10 mg. ($\frac{1}{24}$-$\frac{1}{6}$ gr.). $C_{21}H_{27}NOHCl$. 6-dimethyl-amino-4, 4-diphenyl heptanone-3 hydrochloride.   Mol.wt. 345.90.   M.p. 232-235°. S: sol. W, A; ins. E. A white crystalline powder; odourless; taste bitter.

Available preparations: tablets, sizes 2.5, 5.0, 7.5 mg.; ampuls, sizes, 1 cc. and 2 cc., each ampul containing 10 mg.; vials, size 20 cc. containing 10 mg. per cc.; elixir, containing 1 mg. per cc.; syrup containing 1.3 mg. in 4 cc.

℀ Methadon is a synthetic analgesic drug which produces, in doses of 10 mg., effects very similar to those of 15 mg. of morphine, except that the sedative effects are said to be somewhat less than those of morphine. Methadon has been put under narcotic regulations in Canada and the U.S.A. because repeated administration results in tolerance and addiction. The symptoms following withdrawal of methadon from an addict are usually less severe than the withdrawal symptoms of morphine. It is not clear that methadon has any striking advantages over morphine in medical practice. It may prove to be valuable in treating addicts to morphine or heroin since it relieves the withdrawal symptoms of morphine, but causes less distress when subsequently witheld. Small doses of 1.5 to 2.5 mg. orally are often effective in allaying cough.

Methacholine Chloride U.S.P.   *Methacholinae Chloridum.*   (Acetyl-β-methylcholine Chloride.   T.N. Mecholyl)

DOSES: 0.2 Gm. (3 gr.) oral; 10 mg. ($\frac{1}{6}$ gr.) subcutaneous. $C_8H_{18}ClO_2N$.   Mol.wt. 195.69.   M.p. 170-173°. S: vs. W; fs. A, C. Colourless or white crystals or a white crystalline powder; almost odourless; very deliquescent.

℀ Methacholine Chloride acts like acetylcholine but the effect is more prolonged because it is more slowly destroyed by cholinesterase.

Its uses as a drug are as yet limited and largely experimental. It is a very powerful drug and must be used with care. Some of its applications are: stopping attacks of paroxysmal tachycardia, promotion of intestinal peristalsis postoperatively, prevention of urinary retention postoperatively by stimulating contraction of the bladder, and production of peripheral vasodilatation in peripheral vascular disease. See Carbachol.

Methacholine Chloride Injection U.S.P.
DOSE: 10 mg. (⅙ gr.) parenteral. Size, 10 mg. (⅙ gr.) in 1 cc.

Methacholine Chloride Capsules U.S.P.
Size, 0.2 Gm. (3 gr.).

Methamphetamine Hydrochloride U.S.P. *Methamphetaminae Hydrochloridum.* Methamphetaminium Chloride, Desoxyephedrine Hydrochloride. (T.N. Methedrine, Pervitin)
DOSE: 5 mg. (1/12 gr.). $C_{10}H_{15}N.HCl$. Mol.wt. 185.69. M.p. 171-175°. S: 2 W, 3 A, 5 C; ss. E. White crystals or a white crystalline powder; odourless. Available preparations: ampuls containing 30 mg. in 1.5 cc.; compressed tablets, size 5 mg.

℃ Methamphetamine hydrochloride in oral doses of 5 mg. produces effects resembling those of d-amphetamine sulphate (dexedrine). These include increased alertness, temporary abolition of fatigue and sleepiness, depression of appetite. The effects may persit for 6-12 hours. Larger doses may produce feelings of anxiety, and pounding of the heart. Methedrine, given orally, is recommended for the treatment of narcolepsies. It is also recommended for the treatment or prophylaxis of hypotension during spinal anaesthesia. A usual dose for this purpose is 15 mg. intramuscularly.

Methenamine U.S.P. *Methenamina.* (Hexamethylenamine, Hexamine, Hexamethylenetetramine. T.N. Urotropin)
DOSE: 0.5 Gm. (7½ gr.). $C_6H_{12}N_4$. Mol.wt. 140.19. Sublimes at 260°. S: 1.5 W, 12.5 A, 10 C. Colourless crystals or a white crystalline powder; taste sweetish, afterwards bitter.

℃ In acid solutions hexamine slowly releases formaldehyde. At the maximum acidity of urine the process can proceed sufficiently to cause bacteriostasis. In itself, hexamine is neither antiseptic nor irritant nor toxic but if the urine is kept acid a useful degree of antiseptic action in it can be maintained by oral doses of about 1.0

Gm. every two hours.   No useful anti-infective action can be produced elsewhere in the body because the tissues are not acid enough.   A tablet of hexamine burns with a hot, smokeless flame and can be used to boil a few cc. of water for a hypodermic injection.

Industrial Methylated Spirit, B.P. *Spiritus Methylatus Industrialis.*
(66 O.P., Industrial Methylated Spirits)
Sp.gr. not greater than 0.817.   Alcohol 95% 19, approved Wood Naphtha 1 (commercial methanol).

℃ The B.P. permits the use of industrial methylated spirit in many preparations for external use and in the preparation of various extracts for internal use, provided that the alcohol is removed in the course of manufacture.   In Canada any person using "spirits containing methyl alcohol in any form in any pharmaceutical or medicinal preparation intended for internal use shall be liable to a penalty of five hundred dollars."   (The Excise Act, 1934, para. 319).
Preparations for external use containing methyl alcohol in any form must be labelled *Methyl Hydrate—Poison.*

Methiodal Sodium U.S.P. *Methiodalum Sodicum.* (T. N. Skiodan)
CH_2ISO_3Na.   Mol.wt. 244.0.   S: vs. methyl alcohol; ss. A; ins. acetone, B, E.   A white crystalline powder having a slightly saline taste and sweetish after taste.   Contains 52% Iodine.   Available in 50 cc. bottles of 40% sterile solution.

Methiodal Sodium Injection U.S.P.
10 Gm. (2½ dr.) in 50 cc.; 20 Gm. (5 dr.) in 50 cc.; 40 Gm. (10 dr.) in 100 cc.

℃ Methiodal sodium is a radio-opaque substance designed particularly for use as a contrast medium in radiography of the urinary tract.   It has a diuretic action most evident during the first hour or two after intravenous administration.   About 75% of the substance is eliminated in 3 hours and 90% in 10 hours.   It should not be given intravenously to patients with severe kidney damage or severe liver damage.   Ordinary intravenous doses range from 20-40 Gm. in 40% solution.   For retrograde pyelography, 10-20 Gm. in 20% solution are injected through ureteral catheters.

Methylene Blue B.P. *Methylthioninae Chloridum.* (Methylthionine Chloride)

Doses: B.P. 60-300 mg. (1-5 gr.). $C_{16}H_{18}ClN_3S.3H_2O$. Mol.wt.
373.89. S: 25 W, 65 A. Dark-green crystals or crystalline powder
with a metallic lustre; almost odourless.

Methoxyphenamine Hydrochloride N.N.R. (T.N. Orthoxine Hydrochloride)
Doses: 50-100 mg. orally every 3 or 4 hours if required. $C_{11}H_{17}$
NO.HCl. Mol.wt. 215.72. S: fs. W, A, C; ss. E, B. A white
crystalline powder; odourless and bitter. Available in tablets,
0.1 Gm.

℄ Methoxyphenamine resembles ephedrine in its actions but is
said to be less potent than ephedrine in its pressor effect and stimulating effect on the central nervous system. Its action is said to
be predominantly bronchodilator and inhibitory to smooth muscles.
It is recommended for the treatment of bronchial asthma, allergic
rhinitis and urticaria.

℄ Methylene blue in the blood stream catalyzes the reaction Hb $\rightleftharpoons$
MetHb in either direction. Thus when an excessive amount of
methaemoglobin has been formed in the blood stream, methylene
blue will hasten its removal by reducing agents such as glucose and
ascorbic acid.

In cyanide poisoning, catalysis in the opposite direction occurs and
is of value because cyanide combines with methaemoglobin to form
cyanmethaemoglobin, which is relatively non-toxic. Methylene
blue is given intravenously to hasten the formation of more methaemoglobin to combine with cyanide.

Methylene blue is excreted by the kidneys and colours the urine
blue or green. It has been used to treat cystitis but the antiseptic
and germicidal powers of the dye are feeble.

Methylparaben U.S.P. *Methylparabenum.* (Methyl Parahydroxy-
benzoate)
$C_8H_8O_3$. Mol.wt. 152.14. M.p. 125-128°. S: 400 W, 2.4 A, 8 E,
50 W 80°; ss. B and carbon tetrachloride. Small colourless crystals
or a white crystalline powder; odour faint and characteristic; taste
slightly burning.

℄ Methylparaben is fungistatic in high dilution. It may be used
to preserve liquids from fermentation and fungal growth in concentrations of 0.05-0.2%.

Methyl Salicylate. *Methylis Salicylas.* (Oil of Wintergreen, Gaultheria Oil, Sweet Birch Oil, Betula Oil)

$C_8H_8O_3$. Mol.wt. 152.14. Gm./cc. 1.179-1.184. B.p. 219-224°. S: ss. W, 7 A 70%; sol. A and glacial acetic acid; misc. A 90%. A colourless, yellowish, or reddish liquid having the characteristic odour and taste of gaultheria; produced synthetically or distilled from *Gaultheria procumbens* or *Betula lenta.*

℄ Applied to the skin, methyl salicylate produces local warmth and redness. A considerable proportion may be absorbed and act internally as an analgesic and antipyretic, like other salicylates. It has been given internally in capsules for rheumatic fever but is more commonly used as an external application to inflamed joints, and in liniments for various purposes.

Poisoning may occur from ingestion of overdoses or from absorption of large amounts applied externally. Severe poisoning may result from 30 cc. by mouth. A severe acidosis occurs after 24 hours and should be treated with large doses of sodium bicarbonate or sodium lactate orally, or parenterally if necessary.

Myrrh B.P. *Myrrha.* (Gum Myrrh)

An oleo-gum-resin obtained from the stem of *Commiphora Molmol* and other species of *Commiphora*; odour aromatic; taste aromatic, bitter, and acrid.

℄ Myrrh has antiseptic properties and is used in mouth washes.

Tincture of Myrrh B.P. *Tinctura Myrrhae*

DOSES: B.P. 2-4 cc. (30-60 min.). Myrrh 200 Gm. to make 1000 cc. by maceration. Contains 82-87% v/v of C_2H_5OH.

Naphazoline Hydrochloride U.S.P. *Naphazolinae Hydrochloridum.* (T.N. Privine)

$C_{14}H_{14}N_2HCl$. Mol.wt. 246.73. M.p. 255-260°. S: W, A; ss. C; ins. E. A white crystalline powder; odourless; taste bitter.

Mild Naphazoline Hydrochloride Solution U.S.P. *Liquor Naphazoline Hydrochloridi Mitis*

Contains 45-55 mg. of Naphazoline Hydrochloride in each 100 cc.

Strong Naphazoline Hydrochloride Solution U.S.P. *Liquor Naphazolinae Hydrochloridi Fortis*

Contains 93-107 mg. of Naphazoline Hydrochloride in each 100 cc.

℘ Naphazoline Hydrochloride is a synthetic vasoconstrictor and nasal decongestant. It has very little resemblance chemically to epinephrine and ephedrine. When applied in nasal drops it is used in a strength of 0.1% and is notable for its very powerful and prolonged action. This is both favourable and unfavourable. Symptomatic relief from nasal obstruction may be so satisfactory that there is a temptation to use the drug too often. The result may be to aggravate a state of chronic inflammation in the nose and to induce nose-bleeds.

Neocinchophen U.S.P.   *Neocinchophenum*
DOSE: 0.3 Gm. (5 gr.). C₁₉H₁₇O₂N. Mol.wt. 291.33. M.p. not below 74°. S: nearly insol. W; sol. in hot A; vs. E, C. A white to pale-yellow crystalline powder; odourless; tasteless; affected by light.

℘ Neocinchophen relieves pain and lowers the temperature in fever. It also promotes the excretion of uric acid by the kidney. It is used accordingly to treat acute attacks of gout. Relief is said to be faster than with colchicine. It may also be given to treat other forms of acute and painful arthritis but certain dangers attend its use. The most serious of these is the development of severe and sometimes fatal hepatitis, which may occur very soon after the onset of treatment with neocinchophen.

Neocinchophen Tablets.
Sizes, 0.3 and 0.5 Gm. (5 and 7½ gr.).

Neostigmine Bromide.   *Neostigminae Bromidum*.   (T.N. Prostigmine)
DOSES: B.P. 10-20 mg. (⅙-⅓ gr.); U.S.P. 15 mg. (¼ gr.). C₁₂H₁₉BrN₂O₂. Mol.wt. 303.2. M.p. 167°. S: 1 W; sol. A. A white crystalline powder; odourless; taste bitter.

℘ Neostigmine salts resemble in their actions the salts of physostigmine, i.e. they augment the effects of autonomic nerves with cholinergic endings. This they do by delaying the destruction of acetylcholine by cholinesterase at the nerve endings. They are thus anti-cholinesterases. In ordinary dosage neostigmine has fewer unpleasant side effects, i.e. nausea and vomiting, than has physostigmine. Its main uses are the treatment of myasthenia gravis and postoperative distention of the alimentary tract or of the bladder.

Neostigmine Bromide Tablets U.S.P.

Size, 15 mg. ($\frac{1}{4}$ gr.).

Neostigmine Methylsulphate. *Neostigminae Methylsulphas*

DOSES: B.P. 0.5-2 mg. ($\frac{1}{120}$-$\frac{1}{30}$ gr.) subcutaneous or intramuscular; U.S.P. 0.5 mg. ($\frac{1}{120}$ gr.). $C_{13}H_{22}N_2O_6S$. Mol.wt. 334.38. M.p. 142-145°. S: 10 W; less sol. A. A white, odourless, crystalline powder; taste bitter.

Neostigmine Methylsulfate Injection U.S.P.

Strengths, 0.25 or 0.5 mg. per cc. ($\frac{1}{250}$ or $\frac{1}{120}$ gr. in 15 min.).

Injection of Neostigmine Methylsulphate B.P.

Strength, 0.5 mg. per cc. ($\frac{1}{120}$ gr. in 15 min.).

Nikethamide. *Nikethamidum*. (T.N. Coramine)

DOSES: oral, 0.3-1 Gm. (5-15 gr.); subcutaneous, intramuscular, or intravenous, 0.25-1 Gm. (4-15 gr.). $C_{10}H_{14}N_2O$. Mol.wt. 178.2. F.p. 22-24°. Gm./cc. 1.058-1.063. S: misc. W; sol. A, E, C, acetone. A colourless or yellowish oily liquid or a crystalline solid; almost odourless; taste faintly bitter, followed by a sensation of warmth. Usually sold as a 25% w/v solution in water.

Injection of Nikethamide B.P. Nikethamide Injection U.S.P.

DOSES: subcutaneous, intramuscular, or intravenous, 1-4 cc. (15-60 min.). Strength, about 25%. Sizes, 1.5 and 5 cc.

℘ Nikethamide is a respiratory stimulant which is particularly effective when the respiration is depressed by morphine. Against respiratory depression caused by barbiturates it is less effective than picrotoxin or metrazol. The circulatory effects of nikethamide are not clearly established as very useful. Large doses cause dilatation of coronary arteries and hence the drug has been advocated for chronic heart disease. The evidence for its efficacy in such conditions is dubious.

Nitric Acid B.P. Acidum Nitricum

HNO_3. Mol.wt. 63.02. Gm./cc. 1.41. A fuming, clear, and almost colourless liquid; caustic and corrosive; odour irritating. Contains about 70% w/w HNO_3.

℘ Nitric Acid may be used as a caustic for warts.

Nitrofurazone N.N.R. (T.N. Furacin)

$C_3H_6O_4N_4$. Mol.wt. 198.15. 5-nitro-2-furaldehyde semicarbazone. A lemon-yellow crystalline powder; turns brown-black and decomposes on heating to 236-240°. S: 4200 W, 590 A, 350 propylene glycol. Odourless, and at first almost tasteless, with a bitter after taste; darkens on prolonged exposure to light. Available as: solution, 1:500; soluble dressing, 1:500; ointment, 1:500.

℘ Nitrofurazone is an antibacterial substance for external or topical use. It is bacteriostatic at concentrations of 1:200,000 and bactericidal at 1:50,000 and is effective against a great variety of bacterial forms. Its main use is for application to superficial infections, such as impetigo. Continued application for a month or longer sometimes results in a local reaction due to sensitization.

Nitrogen U.S.P. *Nitrogenium*

N_2. Mol.wt. 28.02. S: 65W, 9 A (20° and 760 mm. pressure). A colourless, odourless and tasteless gas. Non-inflammable.

Nitromersol N.F. (T.N. Metaphen)

For external use only, in solutions of 1:200 to 1:2500. Anhydride of 4-nitro-3-hydroxymercuri-ortho-cresol. $C_7H_5O_3NHg$. Mol.wt. 351.73. S: ins. W, A; sol. dilute alkalis.

In alkaline solutions a soluble hydroxy-mercuri salt is formed.

℘ Nitromersol in dilute solution (1:2500) is relatively non-irritant. It is bacteriostatic and fungistatic. The "tincture" 1:200 is used on intact skin or minor cuts. A disinfecting solution for surgical and dental instruments consists of nitromersol 1:2000 w/v, benzyl alcohol 4 cc. and ethylene glycol 20 Gm. in water to make 100 cc., with sodium hydroxide, and sodium carbonate sufficient to neutralize the nitromersol.

Spirit of Nitrous Ether B.P. *Spiritus Aetheris Nitrosi.* (Sweet Spirit of Nitre)

DOSES: 1-4 cc. (15-60 min.). Gm./cc. 0.833-0.837. S: misc. W. A transparent, faintly yellow liquid; odour and taste characteristic. An alcoholic solution containing 1.25-2.5% w/v of ethyl nitrite, and 84-87% v/v of C_2H_5OH.

℘ Spirit of Nitrous Ether contains ethyl nitrite, which has a vasodilator action. It was once commonly used in mixtures for the symptomatic treatment of fever. It has mild diuretic and antipyretic actions.

Nitrous Oxide. *Oxidum Nitrosum U.S.P. Nitrogenii Monoxidum*
B.P. (Nitrogen Monoxide)

N_2O. Mol.wt. 44.02. S: 1 vol. dissolves in 1.5 cc. W at 20°C;
readily sol. in A, E, and in oils. A colourless gas with a faint odour
and sweetish taste. Contains not less than 95% by vol. of N_2O.

℄ When 100% Nitrous Oxide is inhaled, unconsciousness is
produced in about 30 seconds and, of course, anoxia. Anaesthesia
adequate for some purposes can be maintained by 85-90% N_2O.
with 10-15% oxygen, particularly if the patient is premedicated
with barbiturates or morphine and hyoscine. Muscular relaxation
is, however, poor. This can be remedied by the administration of
curare.

Nitrous Oxide is considered a very safe anaesthetic for short
operations, but there is some danger of acute anoxia due to careless
administration or faulty apparatus.

For dental extractions the gas is often given without premedication.
It should not be used if the patient has heart disease or hypertension.

Nutmeg B.P. *Myristica*
The dried ripe seed of *Myristica fragrans*.

Powdered Nutmeg B.P. *Myristicae Pulvis*
A reddish-brown powder.

Oil of Nutmeg B.P. *Oleum Myristicae*
Oil of Nutmeg is a volatile oil distilled with steam from Nutmeg.

℄ Oil of nutmeg is used only as a flavour but large doses are
convulsant.

Nux Vomica B.P. *Nux Vomica.* (Strychnine Seed)
The dried ripe seeds of *Strychnos Nux-vomica*; contains about
1.2% of strychnine.

Powdered Nux Vomica B.P. *Nucis Vomicae Pulvis*
A yellowish-grey powder.

Prepared Nux Vomica B.P. *Nux Vomica Praeparata*
DOSES: 0.06-0.25 Gm. (1-4 gr.). 0.25 Gm. (4 gr.) contains about
3 mg. ($\frac{1}{20}$ gr.) of strychnine.

Dry Extract of Nux Vomica B.P.   *Extractum Nucis Vomicae Siccum.*
(Extract of Nux Vomica)

DOSES: 15-60 mg. ($\frac{1}{4}$-1 gr.). Dried alcoholic percolate of Nux Vomica adjusted with Calcium Phosphate to contain 4.75-5.25% of strychnine; 60 mg. (1 gr.) contains about 3 mg. ($\frac{1}{20}$ gr.) of strychnine.

Liquid Extract of Nux Vomica B.P.   *Extractum Nucis Vomicae Liquidum*

DOSES: 0.06-0.2 cc. (1-3 min.). An alcoholic percolate adjusted to contain 1.425-1.575% w/v of strychnine; 0.2 cc. (3 min.) contains 3 mg. ($\frac{1}{24}$ gr.) of strychnine. Contains 36-42% v/v of C_2H_5OH.

Tincture of Nux Vomica B.P.   *Tinctura Nucis Vomicae*

DOSES: 0.6-: cc. (10-30 min.). Liquid Extract of Nux Vomica 83.4 cc. diluted to 1000 cc. Contains 0.119-0.131% strychnine; 2 cc. (30 min.) contain 2.5 mg. ($\frac{1}{30}$ gr.) of strychnine. Contains 43-46% v/v of C_2H_5OH.

Strychnine Hydrochloride B.P.   *Strychninae Hydrochloridum*

DOSES: oral, 2-8 mg. ($\frac{1}{32}$-$\frac{1}{8}$gr.); subcutaneous, 2-4 mg. ($\frac{1}{32}$-$\frac{1}{16}$ gr.). $C_{21}H_{22}O_2N_2.HCl.2H_2O$. Mol.wt. 406.9. S: 40 W, 80 A 90% 15.5°. The hydrochloride of an alkaloid obtained from the seed of *Strychnos Nux-vomica* and of other species of *Strychnos*. Colourless prismatic crystals; taste intensely bitter. Contains 82-84% w/w of strychnine alkaloid. *Extremely poisonous.*

Injection of Strychnine Hydrochloride B.P.

Strength, 4 mg. per cc. ($\frac{1}{16}$ gr. in 15 min.).

Solution of Strychnine Hydrochloride B.P.   *Liquor Strychninae Hydrochloridi*

DOSES: 0.2-0.8 cc. (3-12 min.). Strychnine Hydrochloride 1, Alcohol 90% 25, Water to make 100 cc. Contains 0.78-0.86% w/v of strychnine. Contains in 0.8 cc. 8 mg. ($\frac{1}{8}$ gr.) of strychnine hydrochloride and 21-24% v/v of C_2H_5OH.

❡ Strychnine and brucine are the most important alkaloids of nux vomica. Both are intensely bitter. Brucine has effects resembling those of strychnine but is only about one-sixth as toxic. Because of its bitter taste, brucine is sometimes used to denature alcohol. Strychnine is sometimes given to stimulate reflexly the secretion of gastric juice. A dose of 0.3 cc. of the Tincture of Nux Vomica is sufficient to act by its bitter taste but insufficient to produce systemic actions. The main action of strychnine is to facilitate transmission of nerve impulses across synapses. The effect is particularly marked on the synapses of spinal reflexes, so that an effect of small doses is an exaggeration of spinal reflexes while larger doses cause spinal convulsions. Some effects are noticeable elsewhere in the central nervous system. The special senses are made more acute, and the visual fields are enlarged.

Strychnine has been used mostly in tonics, i.e. medicines to hasten convalescence after a serious illness, or to promote a sense of well-being in the vaguely debilitated. Multiple vitamin therapy has largely superseded the old-fashioned strychnine tonic but the latter probably still deserves consideration for the treatment of the aged.

Strychnine was once much used as a "stimulant" in all manner of emergencies, such as circulatory failure, shock, and respiratory failure. Its usefulness is probably restricted to the treatment of severe poisoning by barbiturates.

OINTMENT BASES

℃ The following preparations from Emulsifying Ointment to Ointment of Wool Alcohols (except Emulsifying Wax) are bland ointments often used as bases for medicated ointments. The choice of an appropriate base depends on the consistency desired in the final preparation; the temperature at which it is to be used; whether it should be easily washed off, or on the contrary, resistant to water; whether the medicament is water-soluble, fat-soluble, or insoluble. At one time bases were classified as endermic and epidermic. Endermic bases were designed to favour absorption of the medication, while epidermic bases were designed to retard absorption. Ointments containing lard and wool fat were thought to favour absorption, while the paraffin bases were thought to retard absorption. This is probably true to some extent but cannot be relied on in all cases because absorption is governed by many factors.

In recent years many water-washable or hydrophilic ointments have been developed, largely for cosmetic and industrial purposes. Their medical uses are not yet well established, except perhaps for the application of medication to the scalp. In industry water-washable creams ("invisible gloves") have been used to protect the hands from irritants or absorbable poisons.

Emulsifying Ointment B.P. *Unguentum Emulsificans*
Emulsifying Wax 30, White Soft Paraffin 50, and Liquid Paraffin 20.

Hydrous Emulsifying Ointment B.P. *Unguentum Emulsificans Aquosum*
Emulsifying Ointment 30% with Distilled Water and Chlorocresol.

Emulsifying Wax B.P. *Cera Emulsificans*
Contains Cetostearyl Alcohol, Sodium Lauryl Sulphate, and Distilled Water. A white or pale-yellow waxy solid, becoming plastic when warm; odour faint and characteristic.

ℂ Emulsifying Wax is used in making oil-in-water emulsions or creams.

Hydrophilic Ointment U.S.P. *Unguentum Hydrophilicum*
Methylparaben 0.25, Propylparaben 0.15, Sodium Lauryl Sulfate 10, Propylene Glycol 120, Stearyl Alcohol 250, White Petrolatum 250, Water to make 1000.

℃ Hydrophilic Ointment is an oil-in-water emulsoid and consequently may be described as water-washable.

Hydrophilic Petrolatum U.S.P. *Petrolatum Hydrophilicum*
Cholesterol 30, Stearyl Alcohol 30, White Wax 80, White Petrolatum 860.

℃ Hydrophilic petrolatum is an ointment with characteristics similar to those of Ointment of Wool Alcohols B.P. It will absorb at least an equal volume of water or aqueous solution.

Hydrous Ointment B.P. *Unguentum Aquosum*
Ointment of Wool Alcohols 50, Distilled Water 50.

℃ This preparation is a water-in-oil emulsoid, i.e. not water-washable, nor does it tend to dry out.

Paraffin Ointment B.P. *Unguentum Paraffini*
White Beeswax 2, Hard Paraffin 8, Soft Paraffin, White or Yellow 90.

℃ This base is stiffer than most and might be suitable for general use in tropical climates. In the temperate zone it is suitable for applications which are intended to adhere to a dressing rather than to the skin.

Petrolatum U.S.P.   *Petrolatum.*   **Yellow Soft Paraffin B.P.**
Paraffinum Molle Flavum.   (Petroleum Jelly)
Melting range 38-60°.   S: ins. W, A; sol. E, C.
Yellow soft paraffin is a mixture of semi-solid hydrocarbons obtained from petroleum; it is a yellow, translucent, soft mass, unctuous to the touch, nearly free from odour and taste.

Simple Ointment B.P.   *Unguentum Simplex*
Wool Fat 5, Hard Paraffin 10, and White Soft Paraffin 85.   Yellow Soft Paraffin may be used in a coloured ointment.

℀ Note that Simple Ointment B.P. and White Ointment U.S.P., shown in the next paragraph, are very similar.   For most purposes they would probably be interchangeable.   The purpose of the hard paraffin and white wax in these ointments is to maintain the proper consistency in warm climates.

White Ointment U.S.P.   *Unguentum Album.*   (Simple Ointment)
White Wax 5, White Petrolatum 95.

Yellow Ointment U.S.P.   *Unguentum Flavum*
Yellow Wax 5, Petrolatum 95.

White Petrolatum U.S.P.   *Petrolatum Album.*   **White Soft Paraffin B.P.**   *Paraffinum Molle Album.*   (White Petroleum Jelly)
Melting range 38-60°.   S: ins. W, A; sol. E, C.   White soft paraffin is a mixture of semi-solid hydrocarbons obtained from petroleum and bleached.   It is a white, translucent, soft mass, unctuous to the touch; odourless; tasteless.

Wool Fat.   *Adeps Lanae.*   (Anhydrous Lanolin, Refined Wool Fat)
Melting ranges; 34-40° (B.P.), 36-42° (U.S.P.).   S: ins. W; sps. cold A; sol. E, C.   A fat-like substance prepared from sheep's wool; a tenacious, unctuous substance having only a slight odour.   Can be mixed with about twice its weight of water, without separation.

Hydrous Wool Fat.   *Adeps Lanae Hydrosus.*   (Lanolin)
Wool Fat 70, Water 30.   A yellowish-white ointment-like mass having only a slight odour.

℀ Lanolin is an ingredient of many ointments and so-called "nutrient skin creams."   It is slightly sticky and adherent.

Wool Alcohols B.P.   *Alcoholia Lanae*
M.p. not below 54°.   S: ins. W; sol. A; fs. E, C, light petroleum,

25 abs. A 78°. A fraction of wool fat containing the cholesterols (at least 28%) and other alcohols; a golden-brown solid, somewhat brittle when cold; odour faint.

Ointment of Wool Alcohols B.P. *Unguentum Alcoholium Lanae.*
(T.N. Eucerin)
Wool Alcohols 6 with Hard Paraffin 24, Soft Paraffin, (White or Yellow) 10, and Liquid Paraffin 60.

⟪ Ointment of Wool Alcohols can be made into a fairly stable cream by incorporating with it an equal volume of water to make a water-in-oil emulsion. It is particularly suitable for making penicillin creams. The Hydrophilic Petrolatum of the U.S.P. would appear to have similar properties.

Ointments for the Eye B.P. *Oculenta*
The base for all oculenta is Soft Yellow Paraffin 90, Wool Fat 10. They are prepared with aseptic technique. Ointments for the eye contain as follows, unless otherwise specified by the prescriber:
Atropine Ointment for the Eye. 0.25% Atropine Sulphate.
Atropine with Yellow Mercuric Oxide Ointment for the Eye. 0.125% of Atropine Sulphate, 1% Yellow Mercuric Oxide. *Should not be stored.*
Cocaine Ointment for the Eye. 0.25% of Cocaine Hydrochloride.
Hyoscine Ointment for the Eye. 0.125% of Hyoscine Hydrobromide.
Penicillin Ointment for the Eye. 1000 units per Gm. (Ca salt).
Yellow Oxide of Mercury Ointment for the Eye. 1% of HgO.
Physostigmine (Eserine) Ointment for the Eye. 0.125% of Physostigmine Salicylate.

Ammoniated Mercury Ophthalmic Ointment U.S.P. *Unguentum Hydrargyri Ammoniati Ophthalmicum*
Ammoniated Mercury 30, Liquid Petrolatum 10, White Petrolatum to make 1000 Gm.

Mercury Bichloride Ophthalmic Ointment U.S.P. *Unguentum Hydrargyri Bichloridi Ophthalmicum*
Mercury Bichloride 0.3, Water 20 cc., White Petrolatum to make 1000 Gm.

Oleic Acid. *Acidum Oleicum*
Consists chiefly of $CH_3.(CH_2)_7.CH:CH.(CH_2)_7.COOH$. Mol.wt. 282.45. Gm./cc. 0.893. S: misc. A, C, E, B, fixed and volatile oils;

almost ins. W.   A pale-yellow or brownish-yellow oily liquid; lard-like odour and taste; darkens on exposure to light.

℃ Oleic Acid is used as a solvent for mercuric oxide in preparations for use by inunction and also in liniments as an emulsifying agent with ammonia.

Olive Oil. *Oleum Olivae.* (Sweet Oil)
DOSES: B.P. 15-30 cc. (½-1 fl.oz.);   U.S.P. 30 cc. (1 fl.oz.).   Sp.gr. 0.910-0.915.   S: ss. A; misc. E, C, carbon disulphide and light petroleum.   A pale-yellow or light greenish-yellow oily liquid having a characteristic odour and taste.   A fixed oil from the ripe fruit of *Olea europaea.*

Orange Flower Water U.S.P. *Aqua Aurantii Florum*
A saturated aqueous solution of the odoriferous principles of the flowers of *Citrus Aurantium* prepared by distillation.   A clear or faintly opalescent liquid having the pleasant odour and taste of orange blossoms.

Bitter Orange Peel U.S.P. *Aurantii Amari Cortex.* **Dried Bitter-Orange Peel B.P.** *Aurantii Cortex Siccatus*
The dried rind of the ripe or nearly ripe (B.P.), unripe (U.S.P.) fruit of *Citrus Aurantium.*

Fresh Bitter-Orange Peel B.P. *Aurantii Cortex Recens*
The fresh rind of the ripe or nearly ripe fruit of *Citrus Aurantium.*

Sweet Orange Peel U.S.P. *Aurantii Dulcis Cortex*
The fresh outer rind of the ripe fruit of *Citrus sinensis.*

Concentrated Infusion of Orange Peel B.P. *Infusum Aurantii Concentratum*
DOSES: 2-4 cc. (30-60 min.).   Dried Bitter-Orange Peel and Dilute Alcohol, by maceration.   Contains 21-25% v/v of C_2H_5OH.

Infusion of Orange Peel B.P. *Infusum Aurantii*
DOSES: 15-30 cc. (½-1 fl.oz.).   Concentrated Infusion of Orange Peel 125 cc., diluted to 1000 cc.

Orange Oil U.S.P. *Oleum Aurantii.* (Sweet Orange Oil)
Sp.gr. 0.842-0.846.   An intense yellow-orange to deep-orange liquid having the characteristic odour and taste of fresh sweet orange peel.

Compound Orange Spirit U.S.P. *Spiritus Aurantii Compositus*
Orange Oil 200, with Lemon Oil, Coriander Oil, Anise Oil, and
Alcohol to make 1000. Contains 65-70% v/v C_2H_5OH.

Orange Syrup U.S.P. *Syrupus Aurantii*
Sweet Orange Peel Tincture 5, Citric Acid 0.5, Purified Talc 1.5,
Sucrose 82, Distilled Water to make 100. Contains 2-5% v/v of
C_2H_5OH.

Syrup of Orange B.P. *Syrupus Aurantii*
DOSES: 2:8 cc. (30-120 min.). Tincture of Orange 12.5, Syrup to
make 100.

Tincture of Orange B.P. *Tinctura Aurantii*
DOSES: 2-4 cc. (30-60 min.). Fresh Bitter-Orange Peel and
Alcohol 90%, by maceration. Contains 73-78% v/v of C_2H_5OH.

Sweet Orange Peel Tincture U.S.P. *Tinctura Aurantii Dulcis*
Fresh Sweet Orange Peel 50, Alcohol q.s. to make 100 cc. by
maceration. Contains 73-76% v/v of C_2H_5OH.

(The preparations of orange are highly regarded and used
extensively for flavouring medicines.

Opium. *Opium*
The juice obtained by incision from the unripe capsules of *Papaver
somniferum* and dried by spontaneous evaporation; odour strong and
characteristic; taste bitter. Contains not less than 9.5% anhydrous
morphine.

(Opium contains many alkaloids of which the most important
is morphine. The alkaloids of opium fall into two groups, the
phenanthrene group including morphine and codeine, and the iso-
quinoline group including narcotine and papaverine. The concentrations of these four alkaloids in powdered opium are, roughly,
morphine 10, narcotine 5, papaverine 1, and codeine 0.5 per cent.
Narcotine and papaverine tend to relax smooth muscle, but to
produce an observable effect they must be given in doses considerably
larger than the usual doses of morphine. It is questionable that in
the concentrations found in opium they modify appreciably the
action of the morphine. The actions of opium can accordingly be
considered as those of morphine for all practical purposes.

The usual dose of morphine (15 mg. hypodermically) produces drowsiness and relief of pain which may be described as inattention to a steady pain. Sudden sharp painful stimuli are felt and resented. About 10% of patients may vomit and a higher percentage experience nausea. The pupils are constricted, respiration is decreased in frequency and minute volume. Flushing and slight perspiration is often observed. The muscular tone of the pyloric antrum of the stomach, the small intestine, the colon, and the pyloric sphincter is increased; rhythmic contractions of the stomach may be increased. Emptying of the stomach is, however, delayed (presumably by pyloric contraction). Propulsive activity all along the gastro-intestinal tract is delayed, giving rise to constipation if administration of the drug is continued. Muscular tone is increased in the biliary tract, in the ureters and in the bronchioles. The muscular effects of morphine are thought to be due partly to stimulation of parasympathetic centres in the brain and partly to peripheral cholinergic effects. The effect on the pupil is due almost entirely to stimulation of the third nerve nucleus in the superior colliculus. The cough reflex is depressed by relatively small doses. In cats and in a few humans morphine produces wild excitement rather than sedation. In mice morphine and some of its derivatives produce the *mouse tail reaction* (Straub), in which the tail is held erect, or in a position like the letter S. This reaction may be used for identifying such compounds.

In some persons morphine produces a pleasant and comfortable state called euphoria. Such individuals are particularly prone to become morphine addicts, if given the opportunity. Repeated administration of morphine to anyone leads to the development of *tolerance*, i.e. larger doses can be tolerated without serious ill effects. Repeated administration may also, particularly in susceptible individuals, lead to *addiction*. This means *dependence* on repeated doses of the drug to maintain ordinary mental and physical activity. Withdrawal of the drug leads to intense distress with unmistakable objective signs such as flushing, sweating and tachycardia, and sometimes complete collapse.

In doses of 60-120 mg., morphine causes serious poisoning, characterized by deep stupor and very slow breathing. Death often results from 250 mg. No definite lethal dose can be stated because energetic treatment has often been successful even after enormous doses. Respiratory failure should be treated by repeated injection of Nikethamide or Metrazol.

Emetics should not be given since they usually fail because of the medullary depression produced by the morphine.

The use of morphine should be reserved for preoperative and post-operative sedation, for the relief of the most intense and intractable pain; and to relieve the misery of the dying. In chronic pain its use must be avoided for fear of producing addiction. If it must be given repeatedly, the doses should be spaced as widely as possible.

Morphine takes longer to act than is usually realized. Even after hypodermic injection under favourable conditions the peak of effect in relieving pain is not reached for an hour to an hour and a half. It has happened that a second and third injection of 20-30 mg. have been given when relief of pain has not been observed in fifteen minutes or half an hour after an initial injection of 30 mg. This is particularly likely to occur when the patient is the victim of an accident and is chilled from exposure and has poor circulation in the extremity into which the drug was injected. When admitted to hospital some time later, the patient may then develop signs of morphine poisoning, after he has been warmed, and his circulation has been improved by intravenous fluids.

Morphine is absorbed rapidly from under the tongue. This site of administration may be advantageous on occasion. See also Codeine, Diamorphine Hydrochloride, Ethyl Morphine, Dover's Powder, and Paregoric.

Granulated Opium U.S.P. *Opium Granulatum*
DOSE: 60 mg. (1 gr.). Opium dried and granulated.

Powdered Opium. *Opium Pulveratum. (Pulvis opii I.A.)*
DOSES: B.P. 30-200 mg. ($\frac{1}{2}$-3 gr.); U.S.P. 60 mg. (1 gr.). A light-brown powder containing between 10 and 10.5% anhydrous morphine (U.S.P.); 9.5-10.5% (B.P.). The maximum dose (B.P.) contains about 20 mg. ($\frac{1}{3}$ gr.) of morphine.

Opium Tincture U.S.P. Tincture of Opium B.P. *Tinctura Opii.*
(Laudanum)
DOSES: B.P. 0.3-2 cc. (5-30 min.); U.S.P. 0.6 cc. (10 min.). A tincture standardized to contain 0.95-1.05% w/v anhydrous morphine. The maximum B.P. dose contains about 20 mg. ($\frac{1}{3}$ gr.) of anhydrous morphine. Contains 41-46% v/v (B.P.), 17-19% v/v (U.S.P.) of C_2H_5OH.

(Laudanum was once a popular way of giving opium for diarrhoea, coughs, and to relieve pain. It is seldom used now.

Camphorated Opium Tincture U.S.P. Camphorated Tincture of Opium B.P. *Tinctura Opii Camphorata.* (Paregoric, *Tinctura opii benzoica P.I.*, Compound Tincture of Camphor)

DOSES: B.P. 2-4 cc. (30-60 min.); U.S.P. 4 cc. (1 fl.dr.). Morphine content is 0.045-0.055% (B.P.) or 0.035-0.045% (U.S.P.); 4 cc. of the B.P. tincture contain about 2 mg. of morphine ($\frac{1}{30}$ gr.). In addition, the tincture contains some camphor, benzoic acid, and oil of anise, and 56-60% (B.P.) or 44-46% (U.S.P.) v/v of C_2H_5OH.

⟪ The main use of Paregoric is in cough mixtures to depress the cough reflex. It may also be given for the symptomatic treatment of diarrhoea.

Apomorphine Hydrochloride. *Apomorphinae Hydrochloridum*

DOSES: B.P. subcutaneous, emetic, 2-8 mg. ($\frac{1}{32}$-$\frac{1}{8}$ gr.); U.S.P. 5 mg. ($\frac{1}{12}$ gr.). $C_{17}H_{17}O_2N.HCl.\frac{1}{2}H_2O$. Mol.wt. 312.8. S: 50 W, 50 A, 20 W at 80°; ss. C, E. Minute white or greyish-white crystals, becoming green on exposure to air; odourless; taste bitter.

⟪ Apomorphine, given subcutaneously or by mouth, acts directly on the vomiting centre to produce emesis without much nausea. It is often followed by sleepiness or depression and may on occasion produce this effect without inducing vomiting. It should not be used as an emetic in morphine poisoning or in any other stuporous state as it may increase the depression. Tablets that have turned green should not be used.

Apomorphine Hydrochloride Tablets U.S.P.

Size, 5 mg. ($\frac{1}{12}$ gr.).

Injection of Apomorphine Hydrochloride B.P.

DOSES: subcutaneous, 2-8 mg. ($\frac{1}{32}$-$\frac{1}{8}$ gr.). Strength, 3 mg. per cc. ($\frac{1}{20}$ gr. in 15 min.).

Codeine B.P. *Codeina.* (Morphine Methyl Ether, Methylmorphine)

DOSES: 10-60 mg. ($\frac{1}{6}$-1 gr.). $C_{18}H_{21}O_3N.H_2O$. Mol.wt. 317.4. M.p. 155-156°. S: 120 W, 2 A, 0.5 C, 50 E. Colourless translucent crystals or a white crystalline powder; odourless; taste bitter; efflorescent in dry air.

Codeine Phosphate. *Codeinae Phosphas*

DOSES: B.P. 10-60 mg. ($\frac{1}{6}$-1 gr.); U.S.P. 30 mg. ($\frac{1}{2}$ gr.). Mol.wt.

415.4 (B.P.); 424.38 (U.S.P.). (*Note* B.P. specifies 1 H_2O; U.S.P.—
$1\frac{1}{2}$ H_2O as water of crystallization). S: (U.S.P.) 2.5 W, 325 A; 0.5 W
at 80°. White needle-shaped crystals or white crystalline powder;
odourless; taste bitter. Contains at least 69.5% (B.P.) or 70%
(U.S.P.) of anhydrous codeine.

Codeine Phosphate Tablets U.S.P.
Sizes, 15, 30, 60 mg. ($\frac{1}{4}$, $\frac{1}{2}$, 1 gr.).

Tablets of Codeine Phosphate B.P.
Size, 30 mg. ($\frac{1}{2}$ gr.).

Compound Tablets of Codeine B.P.
Each contains Acetylsalicylic Acid 0.26 Gm. (4 gr.), Phenacetin
0.26 Gm. (4 gr.), and Codeine Phosphate 8.1 mg. ($\frac{1}{8}$ gr.).

Codeine Sulfate U.S.P. *Codeinae Sulfas*
DOSE: 30 mg. ($\frac{1}{2}$ gr.). $(C_{18}H_{21}O_3N)_2.H_2SO_4.5H_2O$. Mol.wt. 786.87.
S: 30 W, 1280 A, 6.5 W at 80°; ins. C, E. White crystals, usually
needle-shaped, or a white crystalline powder; odourless; taste bitter.
Contains about 76% of anhydrous codeine.

Codeine Sulfate Tablets U.S.P.
Sizes, 15, 30, 60 mg. ($\frac{1}{4}$, $\frac{1}{2}$, 1 gr.).

(Codeine and its salts are used in preference to morphine for a
variety of purposes, largely because it has less tendency to induce
addiction. It is, however, on the narcotic list and can be sold only on
prescription, except in certain preparations in which a small amount is
permitted. The main uses of codeine are as a cough sedative and
analgesic. In both these effects it is much weaker than morphine.
It may also be used for its constipating action in the symptomatic
treatment of diarrhoea.

Diamorphine Hydrochloride B.P. *Diamorphinae Hydrochloridum.*
(Diacetylmorphine Hydrochloride, Heroin)
DOSES: 5-10 mg. ($\frac{1}{12}-\frac{1}{6}$ gr.). $C_{21}H_{23}O_5N.HCl.H_2O$. Mol.wt. 423.9.
M.p. 229-233°. S: at 15.5° 2 W, 11 A 90%; ins. E. An alkaloid
produced by the acetylation of morphine. A colourless crystalline
powder; odourless; taste bitter.

℃ Diamorphine acts more rapidly and more intensely but for a shorter time than morphine. Its effects wear off in about $1\frac{1}{2}$ hours. This may explain the claim that Diamorphine is a safer obstetrical analgesic than morphine, in that it has less depressant action on the respiration of the baby when given 2-3 hours before delivery. Diamorphine is the most important drug of addiction and a favourite of the underworld. Its medical use is forbidden in the U.S.A. but permitted in Canada.

Dihydromorphinone Hydrochloride U.S.P. *Dihydromorphinoni Hydrochloridum.* (Dilaudid)

DOSE: 2 mg. ($\frac{1}{30}$ gr.). $C_{17}H_{19}O_3N.HCl$. Mol.wt. 321.80. S: 3 W; sps. A; almost ins. E. A fine, white, crystalline powder. Odourless; affected by light.

Dihydromorphinone Hydrochloride Injection U.S.P.

1 cc. contains 2 mg. (1/30 gr.) Dihydromorphinone Hydrochloride.

Dihydromorphinone Hydrochloride Tablets U.S.P.

Sizes, 1, 2, 4 mg. ($\frac{1}{60}$, $\frac{1}{30}$, $\frac{1}{15}$ gr.).

Ethylmorphine Hydrochloride U.S.P. *Aethylmorphinae Hydrochloridum.* (Dionin)

DOSE: 15 mg. ($\frac{1}{4}$ gr.). $C_{19}H_{23}O_3N.HCl.2H_2O$. Mol.wt. 385.88. M.p. 123°. S: 10 W, 25 A; ss. E, C. A white or faintly yellow microcrystalline powder; odourless.

℃ Dionin resembles codeine in its action and is sometimes used as a cough sedative. Solutions of dionin may be instilled into the conjunctival sac to treat retinal haemorrhage by counter-irritation but the rationale is questionable.

Metopon N. *Methyldihydromorphinone*

DOSES: 6-9 mg. (1/10-1/7 gr.). Metopon is an analgesic drug with a somewhat longer duration of action than morphine. Tolerance to it develops less rapidly than to morphine. For these reasons it may be preferable for the control of pain in incurable cancer. It may be obtained for this one purpose by special application. Available in tablets, each containing 8 mg.

Morphine Hydrochloride B.P. *Morphinae Hydrochloridum*

DOSES: 8-20 mg. ($\frac{1}{8}$-$\frac{1}{3}$ gr.). $C_{17}H_{19}O_3NHCl.3H_2O$. Mol.wt. 375.8. S: at 15.5° 25 W, 50 A 90%; ins. E, C. Colourless, glistening crystals or a crystalline powder; odourless; taste bitter. Contains 74.2-76.2% of anhydrous morphine.

Solution of Morphine Hydrochloride B.P. *Liquor Morphinae Hydrochloridi*

DOSES: 0.3-2 cc. (5-30 min.). Morphine Hydrochloride 10, Dilute Hydrochloric Acid 20, Alcohol 90% 250, Distilled Water to make 1000. Contains 0.72-0.80% w/v of anhydrous morphine. The maximum dose contains about 20 mg. ($\frac{1}{3}$ gr.) of Morphine Hydrochloride. Contains 21-24% v/v of C_2H_5OH.

Suppositories of Morphine B.P.

In each, 15 mg. ($\frac{1}{4}$ gr.) of morphine hydrochloride.

Morphine Sulphate. *Morphinae Sulphas*

DOSES: B.P. 8-20 mg. ($\frac{1}{8}$-$\frac{1}{3}$ gr.); U.S.P. 10 mg. ($\frac{1}{6}$ gr.). $(C_{17}H_{19}O_3N)_2H_2SO_4.5H_2O$. Mol.wt. 758.82. S: 16 W, 570 A, 1 W 80°, 240 A 60°; ins. C, E. White, feathery, silky crystals or a white, crystalline powder; odourless; taste bitter; contains 73.5-75.5% of anhydrous morphine; efflorescent; darkens on prolonged exposure to ight.

Morphine Sulfate Tablets U.S.P.

Sizes, 5, 8, 10, 15, 30 mg. ($\frac{1}{12}$, $\frac{1}{8}$, $\frac{1}{6}$, $\frac{1}{4}$, $\frac{1}{2}$ gr.).

Papaveretum B.P.C. *Papaveretum*. (Opium Concentratum. T.N. Omnopon, Alopon, Pantopon)

DOSES: B.P.C. oral, 10-20 mg. ($\frac{1}{6}$-$\frac{1}{3}$ gr.); subcutaneous, 5-10 mg. ($\frac{1}{12}$-$\frac{1}{6}$ gr.). S: 15 W; more sol. in hot W; less sol. A. A mixture of the hydrochlorides of the alkaloids of opium, containing 47.5-52.5% of anhydrous morphine.

Papaverine Hydrochloride. *Papaverinae Hydrochloridum*

DOSES: B.P. 0.12-0.25 Gm. (2-4 gr.); U.S.P. oral and intravenous 0.1 Gm. (1$\frac{1}{2}$ gr.). $C_{20}H_{21}O_4N.HCl$. Mol.wt. 375.8. M.p. 215-225°. S: 30 W; sol. A, C; ins. E. An alkaloid obtained from opium; white crystals or a white crystalline powder; odourless; taste slightly bitter.

¶ Papaverine, although an alkaloid of opium, has little or no analgesic action. It has a relaxing effect on smooth muscle of all kinds. It may be injected intravenously (or subcutaneously) to relax blood vessels and promote collateral circulation in embolism.

Papaverine Hydrochloride Injection U.S.P.
Size, 30 mg. ($\frac{1}{2}$ gr.) in 1 cc.

Lead Pills with Opium B.P.C. *Pilulae Plumbi cum Opio.* (Pills of Lead and Opium)
DOSES: 1-2 pills. Each pill contains 100 mg. ($1\frac{3}{5}$ gr.) of lead acetate and 15 mg. ($\frac{1}{4}$ gr.) of powdered opium.

⊄ Although discarded by the B.P. 1932, lead and opium pills continue to be used for the symptomatic treatment of diarrhoea.

Extract of Ox Bile B.P. *Extractum Fellis Bovini.* Ox Bile Extract U.S.P. *Extractum Fellis Bovis*
DOSES: B.P. 0.3-1 Gm. (5-15 gr.); U.S.P. 0.3 Gm. (5 gr.). A powder (U.S.P.) or a plastic mass (B.P.) having a bitter taste. S: sol. W, A.

Ox Bile Extract Capsules U.S.P.
Size, 300 mg. (5 gr.).

Ox Bile Extract Tablets U.S.P.
Sizes, 0.2 Gm. (3 gr.); 0.3 Gm. (5 gr.).

⊄ Extracts of ox bile owe their actions to the presence of bile salts which are laxative and also stimulate the liver to produce more bile. They promote digestion and absorption of fats and fat-soluble vitamins. Their use is rational in the chronic nutritional deficiencies associated with biliary fistula. They are also used for chronic constipation. In biliary obstruction their value is dubious.

Oxygen. *Oxygenium*
O_2. Mol.wt. 32. S: 1 vol. dissolves in 32 W, 7 A, at 20° and 760 mm.Hg. A colourless, odourless, tasteless gas. When compressed in cylinders it contains 99% v/v of oxygen U.S.P. or 98% v/v B.P., the residual gas being argon, nitrogen, or hydrogen. *Caution: Use no oil on oxygen equipment.*

⊄ Large quantities of oxygen are used in the modern hospital, in connection with anaesthesia, and in many other applications, such as resuscitation of the new-born, and the treatment of respiratory and circulatory diseases characterized by anoxia. The oxygen content of arterial blood of normal individuals can be raised nearly 15% by breathing 99% oxygen, and a still greater increase can often be achieved if the oxygen saturation of arterial blood is abnormally low. The respiratory minute volume of normal persons may be increased as much as 10% by breathing 99% oxygen. The mechanism of this action is not known. Breathing oxygen at concentrations above 90% for 24 hours has no demonstrable ill effects on humans, but longer exposure may cause pulmonary irritation and sometimes symptoms referable to the central nervous system.

High concentrations of oxygen are best administered by means of masks, and concentrations up to 60% by nasal catheter. Oxygen tents can seldom be relied on to supply oxygen at concentrations above 35%. The only way to ascertain what concentration a patient is getting is by gas analysis.

Oxymel B.P. *Oxymel*
DOSES: 2-8 cc. (30-120 min.). Acetic Acid 15, Distilled Water 15, Purified Honey to make 100 cc.

Pamaquin B.P. *Pamaquinum.* (Pamaquine Naphthoate, T.N. Plasmochin, Plasmoquine)
DOSES: 10-20 mg. ($\frac{1}{6}$-$\frac{1}{3}$ gr.). $C_{42}H_{45}N_3O_7$. Mol.wt. 703.8. S: ins. W; sol. A, acetone. Yellow to orange-yellow, odourless powder; taste, bitter, produces a local anaesthetic effect when placed on the tongue.

℃ Pamaquin is an antimalarial agent of some value in suppressing gametocytes in human carriers of the infection and in preventing recurrences of activity after treatment. It appears to have little or no curative action against an active infection. It is rather toxic, causing epigastric pain, nausea, and vomiting. It also causes methaemoglobinaemia and liver damage and should be discontinued on first appearance of either of these effects.

Pancreatin. *Pancreatinum*
DOSES: B.P. 0.2-0.6 Gm. (3-10 gr.); U.S.P. 0.5 Gm. (7$\frac{1}{2}$ gr.). S: sol. W, giving a slightly turbid solution; ins A 90% and E. Pale, amorphous powder having a meaty odour; prepared from the fresh pancreas of domestic animals used for food; contains trypsin, lipase, and amylase.

℄ Pancreatin is seldom given as a drug but has been used to prepare predigested foods such as peptonized milk, peptonized beef tea, and more recently, various amino-acid concentrates.

Para-Aminobenzoic Acid U.S.P. *Acidum Para-aminobenzoicum*

DOSE: 10 Gm. (2½ dr.). $C_7H_7NO_2$. Mol.wt. 137.13. M.p. 186-189°. S: 170 W, 9 W 100°, 8 A, 50 E; ss. C, G; fs. alkali hydroxides or carbonates. A white or slightly yellow powder; odourless; darkens on exposure to light.

Para-Aminobenzoic Acid Tablets U.S.P.

Size, 0.5 Gm. (7½ gr.).

℄ Para-aminobenzoic acid is effective for the treatment of certain rickettsial infections, including Rocky Mountain Fever, Scrub Typhus and Typhus. Satisfactory results are obtained more frequently if treatment is started during the first week of the disease. Large and frequent doses of the drug are required to maintain effective levels in the blood, e.g. 2 Gm. every two hours. With such large doses, nausea and vomiting are not unusual. The drug is usually given with sodium bicarbonate or in the form of the sodium salt.

Paba is thought to be an essential food factor for humans and has been called vitamin H. Some claims have been made (and also denied) that it prevents greying of the hair. Paba inhibits the bacteriostatic action of most sulphonamide drugs.

Para-aminosalicylic Acid N. (P.A.S.)

DOSES: 3-4 Gm. five times daily. (If the sodium salt is used, the dose is 4-6 Gm. five times daily; 4.14 Gm. of sodium salt (dihydrate) = 3 Gm. of P.A.S.). $NH_2C_6H_3(OH)COOH$. Mol.wt. 153.06. M.p. 140-150°. S: ss. W. A white crystalline powder, odourless, with a slightly acid taste. The sodium salt is freely soluble in water and is stable for a few days if the pH does not exceed 6.8. At higher pH the solution darkens rapidly. The sodium salt (dihydrate) occurs as white crystals, with a bitter taste and a persistent sweet aftertaste. Solutions should be sterilized by filtration, not by heat, since decomposition occurs on heating.

℄ Para-aminosalicylate has been shown to suppress the growth of tubercle bacilli in vivo and in vitro. Favourable effects have been obtained clinically, particularly in pulmonary tuberculosis of the acute toxic type. The improvement in appetite, gain in weight, fall in temperature, seem to exceed what might be expected from the much slower improvement observable in x-rays. For this reason it has been postulated that P.A.S. alters the constitutional response of the patient to the tuberculous infection.

It has been shown that tubercle bacilli in patients treated concurrently with P.A.S. and streptomycin are much less likely to develop resistance to streptomycin.

P.A.S. is usually given as the sodium salt because the acid is poorly absorbed and likely to cause gastro-intestinal irritation. The dose of sodium salt is very large and it is a question whether it is more difficult to swallow the large number of tablets required, or the unpleasant solution of the salt.

Sterile solutions are sometimes injected intrapleurally once or twice weekly for tuberculous empyema.

Hard Paraffin B.P. *Paraffinum Durum*

M.p. 50-57°. S: ins. W, A 90% (cold); sol. E, C. A colourless or white translucent mass, sometimes showing a crystalline structure; odourless; tasteless; slightly greasy to the touch; burns with a luminous flame.

Paraffin U.S.P. *Paraffinum*

M.p. 47-65°C.

Liquid Paraffin B.P. *Paraffinum Liquidum.* **Liquid Petrolatum U.S.P.** *Petrolatum Liquidum.* (Heavy Liquid Petrolatum, White Mineral Oil)

DOSES: B.P. 8-30 cc. ($\frac{1}{4}$-1 fl.oz.); U.S.P. 15 cc. (4 fl.dr.). B.P.—Gm./cc. 0.865-0.890. U.S.P.—Sp.gr. 0.860-0.905. S: ins. W, A; sol. E, C; misc. with most fixed oils but not castor oil. A transparent, colourless, oily liquid; almost odourless and tasteless; obtained from petroleum.

℞ Liquid paraffin is commonly used as a mild laxative or cathartic. It keeps the intestinal contents soft and bulky, thus stimulating peristalsis. It is not decomposed in the intestine or absorbed to any appreciable extent. Prolonged use is inadvisable as it may prevent absorption of fat-soluble vitamins. Extra intake of fat-soluble vitamins may be useful and advisable if mineral oil has to be administered over prolonged periods.

Light Liquid Paraffin B.P. *Paraffinum Liquidum Leve.* (Light White Mineral Oil)

Gm./cc. 0.830-0.870. S: ins. W, A; sol. E, C; misc. with fixed and volatile oils. A transparent, colourless oily liquid; almost odourless and tasteless; obtained from petroleum; lower in viscosity and specific gravity than Liquid Paraffin.

⚓ The Light Liquid Paraffin is preferred for nasal sprays or dressings. Prolonged use in nasal sprays or drops is inadvisable, since small quantities tend to accumulate in the lungs and may cause oil pneumonia.

Emulsion of Liquid Paraffin B.P. *Emulsio Paraffini Liquidi.*
Liquid Petrolatum Emulsion U.S.P. *Emulsum Petrolati Liquidi.* (Mineral Oil Emulsion)

Doses: B.P. 8-30 cc. ($\frac{1}{4}$-1 fl.oz.); U.S.P. 30 cc. (1 fl.oz.). Both preparations contain about 50% v/v of Liquid Paraffin (Liquid Petrolatum) with Acacia, flavours, and preservatives.

Paraldehyde. *Paraldehydum*

Doses: B.P. oral, 2-8 cc. (30-120 min.); rectal, 15-30 cc. ($\frac{1}{2}$-1 fl.oz.); U.S.P. 4 cc. (1 fl.dr.). $C_6H_{12}O_3$. Mol.wt. 132.16. B.p. 120-126°. M.p. not below 11°. Gm./cc. 0.991-0.993. S: 8 W, 17 W 100°; misc. A 90%, E, C and volatile oils. A colourless, transparent liquid, with a strong characteristic odour and a disagreeable taste.

⚓ Paraldehyde is a hypnotic with an excellent reputation for efficiency and safety but a most unpleasant, burning taste. It should be prescribed with a strong covering flavour, e.g. an equal volume of Tincture of Orange, and taken well diluted with water. Paraldehyde is mostly destroyed in the liver but a part is excreted by the kidneys and some by the lungs. It confers an unpleasant odour to the breath for many hours. Administration by rectum is sometimes employed to subdue manic patients and intravenous administration is sometimes resorted to for status epilepticus. Addiction to paraldehyde sometimes occurs.

Pelletierine Tannate B.P. *Pelletierinae Tannas*

Doses: 0.12-0.5 Gm. (2-8 gr.). S: 250 W; sol A; ss. E; ins. C; dissolved by warm dilute acids. The tannates of alkaloids obtained from the bark of the root and stem of the pomegranate, *Punica*

Granatum. A light-yellow, amorphous powder; odourless; taste astringent; it is affected by light.

℃ Pelletierine tannate is used to treat tapeworm infection. It is given on an empty stomach and followed in 2 hours by a saline purge.

PENICILLIN

Most preparations of penicillin are made from amorphous powders of calcium or sodium salts of a mixture of penicillins which have been named F, G, K, and X. Crystalline preparations are also available. Among these crystalline preparations, those of penicillin G are notable for being more stable than others and hence are used in creams and ointments which will retain potency for many months without refrigeration.

Penicillins are particularly effective against gram positive bacteria, staphylococcus, streptococcus, and pneumococcus, and also against the gram negative gonococcus and meningococcus. It is generally ineffective against gram negative bacilli, virus infections, tuberculosis, and fungal infections.

Oral administration of penicillin requires four to five times the dosage of intramuscular administration. It is best given between meals with an antacid. Further information about various modes of administration is given under the preparations that follow. Another method of administration is by aerosol. About 25,000 units per cc. may be nebulized and inhaled at intervals, or more or less continuously through a mask. In the continuous or prolonged forms of administration, weaker solutions are used.

The only toxic effects of penicillin which are of importance are the allergic reactions. Sensitization is said to occur in as many as 10% of patients given topical applications of penicillin.

Although effective against syphilitic infections, the ultimate value of penicillin in the treatment of syphilis will require many years to assess.

Penicillin B.P. *Penicillinum*

DOSE: as prescribed. Penicillin may be either the sodium or calcium salt of the anti-microbial acid obtained from *Penicillium notatum* or related organisms grown under suitable conditions. S: vs. W; ins. fixed oils and liquid paraffin. Complies with tests for sterility and freedom from pyrogens. Potency is not less than

900 units per mg. A pale-yellow to brown powder or masses; amorphous, hygroscopic. Very pure preparations are white and less hygroscopic.

Penicillin Potassium U.S.P. *Penicillinum Potassicum*

USUAL DAILY DOSE: intramuscular, 300,000 units; oral, on a fasting stomach 1,500,000 units. The potassium salt of an antibiotic substance produced by the growth of *Penicillum notatum* or *Penicillium chrysogenum* or each of the substances produced by any other means. It complies with the requirements of the Federal Food and Drug Administration.

Penicillin G Potassium U.S.P. *Penicillinum G. Potassicum.*
(Benzyl Penicillin Potassium, Crystalline Penicillin Potassium G)

USUAL DAILY DOSE: oral on a fasting stomach, 1,500,000 units; intramuscular, 300,000 units. $C_{16}H_{17}KN_2O_4S$. Mol.wt. 372.47. S: vs. W, isotonic sodium chloride and dextrose solutions; sol. A (with inactivation). Colourless or white crystals or a white to slightly yellow powder; almost odourless; hygroscopic. Contains 85% or more $C_{16}H_{17}KN_2O_4S$. Penicillin G Potassium meets all the requirements of the monograph for parenteral and for oral administrations.

Penicillin G Procaine U.S.P. *Penicillinum G Procainicum*

$C_{16}H_{18}N_2O_4S.C_{13}H_{20}N_2O_2H_2O$. Mol.wt. 588.71. The procaine salt of penicillin G complying with the requirements of the Federal Food and Drug Administration. S: 250 W, 120 A, 60 C. White or faintly yellow fine crystals or powder; almost odourless.

Penicillin G Sodium U.S.P. *Penicillinum G Sodicum.* (Benzyl Penicillin Sodium, Crystalline Penicillin Sodium G)

USUAL DAILY DOSE: oral on a fasting stomach, 1,500,000 units; intramuscular, 300,000 units. $C_{16}H_{17}N_2NaO_4S$. Mol.wt. 356.38.

Buffered Crystalline Penicillin U.S.P. *Penicillinum Crystallinum Bufferum*

Crystalline potassium penicillin or crystalline sodium penicillin buffered with 4-5% of Sodium Citrate.

Penicillin for Inhalation U.S.P. *Penicillinum pro Inhalatione*

Crystalline penicillin potassium, crystalline penicillin procaine or crystalline penicillin sodium with or without harmless, suitable diluents, dispensed in a suitable inhaler.

Penicillin Procaine for Aqueous Injection U.S.P. *Penicillinum Procainum pro Injectione Aquosa*

USUAL DAILY DOSE: 300,000 units intramuscular. A sterile dry mixture of penicillin procaine and one or more suitable harmless suspending agents, with or without buffer.

Penicillin Procaine in Oil Injection U.S.P. *Injectio Penicillini Procainici in Oleo*

USUAL DOSE: 300,000 units intramuscular. A sterile suspension of penicillin procaine in Oil, with or without the addition of suitable harmless dispersing or hardening agents.

Penicillin Sodium U.S.P. *Penicillinum Sodicum*

DAILY DOSE: 300,000 units (oral on a fasting stomach), 300,000 units (intramuscular). S: vs. W, isotonic sodium chloride solution, and in dextrose solutions; sol. A but is inactivated by it and by glycerin and by many other alcohols. A brown powder, granules, or scales having a characteristic odour. The potency of sodium penicillin powder in terms of units per mg. is permitted to vary according to the use to which it is to be put.

℆ The dried powder or scales of penicillin sodium or calcium are usually dispensed in sterilized vials into which up to 25 cc. of sterile water or sterile isotonic saline solution may be added to make solutions for intramuscular injections. A convenient size of vial is that containing 200,000 units. When the contents are dissolved in a volume of 20 cc. each cc. contains 10,000 units. A dose of 1½ cc. intramuscularly of this solution every 3 hours will maintain an effective concentration of penicillin in the tissue fluid in an adult.

Cream of Penicillin B.P. *Cremor Penicillini.* (Penicillin Cream)

Penicillin (sodium or calcium salt) q.s. with Emulsifying Wax, Hard Paraffin, Liquid Paraffin, Chlorocresol and Distilled Water. Each Gm. contains, unless otherwise stated, 1000 units of Penicillin.

Sterilised Cream of Penicillin B.P. *Cremor Penicillini Sterilisatus.* Sterilised Penicillin Cream

Same formula as above without chlorocresol, but sterilised as directed in the B.P. by autoclaving the base, cooling to 60°, and adding the penicillin with aseptic precautions.

Injection of Penicillin B.P.

DOSE: as prescribed. Strength, when not specified by the physician, is to be 50,000 units per cc. It should be used within 7 days after preparation. During this time the solution should be kept at a temperature not above 4°C.

Oily Injection of Penicillin B.P.

DOSE: intramuscular, as prescribed. Contains Penicillin (calcium salt) q.s. with White Beeswax and Arachis Oil or Ethyl Oleate to make 100 cc. Strength, 125,000 units per cc. to be supplied when not otherwise specified.

Lozenges of Penicillin. *Trochisci Penicillini*

Each lozenge contains, unless otherwise stated, 500 units of penicillin (calcium salt).

Penicillin Troches U.S.P. *Trochisci Penicillini*

DOSE: 1 troche. Size, 1000 and 5,000 units.

⟨ Troches are intended to be held in the cheek and allowed to dissolve slowly. They are effective for infections of the mouth and throat by micro-organisms which are sensitive to penicillin. Tablets or troches containing more than 3000 units in a recommended oral dose may not be sold in Canada except on prescription.

Ointment of Penicillin B.P. *Unguentum Penicillini*

Penicillin (calcium salt) q.s., in Ointment of Wool Alcohols.
Each Gm. contains, unless otherwise stated, 500 units of Penicillin (calcium salt).

Penicillin Ointment U.S.P. *Unguentum Penicillini*

Penicillin calcium in an ointment base approved by the Federal Food and Drug Administration.

Penicillin Ointment for the Eye B.P. *Oculentum Penicillini*

Contains 1,000 units of Penicillin (calcium salt) per Gm.

Penicillin Tablets U.S.P.

DAILY DOSE: 1,500,000 units on a fasting stomach.

⟨ Tablets of 50,000 and 100,000 units are available. The 50,000 units size, is, perhaps, the most commonly used. Oral therapy requires about five times the dosage usually given by injection. Giving an antacid with the penicillin tablet and giving the tablet between meals is advised to minimize destruction of the penicillin in the digestive tract.

Pentaquine Phosphate U.S.P. *Pentaquinae Phosphas*

USUAL DAILY DOSE: 0.1 Gm. (1½ gr.) $C_{18}H_{27}N_3O.H_3PO_4$. Mol.wt. 399.42. M.p. 188-192°. S: 25 W; insol. C, E; almost ins. A. A yellow crystalline powder; odourless; taste bitter. A new drug for the treatment of malaria.

Pentaquine Phosphate Tablets U.S.P.

Size, 13.3 mg. (1/5 gr.).

Peppermint U.S.P. *Mentha Piperita*

The dried leaf and flowering top of *Mentha piperita* Linn.

Emulsion of Peppermint B.P. *Emulsio Menthae Piperitae*

DOSES: 0.3-2 cc. (5-30 min.). Oil of Peppermint 10 cc., Liquid Extract of Quillaia and Distilled Water to make 100 cc. The Emulsion is equivalent in content of Oil of Peppermint to Spirit of Peppermint.

Peppermint Oil U.S.P. Oil of Peppermint B.P. *Oleum Menthae Piperitae*

DOSES: B.P. 0.06-0.2 cc. (1-3 min.). A volatile oil distilled from the tops of *Mentha piperita*. Gm./cc. 0.897-0.910. S: at 15.5° 4 A 70%. Contains about 45% of free menthol.

Peppermint Spirit U.S.P. Spirit of Peppermint B.P. *Spiritus Menthae Piperitae.* (Essence of Peppermint)

DOSES: B.P. 0.3-2 cc. (5-30 min.); U.S.P. 1 cc. (15 min.).

Both preparations contain about 10% v/v of peppermint oil in 80-82% v/v of C_2H_5OH (B.P.), or 79-85% v/v (U.S.P.).

Concentrated Peppermint Water B.P. *Aqua Menthae Piperitae Concentrata*

DOSES: 0.3-1 cc. (5-15 min.). Oil of Peppermint 2% in 52-56% v/v C_2H_5OH. Used to prepare Peppermint Water B.P.

Peppermint Water U.S.P. *Aqua Menthae Piperitae*

A saturated solution of peppermint oil in distilled water.

❡ The preparations of peppermint are used primarily as flavours. They are also regarded traditionally as having a carminative action and thus are considered by some as suitable medication for "indigestion."

Pepsin B.P. *Pepsinum*

DOSES: 0.3-0.6 Gm. (5-10 gr.). S: sol. W, giving an opalescent solution; ins. A, E. An extract obtained from the mucous membranes of the stomachs of certain animals commonly employed for food. A pale, amorphous powder; odour faintly meaty; taste slightly acid or saline; contains the proteolytic enzyme of the gastric juice. Dissolves not less than 2,500 times its weight of coagulated egg albumen.

ℂ Pepsin is used in a variety of elixirs and solutions which are often prescribed as flavoured vehicles or with the faint hope that they may benefit some types of indigestion. The grounds for such hope are scanty because indigestion is very rarely due to lack of pepsin in the gastric juice.

Pepsin is irreversibly inactivated by alkalis so that it is useless to prescribe it with the ordinary gastric antacids.

Persic Oil U.S.P. *Oleum Persicae.* (Apricot Kernel Oil, Peach Kernel Oil)

Sp.gr. 0.910-0.923. S: ss. A; misc. E, C, B, petroleum benzin. A clear, pale, straw-coloured, oily liquid; almost odourless; taste bland.

Balsam of Peru B.P. **Peruvian Balsam U.S.P.** *Balsamum Peruvianum.* (Peru Balsam)

Gm./cc. 1.140-1.170. S: ins. W, 1 A 90%; ss. E; sol. C. A dark-brown, viscid liquid from the trunk of *Myroxylon Pereirae* (Royle) Klotzsch; odour like vanilla; taste acrid, bitter, and persistent.

ℂ Balsam of Peru has antiseptic properties. It is used in ointments (10%) for pruritus, ringworm, scabies, and pediculosis.

Pethidine Hydrochloride B.P. *Pethidinae Hydrochloridum.* **Meperidine Hydrochloride U.S.P.** (Isonipecaine. T.N. Demerol, Dolantin)

DOSES: B.P. 25-100 mg. ($\frac{2}{5}$-1$\frac{1}{2}$ gr.). U.S.P. average dose, 0.1 Gm. (intramuscular or oral). Available in ampuls of 2 cc. containing 100 mg. of Demerol and also in tablets, for oral use, 50 mg. $C_{15}H_{21}O_2N.HCl$. Mol.wt. 283.8. M.p. 187-189°. S: vs. W; sol. A, C; sps. E, acetone.

Injection of Pethidine Hydrochloride B.P.

DOSES: subcutaneous, 25-100 mg. ($\frac{2}{5}$-1$\frac{1}{2}$ gr.).

℃ Pethidine is an analgesic and antispasmodic. As an analgesic it approaches morphine in effectiveness but is less depressant to respiration. Unlike morphine, it tends to relax smooth muscle by an atropine-like action. It is consequently indicated in colicky pain, e.g. biliary and ureteral colic. Favourable reports have been made on it as an obstetrical analgesic. Amnesia is often secured, particularly when barbiturates are given with it. The duration of action of pethidine is definitely shorter than that of morphine in comparable doses.

Overdoses of pethidine produce convulsions. Tendency to produce addiction is feeble but the drug is included in the Schedule of Narcotic Drugs.

Petroleum Benzin U.S.P. *Benzinum Petrolei.* (Petroleum Ether, Purified Benzin)

Distillation range 35-80°. S: ins. W; fs. A abs.; misc. C, E, B, fixed and volatile oils with the exception of castor oil. A clear, colourless, volatile liquid having an ethereal or faint petroleum-like odour; highly inflammable.

℃ Petroleum Ether is a useful lipoid solvent. In the B.P. *Light Petroleum* is described as a reagent. Two grades with boiling points of 40-50° and 50-60° are distinguished; the corresponding densities are Gm./cc. 0.615-0.685 and 0.665-0.695. When referred to in this text the heavier grade is meant unless otherwise specified.

Phenazone B.P. *Phenazonum.* (Antipyrin)

DOSES: 0.3-0.6 Gm. (5-10 gr.). $C_{11}H_{12}N_2O$. Mol.wt. 188.22. M.P. 111-113°. S: less than 1 W, 1.3 A, 1 C, 43 E. Small colourless crystals or a white crystalline powder; odourless ; taste slightly bitter.

Tablets of Phenazone B.P. (Tablets of Antipyrin)

Size, 0.3 Gm. (5 gr.).

℃ Phenazone is the most soluble of the antipyretic analgesics and can be given in mixtures. It would appear to be a useful substitute for salicylates for persons who do not tolerate the latter. It is said to have, when applied topically, astringent, vasocon-strictor, and local anaesthetic effects and has been incorporated in certain proprietary ear drops. Such local actions are, however, very feeble.

Phenol. *Phenol.* (Carbolic Acid)

F.p. not below 39°. C_6H_5OH. Mol.wt. 94.11. S: 15 W; vs. A, G, E, C, fixed and volatile oils; sol. in soft and liquid paraffins. Colourless or pink, needle-shaped, deliquescent crystals or masses; odour characteristic; taste sweet, pungent.

Liquefied Phenol. *Phenol Liquefactum.* (Liquefied Carbolic Acid)

S: misc. A, E, G. A colourless liquid which may acquire a pinkish hue on keeping; odour characteristic; taste sweetish and pungent. B.P. specifies 77-81.5% w/w phenol (Gm./cc. about 1.058), U.S.P. not less than 88% w/w phenol (Sp.gr. about 1.065).

Glycerin of Phenol B.P. *Glycerinum Phenolis.* (Glycerin of Carbolic Acid)

Phenol 16, Glycerin 84 Gm. Contains about 16% of phenol. *Must be thoroughly mixed! Dilution with water renders Glycerin of Phenol caustic! Liquefied Phenol must not be used in this preparation!*

Lozenges of Phenol B.P. *Trochisci Phenolis*

Each contains about 30 mg. (½ gr.) of Phenol in a base of Acacia and Tragacanth.

Ointment of Phenol B.P. *Unguentum Phenolis.* (Ointment of Carbolic Acid)

2.5-3.1% of Phenol in White Beeswax, Lard, Hard Paraffin and White Soft Paraffin.

℆ Phenol was used by Lister to sterilize surgical instruments, disinfect wounds, and even in an attempt to disinfect air. Many antiseptics of greater efficiency are now available. Phenol, however, is still used to allay itch by its action on sensory endings. It is also used as a standard of reference of potency for other antiseptics (Phenol Coefficient). A 1% aqueous solution of phenol will kill susceptible bacteria in a few minutes and will prevent the growth of most others. A resistant species like B. tuberculosis requires exposure of 24 hours to a 5% solution to be killed. Alcoholic or oily solutions of phenol have little or no antiseptic action because the solvent has such affinity for the phenol that only ineffective amounts of the latter pass into the organism. Solutions in glycerin are also much less active but if water is present in the glycerin the phenol may be unexpectedly active and produce a burn.

It is thought that phenol acts by reacting rather non-specifically with intracellular proteins, coagulating them and thus producing death or inhibition of growth at lower concentrations. Five per cent solutions in water will produce a burning sensation when applied to the skin, followed by numbness and later a whitish necrosis. A 1% solution has sufficient local action on skin or mucous membrane to depress nerve endings and thus to allay itching without much danger of damage.

If phenol is applied to very large areas there is danger of absorption, with systemic effects and possibly poisoning. Similar effects will occur if phenol is taken by mouth accidentally or with suicidal intent. The effects of ingestion are of three kinds, (1) local caustic effects on the alimentary tract, (2) central nervous effects, delirium and convulsions, followed by depression and collapse, (3) renal damage with haematuria and oliguria.

The phenol ointments are used largely as anti-pruritics and so is the suppository. The Glycerin of Phenol and various dilutions of it (Keith's Dressing) have been much used in treating middle ear infection but they are now considered unsafe. The danger of damage to the ear drum is considerable and the moisture encourages fungal infections of the external auditory canal. Burns due to phenol should be treated by washing with alcohol.

Suppositories of Phenol B.P. *Suppositoria Phenolis.* (Suppositories of Carbolic Acid)
Each suppository contains 60 mg. (1 gr.) of Phenol.

Phenolphthalein. *Phenolphthaleinum*
Doses: B.P. 60-300 mg. (1-5 gr.); U.S.P. 60 mg. (1 gr.). $C_{20}H_{14}O_4$. Mol.wt. 318.31. M.p. not under 258°. S: almost ins. W, 15 A, 100 E. A white or yellowish-white, amorphous or crystalline powder; odourless and tasteless.

Tablets of Phenolphthalein B.P.
Size, 0.12 Gm. (2 gr.). To be chewed up before swallowing.

❈ Phenolphthalein is a laxative which acts on the large intestine. Loose stools are produced 6 to 8 hours after an oral dose. A small portion of the drug may be absorbed and excreted in the urine and in the bile. The latter portion may tend to prolong the laxative action. Occasionally a severe dermatitis may result from the use of phenolphthalein. If the urine or faeces are sufficiently alkaline they may be coloured pink or red.

Phenolsulfonphthalein U.S.P. *Phenolsulfonthaleinum.* (Phenol Red)

$C_{19}H_{14}O_5S$. Mol.wt. 354.36. S: 1300 W, 350 A; almost ins. C, E. A bright to dark red crystalline powder; stable in air.

Phenolsulfonphthalein Injection U.S.P. (Phenolsulfonphthalein Ampuls)

Dose: average diagnostic dose 6 mg. ($\frac{1}{10}$ gr.). Phensolsulfonphthalein 6, Sodium Chloride 9, Sodium Bicarbonate 1.43, Distilled Water to make 1000 cc. Strength, 6 mg. ($\frac{1}{10}$ gr.) in 1 cc.

❅ Phenol Red is used to test renal function. Normal kidneys will excrete at least 3 mg. of the 6 mg. dose in one hour. With ureteral catheters in position, the function of each kidney can be tested separately.

Phenylephrine Hydrochloride U.S.P. (T.N. Neosynephrine Hydrochloride)

$C_9H_{14}ClNO_2$. Mol.wt. 203.67. S: sol. A, W. M.p. 139-143°. White odourless crystals having a bitter taste.

Phenylephrine Hydrochloride Injection U.S.P.

10 mg. (1/6 gr.) in 1 cc.; 50 mg. ($\frac{3}{4}$ gr.) in 5 cc.

❅ Phenylephrine Hydrochloride resembles ephedrine in most of its actions and uses. In 0.5% solution it is used in nasal drops or nasal spray as a nasal decongestant. It may be injected to prevent or control hypotension in spinal anaesthesia. For this purpose 5 mg. may be given every 15 minutes as required. Phenylephrine hydrochloride is incompatible with butacaine sulphate. It may be injected with other local anaesthetics to prolong their action by local vasoconstriction but is not highly recommended for this purpose.

Phosphoric Acid B.P. *Acidum Phosphoricum* (Concentrated Phosphoric Acid)

H_3PO_4. Mol.wt. 98.00. Gm./cc. about 1.74. S: misc. W. A colourless syrupy liquid; odourless; contains 88-90% w/w H_3PO_4.

Dilute Phosphoric Acid B.P. *Acidum Phosphoricum Dilutum*
DOSES: 0.3-4 cc. (5-60 min.). Gm./cc. 1.051-1.057. A solution containing 9.5-10.5% w/w H_3PO_4.

℃ Phosphoric Acid well diluted (5 cc. hourly for 12 hours daily) may be used to remove lead from the bones. It increases systemic acidity and provides phosphorus; both factors aid the elimination of lead as soluble acid lead phosphate.

Physostigmine Salicylate. *Physostigminae Salicylas.* (Eserine Salicylate)
DOSES: B.P. 0.6-1.2 mg. ($\frac{1}{100}$-$\frac{1}{50}$ gr.); U.S.P. 2 mg. ($\frac{1}{30}$ gr.). $C_{15}H_{21}O_2N_3.C_7H_6O_3$. Mol.wt. 413.46. M.p. 184-187°. S: 75 W, 16 A, 6 C, 250 E. The salicylate of the alkaloid obtained from *Physostigma venenosum* Balfour (Calabar Bean). White or faintly yellow, shining, odourless crystals; taste bitter; crystals become red when long exposed to light. *Physostigmine Salicylate is extremely poisonous.*

Injection of Physostigmine Salicylate B.P.
Strength, 0.6 mg. per cc. ($\frac{1}{100}$ gr. in 15 min.) Protect from light. Contains 0.05% w/v of Sodium Metabisulphite.

Lamellae of Physostigmine B.P. (Lamellae of Eserine)
Each gelatin disc contains 0.065 mg. ($\frac{1}{1000}$ gr.) of Physostigmine Salicylate.

Physostigmine Ointment for the Eye B.P. *Oculentum Physostigminae*
Contains 0.125% of Physostigmine Salicylate.

℃ Physostigmine inhibits cholinesterases and thus augments the activity of many cholinergic nerves. Adequate doses will restore muscular power in myasthenia gravis, slow the pulse rate, and promote contraction of the intestine and bladder. Applied locally to the eye, a 0.1-0.2 % solution constricts the pupil and contracts the ciliary muscle and thus reduces intraocular tension. The latter is the most important action of the drug and the basis of its use in glaucoma. Physostigmine is seldom used for systemic effects because even ordinary doses often cause nausea and extreme weakness, presumably by actions in the central nervous system. Atropine antagonizes all the effects of physostigmine and is the most effective antidote in case of poisoning.

Picrotoxin. *Picrotoxinum.* (Cocculin)

DOSES: B.P. 0.6-3 mg. ($\frac{1}{100}$-$\frac{1}{20}$ gr.); U.S.P. as prescribed, depending on the severity of the barbiturate poisoning. $C_{30}H_{34}O_{13}$. Mol.wt. 602.57. M.p. 198-200°. S: 350 W, 5 W 100°, 3 A 78°; more readily sol. in dilute acids and alkalis; sps. E, C. A glycoside obtained from the seed of *Anamirta paniculata* Colebrooke (B.P.), or *Anamirta cocculus* (U.S.P.). Flexible, shining, prismatic crystals or a microcrystalline powder; odourless; taste bitter; stable in air but affected by light.

Injection of Picrotoxin B.P. Picrotoxin Injection U.S.P.

DOSES: B.P. intravenous or intramuscular, 0.6-3 mg. ($\frac{1}{100}$-$\frac{1}{20}$ gr.) or more if necessary. See below. Size, 3 mg. ($\frac{1}{20}$ gr.) in 1 cc.

⟨ Picrotoxin is described as a stimulant of the central nervous system. Its most useful action (analeptic) is to alleviate the respiratory depression and coma of poisoning by barbiturates. It is also effective against chloral hydrate. The effects of overdosage are nausea, vomiting, and pallor in the conscious person, followed by twitchings and convulsions. The latter are the only signs of toxic effect of picrotoxin in the comatose victim of barbiturate poisoning. The action of picrotoxin is transient (a matter of minutes); consquently it is important to repeat the administration very frequently (3 mg. every 10 min.), or better still to maintain a continous intravenous drip of 0.5 mg. per minute. The object is to keep the patient on the verge of convulsions till the effects of the barbiturates have worn off. In morphine poisoning picrotoxin is not recommended since morphine augments the convulsant action of picrotoxin.

Pilocarpine Nitrate. *Pilocarpinae Nitras*

DOSES: B.P. 3-12 mg. ($\frac{1}{20}$-$\frac{1}{5}$ gr.); U.S.P. 5 mg. ($\frac{1}{12}$ gr.). $C_{11}H_{16}N_2O_2.HNO_3$. Mol.wt. 271.27. M.p. 170-173° (U.S.P.) or 174-178° (B.P.). S: 4 W, 75 A; ins. C, E. The nitrate of the alkaloid obtained from the dried leaflets of *Pilocarpus microphyllus* Stapf or of *Pilocarpus Jaborandi* Holmes. Shining white crystals or a white crystalline powder; taste bitter.

Pilocarpine Hydrochloride U.S.P. *Pilocarpinae Hydrochloridum*

$C_{11}H_{16}N_2O_2HCl$. Mol.wt. 244.72. M.p. 200-203°. S: 0.3 W, 3 A, 366 C; ins. E. The hydrochloride of the alkaloid obtained from the dried leaflets of *Pilocarpus Jaborandi* Holmes, or of *Pilocarpus microphyllus* Stapf (Fam. *Rutaceae*).

❰ Pilocarpine acts like acetylcholine, stimulating glands and smooth muscles which are innervated by cholinergic nerves. It is not an anticholinesterase but acts directly on effector cells. It is antagonized by atropine which presumably competes with it for combination with some receptor system in the cell.

The glandular effects of pilocarpine are particularly prominent, i.e. sweating, salivation, and bronchial secretion. The drug was used frequently at one period to produce sweating and elimination of non-protein nitrogen in uraemia. The drastic side effects, nausea, diarrhoea, and weakness, have made such treatment unpopular. In 1% solution it is used in the eye for glaucoma but not so commonly as physostigmine.

Posterior Pituitary U.S.P. *Pituitarium Posterius.* (Hypophysis Sicca)

S: only partially sol. in W. The cleaned, dried, and powdered posterior lobe obtained from the pituitary body of domesticated animals which are used as food by man; 1 mg. has not less than 1 U.S.P. Posterior Pituitary Unit. A yellowish or grayish amorphous powder, having a characteristic odour.

Posterior Pituitary Injection U.S.P. *Injectio Pituitarii Posterioris.* (Posterior Pituitary Solution. T.N. Pituitrin)

DOSE: intramuscular 0.3 cc. (1 min.). A sterile aqueous solution containing 10 units of oxytocic activity per cc.

Injection of Pituitary (Posterior Lobe) B.P. *Injectio Pituitarii Posterioris.* (Pituitary (Posterior Lobe) Extract, Pituitary Extract, Posterior Pituitary Injection)

DOSES: subcutaneous or intramuscular, 0.02-0.5 cc. (3-8 min.), (2-5 units). A sterile aqueous extract of the posterior lobe of pituitary bodies of oxen or other mammals. It contains 10 units (oxytocic) per cc. A clear, colourless liquid with a faint odour. The label may also state the vasopressor and antidiuretic activity in appropriate units.

Injection of Oxytocin B.P. *Injectio Oxytocini.* (Oxytocin)

DOSES: subcutaneous or intramuscular, 0.5-1 cc. (8-15 min.), (5-10 units). A clear, colourless liquid, containing oxytocic principle extracted from the posterior lobe of the pituitary bodies of oxen or other mammals. Contains 10 units per cc. of oxytocic activity.

Oxytocin Injection U.S.P.
5 U.S.P. units in 0.5 cc. (8 min.); 10 U.S.P. units in 1 cc. (15 min.).

Injection of Vasopressin B.P. *Injectio Vasopressini.* (Vasopressin)
DOSES: subcutaneous or intramuscular, 0.5-1.5 cc. (8-25 min.). (5-15 units). A clear, colourless, sterile, aqueous solution containing the pressor and antidiuretic principles extracted from the posterior lobe of the pituitary bodies of oxen or other mammals; 1 cc. contains 10 units (pressor).

Vasopressin Injection U.S.P.
Strength 20 units per cc.; sizes 0.5 and 1.0 cc.

❡ Posterior Pituitary Extract has four important actions, (1) oxytocic (stimulation of uterine muscle), (2) vasopressor (constriction of blood vessels), (3) antidiuretic, (4) contraction of intestinal muscle. The most common use of pituitary extract is to produce contraction of the uterus after delivery of the placenta, to prevent post-partum haemorrhage. It may be given with great caution in very small doses initially to start labour or to increase uterine contractions in uterine inertia. Great changes in sensitivity of the uterus to pituitary extract occur prior to parturition. During most of pregnancy the uterus is relatively insensitive to pituitary extract, so that initiation of labour by its use is not feasible. During the last days of pregnancy the sensitivity to pituitary extract increases enormously so that very small doses may initiate an apparently normal labour. Larger doses (1 cc.) at this time may produce such sustained contraction of the uterus that the foetus may be suffocated or the uterus may even rupture itself.

The vasopressor action of pituitary extract shows as pallor after small doses. A few cases of coronary occlusion have been reported after large doses used post-operatively to improve the tone of intestinal muscle and to prevent distension.

The antidiuretic action of pituitary extract is used to control the symptoms of diabetes insipidus.

Citrated Normal Human Plasma U.S.P. *Plasma Humanum Normale Citratum*
DOSE: intravenous, 500 cc. Citrated normal human plasma is the sterile plasma obtained by pooling approximately equal amounts of the liquid portion of citrated blood from eight or more humans

who have been certified by a qualified doctor as free from any disease which is transmissible by blood infusion at the time of drawing the blood. It may be dispensed as liquid plasma, frozen plasma, or as dried plasma. See also Normal Human Serum.

℃ Infusions of plasma are used to restore circulating blood volume after haemorrhage or shock and to restore plasma proteins.

Podophyllum B.P. *Podophyllum.* (Podophyllum Rhizome)
The dried rhizome and roots of *Podophyllum peltatum.*

Powdered Podophyllum B.P. *Podophylli Pulvis*
DOSES: 0.12-0.6 Gm. (2-10 gr.). A light-brown powder.

Indian Podophyllum B.P. *Podophyllum Indicum.* (Indian Podophyllum Rhizome)
The dried rhizome and roots of *Podophyllum hexandrum.*

Powdered Indian Podophyllum B.P. *Podophylli Indici Pulvis*
DOSES: 0.12-0.6 Gm. (2-10 gr.). A light-brown powder.

Resin of Podophyllum B.P. *Podophylli Resina.* (Podophyllum Resin, Podophyllin)
DOSES: 15-60 mg. ($\frac{1}{4}$-1 gr.). S: ins. cold W; partly sol. hot W; sol. A 90%; partly sol. E, C and dilute solution of ammonia. A mixture of resins obtained from Podophyllum or from Indian Podophyllum. An amorphous, pale-yellow to yellowish-brown powder or in brownish-grey masses; odour characteristic; taste bitter and acrid.

℃ Podophyllin is called a drastic purgative because it produces copious watery stools with much griping. It is traditionally used for chronic constipation associated with hepatic dysfunction and is usually given in pills, a number of which are described in the B.P.C.

More recently it has been discovered that podophyllin has the property, like colchicine, of arresting cell division. A 20% solution in alcohol is applied externally to remove soft warts (condyloma acuminatum).

Polyethylene Glycol 400 U.S.P. *Glycol Polyethylenum* 400. (T.N. Carbowax 400)
Represented by the formula $HOCH_2(CH_2OCH_2)_nCH_2OH$ where n varies from 7 to 9. A condensation polymer of ethylene oxide and

water with an average mol.wt. about 400. Sp.gr. 1.110-1.140. S: misc. W, A, acetone and other glycols; sol. in aromatic hydrocarbons but ins. in aliphatic hydrocarbons and ether. A colourless or practically colourless viscous liquid having a slight characteristic odour.

Polyethylene Glycol 400 Monostearate U.S.P. *Glycolis Polyethyleni* 400 *Monostearas*
M.p. 30-34°. S: ins. W; ss. A; fs. CCl_4, C, E, and petroleum benzin. A semi-transparent whitish mass; odourless or nearly so.

Polyethylene Glycol 4000. *Glycol Polyethylenum* 4000. (T.N. Carbowax 4000)
A condensation polymer of ethylene oxide and water represented by the formula $HOCH_2(CH_2OCH_2)_nCH_2OH$. where *n* varies from 70-85. Average mol.wt. about 4000. M.p. 53-56°. S: 4 W, 2.5 A, 2 C; ins. E. A pale creamy white waxy solid or flakes; odourless; tasteless. Resembles hard paraffin in appearance and texture.

Polyethylene Glycol Ointment U.S.P. *Unguentum Glycolis Polyethyleni*
Polethylene Glycol 4000 and Polyethylene Glycol 400 in equal parts.

Polysorbate 80 U.S.P. *Polysorbas* 80. (Polyoxyethylene (20) Sorbitan Mono Oleate. T.N. Tween 80)
A complex mixture of polyoxyethylene ethers of mixed partial oleic esters of sorbitol anhydrides. Sp.gr. 1.06-1.10. S: vs. W; sol. A, cottonseed oil, corn oil, ethyl acetate, methyl alcohol and in toluene; ins. in mineral oils. A lemon to amber coloured oily liquid; odour faint and characteristic; taste warm and somewhat bitter.

ℭ The various compounds of polyoxyethylene listed above are dispersing agents or emulsifying agents used in creams and ointments and also in certain suspensions for intramuscular injection, such as microcrystalline suspensions of testosterone.

Polysorbate 80 is sold under a variety of names for oral administration for the treatment of coeliac disease, and other diarrhoeas characterized by inadequate digestion and absorption of fats. The emulsifying action of the Polysorbate 80 is thought to aid in the digestion of fat. A common dose is 0.5 Gm. three times a day, administered in capsules or flavoured liquids.

POTASSIUM SALTS

In many of its compounds, Potassium serves merely as an indifferent base; in others, however, the presence of potassium may modify the action of the acidic radicle because the body treats very differently the three common cations, K^+, Na^+ and NH_4^+. The level of potassium in blood plasma is normally low (20 mg. per 100 cc.). Ingested potassium is for the most part excreted rapidly by the kidneys. Hence potassium salts are diuretic. Potassium does not, like sodium, favour the formation of oedema fluid. Very large doses of potassium salts, e.g. 20-30 Gm. of KCl, may raise the level of potassium in the plasma sufficiently to produce toxic effects on the heart. If the kidneys are impaired or adrenal cortical function is poor, much smaller doses may induce weak pulse, nausea, and vomiting.

Potassium Acetate B.P., N.F.. *Potassii Acetas*
DOSES: B.P. 1-2 Gm. (15-30 gr.). CH_3COOK. Mol.wt. 98.14. S: 0.5 W, 0.2 W 100°, 3 A. A white powder or granules or white, foliaceous, satiny masses; odourless or with a faint acetous odour; taste sharp, saline, or slightly alkaline; very deliquescent.

℃ Potassium acetate acts as a diuretic since potassium ions are poorly reabsorbed by the kidney. Most of the acetate radicle is oxidized so that the net effect on both the blood and the urine is to increase alkalinity. The salt has been used in the past as an alkalizing diuretic in fevers. More recently it has been used with sulphonamides to alkalize urine or by itself to treat cystitis or pyelitis.

Potassium Acid Tartrate B.P. *Potassii Tartras Acidus.* (Purified Cream of Tartar)
DOSES: 1-4 Gm. (15-60 gr.). $C_4H_5O_6K$. Mol.wt. 188.2. S: at 15.5° 220 W, 16 W 100°; ins. A 90%. Colourless crystals or gritty crystalline powder with a pleasant and acid taste; odourless. Obtained from the deposit occurring during the fermentation of grape juice.

℃ Potassium Acid Tartrate is laxative in action. It may be used in baking with sodium bicarbonate as baking powder.

Potassium Bicarbonate. *Potassii Bicarbonas*
DOSES: B.P. 1-2 Gm. (15-30 gr.). $KHCO_3$. Mol.wt. 100.11.

S: 2.8 W; almost ins. A. Colourless crystals or a white granular powder; odourless; taste saline and slightly alkaline.

℃ Potassium bicarbonate has no obvious advantage over sodium bicarbonate as a gastric antacid but may be used with advantage as a urinary alkalizer and diuretic.

Potassium Bromide. *Potassii Bromidum*
DOSES: B.P. 0.3-1.2 Gm. (5-20 gr.); U.S.P. 1 Gm. (15 gr.). KBr. Mol.wt. 119.01. S: 1.5 W, 250 A, 5 G. White cubical crystals or a white granular powder; stable in air; odourless; taste saline.

Tablets of Potassium Bromide B.P.
Size, 5 gr. To be dissolved in water before administration.

℃ The actions of potassium bromide are due to the sedative effect of the bromide ion (see Sodium Bromide). It may be desirable sometimes to use the potassium salt if the patient is on a low sodium diet.

Potassium Carbonate N.F. *Potassii Carbonas*
$K_2CO_3 1\frac{1}{2}H_2O$. Mol.wt. 165.23. S: 1 W, 0.7 W 100°; ins. A. A white granular powder; odourless; taste strongly alkaline; very deliquescent. Used in Aromatic Rhubarb Syrup.

Potassium Chlorate B.P. *Potassii Chloras*
DOSES: 0.3-0.6 Gm. (5-10 gr.). $KClO_3$. Mol.wt. 122.6. S: at 15.5° 16 W, 30 G, 1700 A. A white powder or colourless crystals; taste cool and saline.

Tablets of Potassium Chlorate B.P.
Size, 0.3 Gm. (5 gr.). Dissolve slowly in the mouth.

℃ The chlorate ion, by liberating nascent oxygen, acts as an antiseptic. In some localities potassium chlorate in solution is used as a mouth wash or gargle. Tablets are available to suck for sore throat. If used too freely and swallowed, methaemoglobinaemia may be produced. Potassium chlorate is liable to spontaneous combustion and tablets should not be carried loosely in the pockets or in a paper container.

Potassium Chloride. *Potassii Chloridum*
DOSES: B.P. 1-2 Gm. (15-30 gr.); U.S.P. 1 Gm. (15 gr.). KCl. Mol.wt. 74.55. S: 2.8 W, 2 W 100°; ins. A, E. Colourless cubical crystals or a white granular powder; odourless; taste saline.

℃ Potassium chloride is a constituent of Ringer's Solution. It is sometimes administered to reveal latent adrenal insufficiency. If this condition is present a rather severe collapse may be produced. Potassium Chloride may be used instead of NaCl as a condiment in "salt free" diets.

Potassium Chloride Tablets U.S.P.
Sizes, 0.3 and 0.5 Gm. (5 and $7\frac{1}{2}$ gr.).

Potassium Citrate B.P.   *Potassii Citras*
DOSES: B.P. 1-2 Gm. (15-30 gr.). COOK.C(OH).(CH$_2$COOK)$_2$. H$_2$O. Mol.wt. 324.4.   S: 1 W, almost ins. A; readily sol. G.   White granular crystals or a crystalline powder; odourless; taste cool, saline; deliquescent.

℃ On absorption the citrate radicle is partly oxidized so that potassium citrate is an alkalizing diuretic, often used in cystitis, gout, and chronic arthritis.   The effervescent salt is pleasant to take. Citrates are more readily absorbed than tartrates and hence are less laxative.

Potassium Hydroxide.   *Potassii Hydroxidum.*   (*Potassa Caustica*, Caustic Potash)
KOH. Mol.wt. 56.10. S: 1 W, 3 A, 2.5 G; vs. A 78°. White or nearly white fused masses, pencils, pellets, sticks, flakes, etc.; very deliquescent.

℃ Potassium hydroxide is powerfully caustic but seldom used for that purpose.   Its chief use is as a pharmaceutical reagent.

Solution of Potassium Hydroxide B.P.   *Liquor Potassii Hydroxidi.* (*Liquor Potassae*, Solution of Potash)
Contains 4.75-5.25% w/v of KOH.

℃ The solution of potassium hydroxide may be used as a cuticle solvent.

Potassium Iodide.   *Potassii Iodidum*
DOSES: B.P. 0.3-2 Gm. (5-30 gr.); U.S.P. 0.3 Gm. (5 gr.). KI. Mol.wt. 166.02. S: 0.7 W, 0.5 W 100°, 22 A, 2 G. Cubical crystals; colourless, transparent or somewhat opaque or a white granular powder; odourless; taste saline and slightly bitter.

℃ Potassium or sodium iodide has an extraordinary variety of uses in medicine.   It is usually immaterial which salt is used since the effects are presumably due to the iodide ion. Potassium iodide in the Aqueous Solution of Iodine serves to hold the iodine in solution. Iodides are added to table salt to prevent goitre or to treat simple colloid goitre. Potassium iodide is often given to suppress the symptoms of hyperthyroidism, in preparation for operation or in conjunction with derivatives of thiouracil, or for the treatment of thyroid storm. In cough mixtures potassium iodide is often included to thin the bronchial secretions and to facilitate expectoration. Sodium iodide is sometimes given intravenously in acute intractable asthma. Good results have been reported but the rationale is uncertain. Perhaps it acts by thinning sticky bronchial secretions.

Syphilitic gummata, now seldom seen, are said to disappear rapidly under the influence of potassium iodide. By analogy, iodides have been used in other chronic inflammations, in hypertension and chronic vascular disease but with less obvious effect.

An occasional person has an idiosyncrasy to iodides often manifested in the form of rash or urticaria. Very occasionally a patient may develop oedema of the glottis and die.

Potassium Nitrate. *Potassii Nitras.* (Saltpetre, Nitre)

DOSES: 0.3-1 Gm. (5-15 gr.). KNO_3. Mol.wt. 101.10. S: 3 W, 0.5 W 100°, 620 A. Colourless, transparent prisms or a white crystalline powder; odourless; taste saline and cooling; slightly hygroscopic.

℄ Potassium nitrate is more effective as a diuretic than other salts of potassium, presumably because the nitrate ion, as well as the potassium ion, is poorly reabsorbed by the kidney. The salt is rather irritant to the alimentary tract and should be taken well diluted. Blotting paper may be soaked in a solution of potassium nitrate, dried and ignited and the fumes inhaled for asthma. Nitric oxide so liberated forms nitrite ions in the respiratory tract. This relaxes the bronchiolar muscle.

Potassium Permanganate. *Potassii Permanganas*

DOSES: B.P. 60-200 mg. (1-3 gr.). $KMnO_4$. Mol.wt. 158.0. S: 15 W, 3.5 W 100°. Dark purple, slender crystals having a metallic lustre; may have a dark bronze-like appearance; taste sweet and astringent.

℄ Potassium permanganate in solution has a variety of uses, all dependent on its oxidizing power. In 3-5% solution it may be applied to the rash produced by poison ivy. It oxidizes any residual oily irritant and is said to hasten healing. Very small amounts, just enough to make the water pink, may be used to disinfect drinking water.

Dilute solutions (1:1000) may be used to treat infected ulcers or for urethral irrigations; 1:4000 solutions are used as a vaginal douche.

The pure crystals are rubbed into snake bites to cauterize them and destroy the venom.

Sodium Potassium Tartrate B.P. *Sodii et Potassii Tartras.* (Rochelle Salt)

DOSES: B.P. 8-16 Gm. (120-240 gr.); $KNaC_4H_4O_6.4H_2O$. Mol. wt. 282.23. S: 1 W; ins. A. Colourless crystals or a white crystalline powder having a cool saline taste; efflorescent in warm dry air.

ℂ Tartrates are poorly absorbed from the alimentary tract and consequently act as laxatives. Rochelle Salt is commonly given for this purpose in the form of Seidlitz Powders.

Proflavine Hemisulphate B.P. *Proflavinae Hemisulphas.* (Neutral Proflavine Sulphate, Proflavine)

$(C_{13}H_{11}N_3)_2H_2SO_42H_2O$. Mol.wt. 552.6. S: 150 W 15.5°, 1 W 100°, 32 G; ss. A 90%; ins. E, C. An orange to red hygroscopic crystalline powder; odourless; taste bitter.

ℂ Proflavine, like acriflavine, is germicidal in very dilute solution, 1:150,000. Both are slowly germicidal, taking a matter of hours to kill but proflavine is rather more rapid in action. It is used in strengths of about 1:1000 to treat septic wounds or ulcers or to irrigate the bladder. It is relatively non-toxic to tissues.

Propylene Glycol U.S.P. *Glycol Propylenum*

$C_3H_8O_2$. Mol. wt. 76.09. Sp.gr. 1.035-1.037. S: misc. W, acetone, C; sol. E; dissolves many essential oils but is immiscible with fixed oils. A colourless, viscous liquid having a slight acrid taste; odourless. It may be used as a vehicle for certain injections, e.g. progesterone, and phenobarbitone.

Propylparaben U.S.P. *Propylparabenum.* (Propyl Parahydroxy-benzoate)

$C_3H_7.COO.C_6H_4OH$. Mol.wt. 180.20. Mp. 95-98°. S: 2000 W; sol. A, E, acetone. Small colourless crystals or a white powder.

℃ Propylparaben is fungistatic and bacteriostatic in dilute solution (less than 1:2000) and is used as a preservative for solutions, creams and ointments.

Pyroxylin. *Pyroxylinum.* (Soluble Guncotton)
S: dissolves slowly and completely in 25 parts of a solution of 3 volumes of ether and 1 volume of alcohol, giving a clear, almost colourless, solution. Contains chiefly cellulose tetranitrate; a white, matted mass of filaments resembling cotton wool; *highly inflammable.*

℃ Pyroxylin is used to make collodion.

Quassia B.P. *Quassia.* (Quassia Wood, Jamaica Quassia)
The stem wood of *Picraena excelsa* (Sw.) Lindl, consisting usually of yellowish-white chips or raspings of logs; odourless; taste persistently bitter.

Powdered Quassia B.P. *Quassiae Pulvis*
A pale buff powder.

Concentrated Infusion of Quassia B.P. *Infusum Quassiae Concentratum*
DOSES: 2-4 cc. (30-60 min.). Quassia 8 Gm. to make 100 cc. Contains 21-24% v/v of C_2H_5OH. When diluted with 7 times its volume of distilled water it yields a preparation approximately equivalent in strength but not in flavour to the fresh infusion.

Fresh Infusion of Quassia B.P. *Infusum Quassiae Recens*
DOSES: 15-30 cc. ($\frac{1}{2}$-1 fl.oz.). Quassia 1, cold Distilled Water 100.

Infusion of Quassia B.P. *Infusum Quassiae*
DOSES: 15-30 cc. ($\frac{1}{2}$-1 fl.oz.). Concentrated Infusion of Quassia 12.5, Distilled Water to make 100 cc.

Tincture of Quassia B.P. *Tinctura Quassiae*
DOSES: 2-4 cc. (30-60 min.). Quassia 10, Alcohol 45% 100, by maceration. Contains 43-45% v/v of C_2H_5OH.

℃ Quassia is called a simple bitter because it contains no tannic acid or other astringents. It contains the bitter principles alpha and beta picrasmin, which are said to be toxic to insects and useful as insecticides. Little is known of the pharmacology of these substances but they seem to be relatively harmless to humans since large doses of the galenical preparations taken by mouth produce only vomiting, dizziness, and weakness. Infusions of quassia are used as rentention enemas to treat pin worms in children. After the rectum has been emptied by an ordinary enema, about half a pint of infusion is injected and retained as long as possible. The infusion, according to some authorities, should be made freshly from 1 part of chips to 20 parts of cold water.

The tincture is used mainly in bitter tonics.

Quillaia B.P. *Quillaia.* (Quillaia Bark, Soap Bark)

The dried inner bark of *Quillaja saponaria* or other species of *Quillaja*; odourless; dust strongly sternutatory; taste, acrid and astringent.

Powdered Quillaia B.P. *Quillaiae Pulvis*

A pale buff powder with a pink tinge.

Liquid Extract of Quillaia B.P. *Extractum Quillaiae Liquidum*

Quillaia 100 Gm. to make 100 cc., by percolation. Contains 28-34% v/v of C_2H_5OH.

⟪ Liquid Extract of Quillaia is used as an emulsifying agent.

Quinacrine Hydrochloride. see **Mepacrine**

Quinidine Sulphate. *Quinidinae Sulphas*

DOSES: B.P. 60-300 mg.(1-5 gr.); U.S.P. 0.2 Gm. (3 gr.). $(C_{20}H_{24}N_2O_2)_2.H_2SO_4.2H_2O.$ Mol.wt. 782.92. S: 100 W, 15 W 100°, 10 A; sol. C; almost ins. E. The sulphate of the alkaloid quinidine, obtained from the bark of various species of *Cinchona* and their hybrids (and from *Remijia pedunculata* U.S.P.). It may be prepared from quinine. Colourless, needle-like crystals; odourless; taste intensely bitter; efflorescent; darkens on exposure to light; contains 82-87% of quinidine alkaloid.

Quinidine Sulfate Capsules U.S.P.

Size, 200 mg. (3 gr.).

Quinidine Sulfate Tablets U.S.P.

Sizes, 100, 200 and 300 mg. (1½, 3 and 5 gr.).

⟪ Quinidine is the dextro-isomer of quinine and has many similar actions but has a much greater effect on muscle, particularly cardiac muscle. It prolongs the refractory period and decreases the excitability of cardiac muscle. Unlike digitalis, it does not increase the force of muscular contraction. Quinidine is given to stop or to prevent cardiac arrhythmias characterized by rapid heart rate, provided that the ventricular muscle is relatively healthy and efficient, e.g. paroxysmal tachycardia, paroxysmal auricular flutter, or paroxysmal auricular fibrillation. It is contraindicated if delayed conduction or heart block is present.

Some people react badly to quinidine so that a test dose of 0.2 Gm. should be given on the first occasion and repeated in two hours. If no ill effects follow, such as nausea, vomiting, convulsions, more serious cardiac irregularities, or respiratory distress, within another two hours full doses may be given.

Quinine Bisulphate B.P. *Quininae Bisulphas.* (Quinine Acid Sulphate)

DOSES: B.P. 0-3-0.6 Gm. (5-10 gr.). $C_{20}H_{24}N_2O_2H_2SO_4.7H_2O$. Mol wt. 548.60. S: 10 W, 25 A, 15 G, 625 C, 1 W 100°, 1 A 78°. The bisulphate of the alkaloid quinine obtained from the bark of various species of *Cinchona*; white or colourless needles or a white crystalline powder; odourless; taste intensely bitter; efflorescent; turns yellow on exposure to light; contains 58-62% of quinine alkaloid.

Tablets of Quinine Bisulphate B.P.

Size, 0.3 Gm. (5 gr.).

Quinine Dihydrochloride. *Quininae Dihydrochloridum.* (Acid Quinine Hydrochloride, Quinine Acid Hydrochloride)

DOSES: B.P. oral or intravenous, 0.3-0.6 Gm. (5-10 gr.); U.S.P. 1 Gm. (15 gr.). $C_{20}H_{24}N_2O_2.2HCl$. Mol.wt. 397.34. S: 0.6 W, 12A. A white or colourless, odourless powder having an intensely bitter taste. It is affected by light. Contains 79-82% of quinine alkaloid.

Injection of Quinine Dihydrochloride B.P.

Strength, 0.3 Gm. in 5 cc. (5 gr. in 75 min.). To be diluted with at least 10 times its volume of Injection of Sodium Chloride before administration and injected slowly into a vein.

Quinine Ethyl Carbonate B.P. *Quininae et Aethylis Carbonas.* (Euquinine)

DOSES: 0.3-0.6 Gm. (5-10 gr.). $C_{20}H_{23}O_2N_2CO_2.C_2H_5$. Mol.wt. 396.47. M.p. not below 90°. S: ss. W, 3 A, 1 C, 10 E; readily sol. in dil. acids. Fine, white, soft needles usually matted together;

odourless; practically tasteless but when chewed has a bitter taste; contains 80-82% of anhydrous quinine.

Quinine Hydrochloride. *Quininae Hydrochloridum*

DOSES: B.P. 0.3-0.6 Gm. (5-10 gr.); U.S.P. 0.6 Gm. (10 gr.); intramuscular, 0.2 Gm. (3 gr.). $C_{20}H_{24}N_2O_2.HCl.2H_2O$. Mol.wt. 396.91. S: 16 W, 1 A, 1 C, 7 G, 350 E, 0.5 W 100°. The hydrochloride of quinine. White or colourless glistening needles having a very bitter taste; odourless; efflorescent in warm air; contains 81-83% anhydrous quinine.

Tablets of Quinine Hydrochloride B.P.

Size, 0.3 Gm. (5 gr.).

Quinine Sulphate. *Quininae Sulphas*

DOSES: B.P. 0.3-0.6 Gm. (5-10 gr.); U.S.P. 0.6 Gm. (10 gr.). $(C_{20}H_{24}N_2O_2)_2.H_2SO_4.2H_2O$. Mol.wt. 782.92. S: 810 W, 120 A, 35 W 100°, 10 A 78°; ss. C, E; fs. in a solution containing 2 vol. C and 1 vol. dehydrated A. The sulphate of quinine. White, fine, usually lustreless needle-like crystals; odourless; taste intensely bitter; may turn slightly brown on exposure to light; contains 82-84% of quinine alkaloid.

Quinine Sulfate Capsules U.S.P.

Sizes, 120, 200, and 300 mg. (2, 3, and 5 gr.).

Quinine Sulfate Tablets U.S.P.

Sizes, 0.12, 0.2 and 0.3 Gm. (2, 3 and 5 gr.).

℀ The cinchona alkaloids have been used to treat fevers for over 300 years. Of these, quinine and its various salts are the best known. Its main useful action is to kill or suppress the growth of malarial parasites at concentrations not unduly toxic to the host. It has been used for many fevers of non-malarial origin and sometimes seems effective. It is thought by some that quinine acts as an antipyretic in fevers, like salicylates, lowering the febrile temperature by increasing vasodilation. However, any such action must be considered of secondary importance in the use of quinine. Although quinine is rather depressant to most muscles, it is said to stimulate uterine muscle to rhythmic contraction and is sometimes used, together with castor oil, to initiate labour.

Although many new antimalarials have been introduced in recent years, quinine and its salts retain an important position in the treatment of malaria. The choice of salt for administration seems to be a matter of personal preference. The acid salts, the bisulphate and the dihydrochloride are very soluble and hence may be absorbed more rapidly than the others. They would, of course, be the ones to use in mixtures. Administration is usually by mouth but sometimes in very sick patients intravenous injection may be advisable. Note that the Injection of Quinine and Urea Hydrochloride is not for the treatment of malaria but for sclerosing varicose veins or haemorrhoids.

Overdoses of quinine give rise to a symptom complex known as *cinchonism*, characterized by headache and ringing in the ears. In severe cases deafness, confusion, and delirium may ensue. Eight to 10 Gm. is considered a fatal dose. Urticarial and erythematous reactions to small doses are not uncommon.

Injection of Quinine and Urethane B.P.

DOSES: intravenous, *as a sclerosing agent*, 0.5-5 cc. (8-75 min.). Contains Quinine Hydrochloride 12.5 Gm., Urethane 6.25 Gm. and Water for Injection to make 100 cc. Solid matter may separate on standing. It should be redissolved by warming. The syringe should be previously warmed.

Quinine and Urethane Injection U.S.P. (Quinine Hydrochloride and Ethyl Carbamate Injection U.S.P. XII)

Quinine Hydrochloride 250 mg. (4 gr.) and Urethane 120 mg. (2 gr.) in 2 cc.

℀ The Injection of Quinine and Urethane is used to sclerose varicose veins.

Raspberry Juice U.S.P. *Succus Rubi Idaei*

The juice expressed from the ripe fruit of varieties of *Rubus idaeus* (Linn.) or *Rubus strigosus* (Michaux). Sp.gr. 1.025-1.045. A red to reddish orange liquid with aromatic characteristic odour and characteristic sour taste.

Raspberry Syrup U.S.P. *Syrupus Rubi Idaei*

Raspberry Juice 475, Sucrose 800, Alcohol 20, Water to make 1000 cc. Contains 1%-2% C_2H_5OH.

Resorcinol. *Resorcinol.* (Resorcin, Metadihydroxybenzene)

C_6H_4-1: 3-$(OH)_2$. Mol.wt. 110.11. M.p. 109-111°. S: 1 W, 1 A;

fs. G, E; ss. C.   White or nearly white needle-shaped crystals or powder having a slight characteristic odour; taste sweetish, then bitter; turns pink on exposure to light.

℃ Resorcinol is an antiseptic and antipruritic, often used in the treatment of various skin diseases.   A 1% aqueous solution is used for dandruff.   Ointments varying in strengths from 5-20% are used for psoriasis.   *Caution: Resorcinol discolours blond hair.*

Rhubarb B.P.   *Rheum*
The dried rhizome of various species of *Rheum* grown in China and Tibet, but not *Rheum Rhaponticum* (common rhubarb).

Powdered Rhubarb B.P.   *Rhei Pulvis*
DOSES: 0.2-1 Gm. (3-15 gr.).   Orange-yellow to brown powder.

Compound Pill of Rhubarb B.P.   *Pilula Rhei Composita.*   (Compound Rhubarb Pill)
DOSES: 0.25-0.5 Gm. (4-8 gr.).   Rhubarb 25, Aloes 20, with Myrrh, Hard Soap, Oil of Peppermint, and Syrup of Liquid Glucose to make about 100 Gm.

Compound Tincture of Rhubarb B.P.   *Tinctura Rhei Composita*
DOSES: 2-4 cc. (30-60 min.).   Rhubarb 100 Gm., with Cardamom, Coriander, Glycerin and Alcohol to make 1000 cc., by percolation. Contains 48-53% v/v of C_2H_5OH.

Compound Powder of Rhubarb B.P.   *Pulvis Rhei Compositus.*   (Gregory's Powder)
DOSES: 0.6-4 Gm. (10-60 gr.).   Rhubarb 25, Heavy Magnesium Carbonate 32.5, Light Magnesium Carbonate 32.5, with Ginger to make 100 Gm.

℃ The various preparations of rhubarb are used for their cathartic action, which is due to emodin or other anthracene derivatives. The action is principally on the large intestine and movements occur 8 to 12 hours after administration.   Rhubarb contains much tannic acid which is said to produce some constipation after the laxative action is over.   Some persons develop dermatitis if given preparations of rhubarb.

Ringer's Solution U.S.P.   *Liquor Ringeri.*   (Isotonic Solution of Three Chlorides U.S.P. XII)
Three grades are recognized, (1) non-sterile, (2) sterile, not for

parenteral use, (3) sterile, for parenteral use. The last meets a requirement for freedom from pyrogens. Sodium Chloride 8.6, Potassium Chloride 0.3, Calcium Chloride 0.33, Distilled Water recently boiled to make 1000 cc. Unless otherwise specified, Sterile Ringer's Solution for Parenteral Use made with Water for Injection must be dispensed.

Compound Injection of Sodium Chloride B.P. (Ringer's Solution for Injection, Compound Solution of Sodium Chloride)
Sodium Chloride 8.6 Gm., Potassium Chloride 0.3 Gm., Hydrated Calcium Chloride 0.48 Gm., Water for Injection to make 1000 cc.

ℂ For the maintenance of body fluids and electrolytes, it has been the custom in the past to administer continuous intravenous infusions of isotonic solutions of sodium chloride rather than Ringer's solution, because it was felt that the body could easily supply the small amount of other electrolytes required. This may be so most of the time, but probably not always. Ringer's solution should be preferable. The non-sterile solution might be given orally, and the sterile solution not for parenteral use might be used externally.

Lactated Ringer's Solution U.S.P. *Liquor Ringeri Lacticus*
A clear, colourless or not more than slightly coloured liquid, sterilized for injection, containing in each 100 cc., between 18 and 22 mg. $CaCl_2.2H_2O$, 27 and 33 mg. KCl, 570 and 630 mg. NaCl and 290 and 330 mg. sodium lactate ($NaC_3H_5O_3$). Concentrated solutions suitable for dilution are available.

Compound Injection of Sodium Lactate B.P. (Hartmann's Solution for Injection, Ringer-Lactate Solution for Injection)
Lactic Acid 2.4 cc., Sodium Hydroxide q.s., Sodium Chloride 6 Gm., Potassium Chloride 0.4 Gm., Hydrated Calcium Chloride 0.4 Gm., Water for Injection to make 1000 cc. Adjusted to pH of about 7.0.

ℂ When acidosis, as well as dehydration, is to be corrected, Lactated Ringer's Solution is indicated. The lactate ion is oxidized, leaving extra basic ions to neutralize fixed acids.

Ricinoleic Acid B.P. *Acidum Ricinoleicum*
Gm./cc. 0.940-0.943. S: ins. W; sol. A, E. A yellow or yellowish-brown viscous liquid; odour and taste characteristic.

℃ Ricinoleic Acid forms a soap which is said to be more antiseptic than other soaps and is used to emulsify chloroxylenol in Solution of Chloroxylenol (Dettol, Roxenol).

Rose Oil U.S.P. *Oleum Rosae.* (Otto of Rose)
Sp.gr. 0.848-0.863 at 30°. S: 1 C. The volatile oil distilled with steam from the fresh flowers of *Rosa gallica, Rosa damascena, Rosa alba, Rosa centifolia* and varieties of these species. A colourless or yellowish liquid having the characteristic odour and taste of rose. At 25° it is a viscous liquid and on cooling becomes a translucent crystalline mass.

℃ Rose oil is used only for its perfume.

Stronger Rose Water U.S.P. *Aqua Rosae Fortior*
A saturated solution of the odoriferous principles of the flowers of *Rosa centifolia* prepared by distilling the fresh flowers with water and separating the excess volatile oil.

℃ Rose water confers a pleasant odour in creams and lotions.

Rose Water U.S.P. *Aqua Rosae*
Stronger Rose Water 1, Distilled Water 1.

Rose Water Ointment U.S.P. *Unguentum Aquae Rosae*
Spermaceti 125, White Wax 120, Expressed Almond Oil 560 Gm., Sodium Borate 5, Rose Water 50, Distilled Water 140, Rose Oil 0.2 cc., to make 1000 Gm.

℃ Rose Water Ointment is a typical cold cream, containing about 20% of water. It is used to thin or dilute other ointments.

Petrolatum Rose Water Ointment U.S.P. *Unguentum Aquae Rosae Petrolatum*
Spermaceti 125, White Wax 120, Liquid Petrolatum 560, Sodium Borate 5, Rose Water 50, Distilled Water 140, Rose Oil 0.2 to make about 1000 Gm; a cheaper formula for cold cream.

Oil of Rosemary. *Oleum Rosmarini*
Gm./cc. 0.895-0.914. S: 10 A 80%, 1 A 90%. The volatile oil distilled from the fresh flowering tops of *Rosmarinus officinalis*.

℃ Oil of Rosemary is used in scalp lotions for a supposed favourable effect on the growth of hair. It has a rubefacient action.

Saccharin. *Saccharinum.* (Gluside, Benzosulfimide)

$C_7H_5O_3NS$. Mol.wt. 183.18. M.p. 226-230°. S: 290 W, 31 A, 25 W 100°; ss. E, C; readily sol. in alkaline solutions. White crystals or a white crystalline powder; odourless or having a faint aromatic odour. In dilute solution it is 300-500 times as sweet as sucrose.

Saccharin Sodium. *Saccharinum Sodicum.* (Soluble Gluside, Sodium Benzosulfimide, Soluble Saccharin)

$C_7H_4O_3NS.Na.2H_2O$. Mol.wt. 241.20. S: 1.5 W, 50 A. White crystals or a white crystalline powder; odourless or with a faint aromatic odour; taste intensely sweet; efflorescent.

Saccharin Sodium Tablets U.S.P.

Sizes, 15, 30, 60 mg. ($\frac{1}{4}$, $\frac{1}{2}$, 1 gr.). One 60 mg. (1 gr.) Saccharin Sodium Tablet is equivalent in sweetening power to approximately 30 Gm. Sucrose.

℄ Soluble saccharin is used more often than saccharin for sweetening liquids. Careful studies have revealed no harmful effects from long-continued use. One part of saccharin in 3000 of final solution gives sufficient sweetness for most purposes.

Salicylic Acid. *Acidum Salicylicum.* (Orthohydroxybenzoic Acid)

$OH.C_6H_4.COOH$. Mol.wt. 138.12. M.p. 158-161°. S: 460 W, 3 A, 45 C, 3 E, 135 B, 15 W 100°. White needles or a fine, fluffy, crystalline powder; taste sweetish, afterwards acrid.

℄ Salicylic Acid is bacteriostatic and fungistatic; 1-2% in alcohol may be applied to the feet to combat fungus infections or malodorous perspiration. A 10% solution in collodion softens callouses and corns. For systemic actions see Sodium Salicylate.

Salicylic Acid Plaster U.S.P. *Emplastrum Acidi Salicylici*

A plaster prepared by spreading a uniform mixture of Salicylic Acid in a suitable base on paper, cotton cloth or other suitable backing material. The salicylic acid content must be 90%-110% of the labelled amount. This plaster may be used to destroy warts or corns. The B.P.C. specifies 18%-22% of salicylic acid in the adhesive mass for such purposes.

Ointment of Salicylic Acid B.P. *Unguentum Acidi Salicylici.* (Salicylic Acid Ointment)

Salicylic Acid 2, Ointment of Wool Alcohols 98.

⟪ This ointment is sometimes used for the treatment of epidermophytosis.

Santonin B.P. *Santoninum*
Doses: 60-200 mg. (1-3 gr.). $C_{15}H_{18}O_3$. Mol.wt. 246.3. M.p. 171-174.° S: almost ins. W, 50 A 90%, 2.5 C 15.5°. The bitter principle prepared from the dried unexpanded flowerheads of *Artemisia cina* and other species. Colourless, flat, rhombic prisms or a white crystalline powder; becomes yellow when exposed to air.

⟪ Santonin is an anthelmintic which is particularly effective against roundworms (ascaris), but also used for pinworms (oxyuris) and threadworms (trichuris). Its use is said to be decreasing since newer and safer agents, such as hexylresorcinol, have become available. The drug is usually administered in the form of a powder on an empty stomach in the morning. No breakfast is allowed and a saline purge is given 2 hours after the santonin. A fairly common symptom of mild toxic action by santonin is xanthopsia, yellow vision. More severe poisoning is characterized by further derangement of vision, taste and smell, mental confusion, and convulsions.

Sarsaparilla U.S.P. *Sarsaparilla*
The dried root of *Smilax aristolochiaefolia*, *Smilax Regelii* or of undetermined species of *Smilax*. Almost odourless; taste somewhat sweetish, acrid, and mucilaginous.

Sarsaparilla Fluidextract U.S.P. *Fluidextractum Sarsaparillae*
Sarsaparilla 1000 Gm., by maceration and percolation with diluted alcohol to make 1000 cc. Contains 37-42% v/v of C_2H_5OH.

Compound Sarsaparilla Syrup U.S.P. *Syrupus Sarsaparillae Compositus*
Sarsaparilla Fluidextract 200, Glycyrrhizae Fluidextract 15, Sassafras Oil 0.2, Anise Oil 0.2, Methyl Salicylate 0.2, Alcohol 19.4, Syrup 765. To make about 1000 cc. Contains 8.5-11% v/v of C_2H_5OH.

⟪ This syrup has good covering power for disagreeable drugs because it has a strong and persistent taste. The **Compound Syrup of Sassafras C.F.** is very similar.

Oil of Sassafras C.F. Sassafras Oil U.S.P. *Oleum Sassafras*
DOSES: C.F. 0.06-0.2 cc. (1-3 min.). S: 2 A 90%. The volatile oil distilled from the root of *Sassafras* (*variifolium* C.F., *albidum* U.S.P.). A yellow to reddish-yellow liquid having the characteristic odour and taste of safrol.

Senega B.P. *Senega.* (Senega Root)
The dried root of *Polygala Senega*; taste sweet at first, then acrid; odour resembling methyl salicylate.

Powdered Senega B.P. *Senegae Pulvis*
A grey powder.

Concentrated Infusion of Senega B.P. *Infusum Senegae Concentratum*
DOSES: 2-4 cc. (30-60 min.). Senega 40, with Dilute Solution of Ammonia and Alcohol to make 100, by percolation. Contains 20-24% v/v of C_2H_5OH. When diluted with 7 vols. of water it approximates a fresh infusion in strength but not in flavour.

Infusion of Senega B.P. *Infusum Senegae*
DOSES: 15-30 cc. ($\frac{1}{2}$-1 fl.oz.). Concentrated Infusion of Senega 12.5, Distilled Water to make 100 cc.

Liquid Extract of Senega B.P. *Extractum Senegae Liquidum*
DOSES: 0.3-1 cc. (5-15 min.). Senega 100 Gm. with Dilute Solution of Ammonia q.s. and Alcohol to make 100 cc., by percolation, evaporation, and re-solution. Contains 38-44% v/v of C_2H_5OH.

Tincture of Senega B.P. *Tinctura Senegae*
DOSES: 2-4 cc. (30-60 min.). Liquid Extract of Senega 20 cc. in 100 cc. Contains 55-58% v/v of C_2H_5OH.

℄ Senega is used mainly as a expectorant. The action is due to saponins which irritate the mucosa of the alimentary tract and reflexly stimulate bronchial secretions.

Senna Fruit B.P. *Sennae Fructus.* (Senna Pod)
DOSES: 0.6-2 Gm. (10-30 gr.). The dried ripe fruits (pods) of *Cassia acutifolia* and of *Cassia angustifolia*.

Senna Leaf B.P. *Sennae Folium.*
DOSE: U.S.P. 2 Gm. (30 gr.). The dried leaflets of *Cassia*

acutifolia and of *Cassia angustifolia*. Taste mucilaginous and slightly bitter.

Powdered Senna Leaf B.P. *Sennae Foliae Pulvis*
DOSES: 0.6-2 Gm. (10-30 gr.). A green to yellowish-green powder.

Liquid Extract of Senna B.P. *Extractum Sennae Liquidum*
DOSES: 0.6-2 cc. (10-30 min.). Senna Fruit 100 Gm., Oil of Coriander, Alcohol, Chloroform Water, and Distilled Water to make 100 cc., by maceration. Contains 21-24% v/v of C_2H_5OH.

Concentrated Infusion of Senna B.P. *Infusum Sennae Concentratum*
DOSES: 2-8 cc. (30-120 min.). Senna Fruit 80, Strong Tincture of Ginger and Alcohol to make 100 cc., by percolation. Contains 20-24% v/v of C_2H_5OH.

Infusion of Senna B.P. *Infusum Sennae*
DOSES: 15-60 cc. ($\frac{1}{2}$-2 fl.oz.). Concentrated Infusion of Senna 12.5, Distilled Water to make 100 cc.

Compound Mixture of Senna B.P. *Mistura Sennae Composita.*
(Black Draught)
DOSES: 30-60 cc. (1-2 fl.oz.). Magnesium Sulphate 25 Gm., Liquid Extract of Liquorice 5, Compound Tincture of Cardamom 10, Aromatic Spirit of Ammonia 5, with Infusion of Senna to make 100 cc.

⟨ Senna is a cathartic. The active principle is thought to belong to the anthracene group which acts mainly on the large bowel. Laxative effects occur 10 to 12 hours after administration. Senna is said to be the active ingredient of Castoria.

Syrup of Senna B.P. *Syrupus Sennae*
DOSES: 2-8 cc. (30-120 min.). Liquid Extract of Senna 25, Syrup to make 100.

Scopolamine. See Hysocine.

Sesame Oil. *Oleum Sesami*
Gm./cc. 0.916-0.919. Sp.gr. 0.916-0.921. S: ss. A; misc. E, C, petroleum benzin, carbon disulfide. The fixed oil obtained from the seed of one or more cultivated varieties of *Sesamum indicum*. A pale-yellow liquid having a slight odour and bland taste.

ⵁ Sesame oil is an accepted substitute for olive oil in soaps and liniments. It is also used in the manufacture of margarine. Sesame oil is being used increasingly as a vehicle in oily injections. It is said to be non-allergenic.

Sex Hormone-like Drugs are presented in the following order:— androgens, oestrogens, gonadotrophins, progestins.

ANDROGENS

Methyltestosterone. *Methyltestosteronum*
DOSES: B.P. daily for men, 25-50 mg. ($\frac{2}{5}$-$\frac{3}{4}$ gr.); daily for women, 5-20 mg. ($\frac{1}{12}$-$\frac{1}{3}$ gr.); U.S.P. oral, 10 mg. ($\frac{1}{6}$ gr.), sublingual, 5 mg. ($\frac{1}{12}$ gr.). $C_{20}H_{30}O_2$. Mol.wt. 302.44. M.p. 161-167°; S: ins. W; sol. A, methanol, E, other organic solvents; sps. in vegetable oils. White or slightly yellow crystals or crystalline powder; odourless; tasteless; affected by light.

Methyltestosterone Tablets U.S.P.
Sizes, 10 and 25 mg.

Tablets of Methyltestosterone B.P.
Size, 5 mg. ($\frac{1}{12}$ gr.).

Testosterone U.S.P. *Testosteronum*
DOSE: 0.3 Gm. (5 gr.) by implantation. $C_{19}H_{28}O_2$. Mol.wt. 288.41. M.p. 152-156°. S: ins. W, 6 A abs. 2 C, 100 E; sol. in dioxan and in vegetable oils. White or creamy white crystals or a crystalline powder; odourless.

Testosterone Pellets U.S.P.
Size, 75 mg. (1$\frac{1}{4}$ gr.); for subcutaneous implantation.

Testosterone Propionate. *Testosteroni Propionas*
DOSES: B.P. intramuscular, 5-25 mg. ($\frac{1}{12}$-$\frac{2}{5}$ gr.) daily; U.S.P. 25 mg. ($\frac{3}{8}$ gr.) intramuscularly. $C_{22}H_{32}O_3$. Mol.wt. 344.48. M.p. 118-122°. S: ins. W; fs. A, E; sol. in vegetable oils. White or slightly yellow crystals or a crystalline powder; odourless; stable in air.

Injection of Testosterone Propionate B.P.
Strength, 10 mg. per cc. ($\frac{1}{6}$ gr. in 15 min.). A sterile solution in Ethyl Oleate or a suitable oil.

Testosterone Propionate Injection U.S.P.

Sizes, 5, 10, 25 mg. (1/12, 1/6, ⅜ gr.) in 1 cc.; 250 mg. (4 gr.) in 10 cc.

⫶ Androgenic substances have the actions of male sex hormone. They cause the development of secondary sex characteristics in the male and maturation of the genitalia. They maintain spermato-genesis. The two most useful are methyltestosterone and testo-sterone. Both are prepared synthetically. Androsterone is another androgen which is found in the urine of males. It is much less active than the other two. Methyltestosterone is active by mouth or sublingually, while testosterone must be injected. It may also be given through the skin by inunction.

The most obvious use of androgens is to replace testicular function after castration or atrophy of the testicles. For such applications testosterone is injected in oily solution or a pellet of 75 mg. may be implanted under the skin for a prolonged effect. Another use is for elderly men who may be suffering symptoms of the male climacteric. For such, methyltestosterone sublingually seems to be preferred. Androgenic therapy is reported to relieve symptoms of prostatic enlargement. It may also be administered to women for a variety of complaints such as dysmenorrhoea. Overdosage, e.g. more than 300 mg. of testosterone a month, will produce virilism in women. The use of androgens in women is in its experimental stage. One other use in women is to check lactation.

OESTROGENIC SUBSTANCES

Oestrogenic substances fall into two groups (a) synthetic, (b) natural. In the synthetic group are stilboestrol, dienoestrol, and hexoestrol, while the natural group includes oestrone, oestradiol, oestriol, and their esters. It seems that, for all practical purposes, the synthetic materials imitate exactly the actions of the natural materials. Under experimental conditions, some differences can be demonstrated. For example, stilboestrol will not antagonize the action of androgens on the growth of the comb in capons, as natural oestrogens do.

The oestrogens are powerful drugs producing many changes in the body. The main effects are:

(1) Maturation of vagina and uterus.

(2) Maturation of the breasts.

(3) Proliferation of the endometrium.

(4) Thickening and cornification of vaginal epithelium.

(5) Sensitization of uterine muscle to oxytocic hormone of the posterior pituitary.

(6) Retention of fluid in certain parts of the body, including subcutaneous tissue.

(7) Carcinogenesis in susceptible strains of animals.

The most important use of oestrogens is to treat menopausal symptoms, certain types of functional bleeding, and certain types of painful menstruation. A variety of other uses are experimental, e.g. palliative treatment of carcinoma of the prostate. At one time oestrogens were applied locally to treat vulvovaginitis in young children by producing cornification of the vagina. This use has been rendered unnecessary since the advent of penicillin, except when infection is due to resistant organisms.

Dienoestrol B.P.   *Dienoestrol.*   (Dihydroxydiphenylhexadiene)

DOSES: 0.1-5 mg. ($\frac{1}{600}$-$\frac{1}{12}$ gr.) daily. $C_{18}H_{18}O_2$. Mol.wt. 266.3. M.p. 233-234°. S: ins W; sol. A 90%, acetone, E; ss. B; sol. in solutions of NaOH in H_2O. A colourless crystalline powder; odourless.

Tablets of Dienoestrol B.P.

Size, 0.1 mg. ($\frac{1}{600}$ gr.).

❡ Dienoestrol is a synthetic oestrogen of somewhat greater potency than stilboestrol.

Diethylstilbestrol U.S.P.   *Diethylstilbestrol.*   **Stilboestrol B.P.** *Stilboestrol*

DOSES: B.P. 0.5-2 mg. ($\frac{1}{120}$-$\frac{1}{30}$ gr.) daily; U.S.P. 0.5 mg. ($\frac{1}{120}$ gr.). $C_{18}H_{20}O_2$. Mol.wt. 268.34. M.p. 168-172°. S: almost ins. W; sol. A, C, E, fatty oils and in dilute alkali hydroxides. A white, odourless, crystalline powder.

❡ Stilboestrol is a synthetic substance of relatively simple structure which nevertheless imitates the actions of oestrogenic hormones of the ovary. It is active by mouth. To control menopausal symptoms a daily dose of 0.5 to 1 mg. is adequate; larger doses may cause nausea and vomiting or gain in weight due to retention of fluid.

Diethylstilbestrol Injection U.S.P.

Strengths, 0.5 mg. ($\frac{1}{120}$ gr.) in 1 cc., 1 mg. ($\frac{1}{60}$ gr.) in 1 cc. in a suitable oil, for intramuscular injection.

Diethylstilbestrol Capsules U.S.P.

Sizes, 0.1, 0.5 and 1 mg. ($\frac{1}{600}$, $\frac{1}{120}$, $\frac{1}{60}$ gr.).

Diethylstilbestrol Tablets U.S.P.

Sizes, 0.1, 0.5, 1 mg. ($\frac{1}{600}$, $\frac{1}{120}$, $\frac{1}{60}$ gr.).

Tablets of Stilboestrol B.P.

Size, 0.5 mg. ($\frac{1}{120}$ gr.).

Stilboestrol Dipropionate Can. Supp. *Stilboestrolis Dipropionas.*
(Diethylstilboestrol Dipropionate)

Doses: 1-5 mg. ($\frac{1}{60}$-$\frac{1}{12}$ gr.) intramuscularly. $C_{24}H_{28}O_4$. Mol.wt. 380.2; M.p. 103-106°. S: ins. W; sol. A, C, E, B and in fatty oils. A white powder or colourless or pale cream crystalline plates; odourless.

Hexoestrol B.P. *Hexoestrol*

Doses: 1-5 mg. ($\frac{1}{60}$-$\frac{1}{12}$ gr.) daily. $C_{18}H_{22}O_2$. Mol.wt. 270.4. M.p. 185-188°. S: ins. W; sol. A 95%, acetone; ss. C; sol. E, vegetable oils and dilute solutions of NaOH in H_2O. Colourless crystals or crystalline powder; odourless.

Tablets of Hexoestrol B.P.

Size, 1 mg. ($\frac{1}{60}$ gr.).

⟪ Hexoestrol is a synthetic oestrogen which is a little less potent than stilboestrol.

Estradiol U.S.P. *Estradiol.* (Dehydrotheelin, Oestradiol, Alpha-estradiol)

Dose: 0.2 mg. ($\frac{1}{300}$ gr.). M.p. 173-179°. S: almost ins. W; sol. A, in acetone, dioxane, solutions of fixed alkali hydroxides; sparingly sol. in vegetable oils. White or yellow small crystals or a crystalline powder; odourless and stable in air.

Estradiol Tablets U.S.P.

Sizes, 0.1 and 0.2 mg. (1/600 and 1/300 gr.).

⟪ Oestradiol, oestrone, and their esters are known as natural oestrogenic materials. They are usually prepared commercially from pregnant mares' urine. They are much more expensive than the derivatives of stilboestrol and have no obvious advantages over the latter.

Estradiol Benzoate U.S.P. *Estradiolis Benzoas.* Oestradiol Monobenzoate B.P. *Oestradiolis Monobenzoas.* (Dihydroxyoestrin Monobenzoate)

DOSES: B.P. intramuscular, daily, 1-5 mg. $(\frac{1}{60}-\frac{1}{12}$ gr.) (10,000-50,000 units); U.S.P. 1 mg. $(\frac{1}{60}$ gr.), intramuscularly. $C_{18}H_{23}O.C_7H_5O_2$. Mol.wt. 376.47. M.p. 190-196°. S: almost ins. W; sol. A, acetone, dioxane; ss. E; sps. in vegetable oils. The benzoate of alpha-estradiol. White or slightly yellow to brownish crystalline powder; odourless; stable in air. The B.P. unit of oestrogenic activity (benzoate standard) is the specific oestrus producing activity contained in 0.0001 mg. of the standard preparation of the monobenzoate of dihydroxyoestrin.

Estradiol Benzoate Injection U.S.P.

1 cc. contains 0.166, 0.333, 1 or 1.66 mg (1/400, 1/200, 1/60 or 1/40 gr.); 10 cc. contain 1.66 or 3.33 mg. (1/40 or 1/20 gr.) in oil.

Injection of Oestradiol Monobenzoate B.P.

Strength, 1 mg. per cc. $(\frac{1}{60}$ gr. in 15 min.). A sterile solution in Ethyl Oleate or a suitable oil.

Oestriol Glycuronate N. (T.N. Emmenin)

This orally active oestrogen is assayed in Collip units, which are hard to equate to international units. It is usually given in doses of 120 units, i.e. one tablet or 1 teaspoonful of Emmenin Liquid. Such dosage is considered to be decidedly less potent than 0.5 mg. of stilboestrol.

Estrone U.S.P. *Estronum.* Oestrone B.P. *Oestronum.* (Theelin) Ketohydroxyoestrin)

DOSES: B.P. 1-10 mg. $(\frac{1}{60}-\frac{1}{6}$ gr.) daily; U.S.P. 1 mg. $(\frac{1}{60}$ gr., intramuscularly. $C_{18}H_{22}O_2$. Mol.wt. 270.36. M.p. 254-262°. S: ss. W; sol. A, acetone, dioxane and oils and aqueous solutions of NaOH. White crystals or a white crystalline powder; odourless; stable in air. The B.P. unit of oestrogenic activity (oestrone standard) is the specific oestrus producing activity contained in 0.0001 mg. of the standard oestrone.

Estrone Injection U.S.P.

1 cc. contains 0.1, 0.2, 0.5 or 1 mg. (1/600, 1/300, 1/120 or 1/60 gr.) in oil.

Tablets of Oestrone B.P.

Size, 1 mg. ($\frac{1}{60}$ gr.).

GONADOTROPHINS

Three classes of gonadotrophins are recognized, (*a*) anterior pituitary gonadotrophins, (*b*) serum gonadotrophins (from the serum of pregnant mares), (*c*) chorionic gonadotrophins (from the urine of pregnant women).

Chorionic gonadotrophins produce changes in the ovaries of rodents and are the basis of the various pregnancy tests. They have no demonstrable action on female sex organs in the human and hence are presumably useless for the treatment of feminine disorders. They do, however, have definite effects on human males, stimulating interstitial cells of the testes and so increasing production of androgenic hormone and thus the development of secondary sex characteristics. Chorionic gonadotrophins may be used to cause descent of undescended testes, provided no mechanical obstruction exists.

Serum gonadotrophins are thought to be identical with anterior pituitary gonadotrophins but this opinion is subject to change on further evidence. Their use is experimental as yet, and they are expensive.

Chorionic Gonadotrophin B.P. *Gonadotrophinum Chorionicum*

S: sol. in W. A white or fawn powder. A sterile preparation containing the gonad-stimulating substance obtained from the urine of pregnant women. The international unit is the activity of 0.1 mg. of Standard Powder.

Injection of Chorionic Gonadotrophin B.P.

DOSES: intramuscular, 100-500 units. Supplied dry in sealed containers. Fresh solutions in Water for Injection containing 0.5% phenol are to be made up immediately before administration.

Serum Gonadotrophin B.P. *Gonadotrophinum Sericum*

A white powder; sol. in W. A sterile preparation which contains the follicle-stimulating substance obtained from the serum of pregnant mares. The international unit is the activity of 0.25 mg. of Standard Powder.

Injection of Serum Gonadotrophin B.P.

DOSES: intramuscular, 200-1000 units. Supplied dry in sealed containers. Fresh solutions in Water for Injection containing 0.5% phenol are to be made up immediately before administration.

PROGESTINS

⦅The progestin preparations produce secretory (progestational) changes in the uterine mucosa and engorgement of the breasts. They also desensitize uterine muscle to pituitrin. These actions should be useful in treating threatened abortion or habitual abortion, and progestins are usually administered in these conditions, but too often without decided benefit. Note that the ethisterone is active by mouth.

Ethisterone. *Aethisteronum.* (Pregneninolone, Ethinyltestosterone. T.N. Pranone)
DOSES: B.P. 5-25 mg. ($\frac{1}{12}$-$\frac{2}{5}$ gr.) daily; U.S.P. 10 mg. ($\frac{1}{6}$ gr.). $C_{21}H_{28}O_2$. Mol.wt. 312.43. M.p. (U.S.P.) 266-273°, (B.P.) 269-275°. S: ins. W; ss. A, C, E, vegetable oils and in some other organic solvents. White or slightly yellow crystals or a crystalline powder; odourless; tasteless; stable in air; affected by light.

Tablets of Ethisterone B.P. (Tablets of Pregneninolone. Tablets of Ethinyltestosterone)
Size, 5 mg. ($\frac{1}{12}$ gr.).

Ethisterone Tablets U.S.P.
Sizes, 5 and 10 mg. ($\frac{1}{12}$ and $\frac{1}{6}$ gr.).

Progesterone. *Progesteronum*
DOSES: B.P. intramuscular, 2-20 mg. ($\frac{1}{30}$-$\frac{1}{3}$ gr.) daily; U.S.P. intramuscular, 5 mg. ($\frac{1}{12}$ gr.). $C_{21}H_{30}O_2$. Mol.wt. 314.45. M.p. alpha form 127-131°; beta form 121°; S: ins. W; sol. A, acetone, dioxane; sps. vegetable oils. A white crystalline powder; stable in air. May be prepared from the corpora lutea of the ovaries of sows or other mammals or from stigmasterol, pregnanediol, or cholesterol. One international unit is the activity of 1 mg. of the Standard Powder.

Injection of Progesterone B.P.

Strength, 5 mg. per cc. ($\frac{1}{12}$ gr. in 15 min.). A sterile solution in Ethyl Oleate or a suitable oil.

Progesterone Injection U.S.P.

1, 2, 5 and 10 mg. (1/60, 1/30, 1/12 and 1/6 gr.) in 1 cc. of a suitable oil.

Purified Siliceous Earth U.S.P. *Terra Silicea Purificata.* (Purified Kieselguhr, Purified Infusorial Earth)

S: ins. W, acids or dilute solutions of alkali hydroxides. A form of silica (SiO_2) consisting of the frustules and fragments of diatoms purified by boiling with diluted hydrochloric acid, washing and calcining. A fine white, light-grey, or pale-buff gritty powder. Readily absorbs moisture and retains about four times its weight of water without becoming fluid.

⟪ Kieselguhr is often used in dusting powders for its water absorbing qualities. It is also used for filtering and clarifying solutions.

Silver Nitrate. *Argenti Nitras*

$AgNO_3$. Mol.wt. 169.89. S: 0.4 W, 30 A, slightly more than 0.1 W at 100°, 6.5 A at 78°; ss. E. Colourless or white crystals; taste bitter and metallic; darkens on exposure to light.

Silver Nitrate Ophthalmic Solution U.S.P. *Liquor Argenti Nitratis Ophthalmicus*

A solution of Silver Nitrate in a buffered water medium containing 0.95%-1.05% $AgNO_3$, preserved in wax composition capsules containing about 5 drops of solution.

⟪ Silver Nitrate precipitates proteins and kills bacteria. A 1-2% solution is instilled into eyes of new-born infants to prevent ophthalmia neonatorum (gonococcal infection). Sticks of toughened silver nitrate are used to touch ulcers to promote healing, and cuts, to prevent bleeding.

A solution of 1:1000 may be used in the eye for astringent and germicidal action but is irritant. Prolonged use is inadvisable since reduced silver may be deposited in the tissues, causing a permanent darkening of the skin (argyria).

A concentrated solution (25-35%) is a useful caustic and obtundent for treating sensitive dentine. Ammoniacal silver nitrate solution containing about 30% of reducible silver is just as effective, and often used in preference to the foregoing.

Toughened Silver Nitrate B.P. *Argenti Nitras Induratua.* (Toughened Caustic, Moulded Silver Nitrate, Fused Silver Nitrate, Silver Nitrate Pencils, Lunar Caustic)
Silver Nitrate 95, Potassium Nitrate 5, fused and moulded into white rods.

Silver Protein B.P. *Argentoproteinum.* (Strong Protein Silver, Silver Proteinate. T.N. Protargol)
S: slowly soluble in 2 W; ins. A, C, E. A brown odourless powder; somewhat hygroscopic; decomposes in light; contains about 7.5-8.5% silver.

℄ The Strong Protein Silver Solution is germicidal and about as irritant as 0.1% silver nitrate but rather more effective as a bacteriostatic agent in the presence of sodium chloride in solution, because all the silver is not rapidly precipitated as silver chloride. Argyria may result from prolonged use of any silver preparation. Linen may be badly stained by these solutions.

Curd Soap B.P. *Sapo Animalis*
A sodium soap made from purified solid animal fats. S: sps. cold W; completely sol. hot W; almost completely sol. A 90%. A yellowish-white or greyish-white substance; nearly odourless; easily moulded when heated and becoming horny and pulverizable when dried.

℄ Curd soap is used in pills to hold resins or volatile oils.

Hard Soap B.P. *Sapo Durus*
S: slowly dissolves in W and in A. A sodium soap made from suitable vegetable oils. A greyish-white, yellowish-white, or greenish-white solid in bars or in powder; odour faint and free from rancidity.

Powdered Hard Soap B.P. *Saponis Duri Pulvis*

Liniment of Soap B.P. *Linimentum Saponis*
Soft Soap 80, Camphor 40, with Oil of Rosemary, Distilled Water and alcohol to make 1000 cc. Contains 61-65% v/v of C_2H_5OH.

Medicinal Soft Soap U.S.P. *Sapo Mollis Medicinalis.* (Soft Soap, Green Soap)

The Vegetable Oil 380 Gm., Oleic Acid 20 Gm., Potassium Hydroxide 91.7 Gm., Glycerin 50 cc., Distilled Water to make about 1000 Gm. A soft, unctuous, yellowish-white to brownish or greenish-yellow transparent or translucent mass; odour slight and characteristic. Coconut oil and palm kernel oil are excluded. Glycerin is not removed.

Soft Soap B.P. *Sapo Mollis*

S: sol. W, A 90%. A potassium or sodium soap made from suitable vegetable oils. A yellowish-white to green or brown unctuous substance.

⟪ The detergent (physical cleansing) qualities of soap are more important than its antiseptic power. Soaps do, however, possess appreciable germicidal properties. Lathers or 1% solutions will kill many organisms in a few minutes. Staphylococci and colon bacilli are very resistant and spores are not harmed. Ordinary soaps, in the way they are commonly used, are just as effective as medicated "germicidal" soaps, according to many careful investigators.

Surgical Solution of Chlorinated Soda B.P. *Liquor Sodae Chlorinatae Chirurgicalis.* (Dakin's Solution)

An aqueous solution containing 0.5-0.55% w/v of available chlorine, made from Chlorinated Lime, Sodium Carbonate and Boric Acid.

⟪ Dakin's Solution was once much used for the continuous irrigation of infected wounds. It has the property of dissolving dead tissue. Surrounding skin must be protected from its irritant action.

Soda Lime. *Calx Sodica*

A mixture of calcium hydroxide with sodium or potassium hydroxide or both, intended for absorption of CO_2 in metabolism tests, anaesthesia, or oxygen therapy. White or greyish-white granules, or may be coloured if an indicator has been added. Absorbs about 20% of its weight as carbon dioxide.

Sodium Acid Phosphate B.P. *Sodii Phosphas Acidus.* Sodium Biphosphate U.S.P. *Sodii Biphosphas.* (Sodium Dihydrogen Phosphate, Monosodium Orthophosphate)

Doses: B.P. 2-4 Gm. (30-60 gr.); U.S.P. 0.6 Gm. (10 gr.).

$NaH_2PO_4.H_2O$ (U.S.P.) or $NaH_2PO_4.2H_2O$ (B.P.).   Mol.wt. 138.01 (U.S.P.) or 156.1 (B.P.).   S: fs. W; ins. A.   Colourless crystals or a white crystalline powder; taste acid and saline.   The aqueous solution is acid to litmus paper and effervesces with sodium carbonate.

₵ Sodium acid phosphate is sometimes given to acidify the urine, often with hexamine.   Ammonium chloride is, however, more effective.   The phosphate is somewhat laxative.

Sodium Aurothiomalate B.P.   *Sodii Aurothiomalas.*   (T.N. Myochrisine)

DOSES: intramuscular, 10 mg. increasing gradually to 100 mg. ($\frac{1}{6}$-1$\frac{1}{2}$ gr.) weekly.   S: vs. W.   A fine, pale-yellow powder having a slight odour.   Hygroscopic.   Contains 44.5-46.0% of gold.

Injection of Sodium Aurothiomalate B.P.

Strength, 10 mg. per cc. ($\frac{1}{6}$ gr. in 15 min.).

₵ Sodium aurothiomalate or other salts of gold are used in the treatment of lupus erythematosus and rheumatoid arthritis.   The gold salts are very toxic and their therapeutic value is not thoroughly established.   The toxic effects are varied and severe and include fever, vomiting, dermatitis, and hepatitis.   Bal is an antidote.

Sodium Benzoate.   *Sodii Benzoas*

DOSES: B.P. 0.3-2 Gm. (5-30 gr.). $NaC_7H_5O_2$. Mol.wt. 144.11. S: 2 W, 75 A, 50 A 90%.   A white amorphous, granular, or crystalline powder; stable in air; almost odourless; taste, unpleasant sweetish, and saline.

₵ Sodium benzoate is used as a food preservative.   It is only active in this respect in neutral or acid medium in which some free benzoic acid is liberated.   The small amounts permitted in the preservation of food are regarded as entirely harmless.   Sodium benzoate is rarely given for systemic action but it does have actions like the salicylates, i.e. antipyretic and analgesic.   It is excreted in combination with glycocoll (glycine) as hippuric acid.

Sodium Bicarbonate.   *Sodii Bicarbonas.*   (Baking Soda)

DOSES: B.P. 1-4 Gm. (15-60 gr.);   U.S.P. 2 Gm. (30 gr.). $NaHCO_3$.   Mol.wt. 84.02.   S: 10 W; ins. A.   A white crystalline powder; odourless; taste saline.   Aqueous solutions are slightly alkaline to litmus when freshly prepared. The alkalinity increases if the solutions are left standing, are agitated, or are boiled.

Compound Tablets of Sodium Bicarbonate B.P. (Soda Mint Tablets)

DOSES: 2-6 tablets. Sodium Bicarbonate 324, Oil of Peppermint 4 cc., to make 1000 tablets. Size 0.32 Gm. (5 gr.). Dissolve slowly in the mouth.

Sodium Bicarbonate Tablets U.S.P.

Sizes, 300 and 600 mg. (5 and 10 gr.).

Injection of Sodium Bicarbonate B.P.

Strength when not otherwise specified, 5% w/v.

⟨ Sodium bicarbonate has many uses as a household remedy. It gives rapid relief from symptoms of gastric hyperacidity but is not good for sustained suppression of acidity because an excess may cause the gastric contents to become definitely alkaline and thus provoke further secretion of acid, which quickly neutralizes the excess bicarbonate. It is also given often with sulphonamides to alkalinize the urine or with salicylates to reduce their toxicity (probably by hastening their excretion). It may be given orally or intravenously to combat systemic acidosis as in methyl alcohol poisoning. Sustained administration of sodium bicarbonate in large doses occasionally leads to alkalosis and tetany but only if impaired kidney function, dehydration, or loss of acid by vomiting has reduced the power of the body to regulate its acid base balance. A paste of sodium bicarbonate in water applied to insect bites or itchy skin eruptions often relieves discomfort.

Sodium Bisulphite U.S.P. *Sodii Bisulfis.* (Sodium Hydrogen Sulfite, Sodium Acid Sulfite)

$NaHSO_3$. Mol.wt. 104.07. S: 4 W; ss. A. A white granular powder; odour resembling that of sulfur dioxide; unstable in air; a substance which may be used in tablets or injections to inhibit oxidation.

Sodium Borate. See Borax.

Sodium Bromide. *Sodii Bromidum*

DOSES: B.P. 0.3-1.2 Gm. (5-20 gr.); U.S.P. 1 Gm. (15 gr.). $NaBr$. Mol.wt. 102.91. S: 1.2 W, 16 A. White or colourless cubic crystals or a white granular powder; odourless; taste saline and slightly bitter; deliquescent in moist air.

⁋ The actions of sodium bromide are due mainly to the bromide ion which has a characteristic type of sedative action on the central nervous system which may be loosely described as inducing apathy and depressing motor activity by actions on the higher centres of the nervous system. Such effects are produced in a mild form by doses of 1-2 Gm. Larger doses will depress reflexes and cause general stupor but a general anaesthesia is not attained. In ordinary doses bromides will not compel sleep but will favour it. Ordinary doses decrease the electrical excitability of the motor cortex and decrease the effect of convulsant drugs. Consequently the drug may be described as an anti-convulsant.

Bromides are excreted almost entirely in the urine. The rate of excretion depends on the intake of salt and water. If salt intake is restricted, chloride and bromide ions are retained by the kidneys. If salt intake is high, the excretion rate of bromide and chloride is high.

Bromides are used to treat epilepsy, to relieve sleeplessness due to motor restlessness, to pacify patients with mental disturbances.

Acute fatal poisoning with bromides is practically unknown but chronic poisoning is often reported, usually as a result of prolonged treatment of epileptics and psychotics. Even small doses tend to accumulate, particularly when food intake is low. When blood levels rise above 100 mg. per cent, toxic symptoms may occur and above 200 mg. per cent are frequently serious. Chronic poisoning is frequently characterized by acne-like skin eruptions, pruritus, dullness, loss of appetite, and foul breath. Treatment is by withdrawing the bromide and increasing the chloride intake.

Sodium Carbonate B.P. *Sodii Carbonas.* (Washing Soda)
$Na_2CO_3.10H_2O$. Mol.wt. 286.2. S: 2 W 15.5°; ins. A 90%. Transparent, colourless, rhomboid crystals; odourless; taste strongly alkaline; efflorescent. Aqueous solutions are very alkaline to litmus.

Exsiccated Sodium Carbonate B.P. *Sodii Carbonas Exsiccatus.*
(Anhydrous Sodium Carbonate)
Mol.wt. 106.0. S: readily sol. in W. A white powder; odourless; taste strongly alkaline.

⁋ Sodium carbonate is seldom used medicinally but is an ingredient of many preparations. It is sufficiently alkaline to be somewhat caustic or at least irritant.

Sodium Chloride. *Sodii Chloridum*
NaCl. Mol.wt. 58.45. S: 2.8 W, 10 G, 2.7 W 100°; ss. A. Colourless, transparent, cubical crystals or a white crystalline powder; odourless; taste saline.

Injection of Sodium Chloride B.P. (Physiological Solution of Sodium Chloride, Physiological Saline Solution, Normal Saline Solution)
Sodium Chloride 9 Gm., Water for Injection to make 1000 cc. See also Ringer's Solution.

⟪ Sodium chloride in hypertonic solution acts as an emetic by irritating the stomach (1 tablespoonful in a glass of warm water; about 10% solution). Isotonic solutions are given intravenously, or less often nowadays, subcutaneously or by rectal drip to maintain or restore body fluids. Increased amounts of sodium chloride are given in the diet of patients with Addison's disease to maintain the sodium content of the plasma. Sodium chloride intake is restricted in oedema.

Isotonic Solution of Sodium Chloride U.S.P. *Liquor Sodii Chloridi Isotonicus*
Sodium Chloride 9, Distilled Water to make 1000 cc. A clear, colourless solution, having a slightly saline taste; pH lies between 5-7. Three grades are specified, (1) unsterilized, (2) sterilized, (3) for injection (made with Water for Injection).

⟪ When Isotonic Solution of Sodium Chloride is prescribed it should be specified whether a non-sterile preparation is required, or a sterilized one for external use, or a sterilized one for injection (parenteral use). For the last-named use the U.S.P. requires that the solution meet the tests for sterility and freedom from pyrogens, and other requirements for injections. Unless otherwise specified this quality is to be supplied.

Sodium Citrate. *Sodii Citras*
DOSES: B.P. 1-4 Gm. (15-60 gr.); U.S.P. 1 Gm. (15 gr.). $Na_3C_6H_5O_7.2H_2O$. Mol.wt. 294.12. S: 1.5 W, 0.6 W 100°; ins. A. White granular crystals or a crystalline powder; odourless; taste saline and cooling.

Tablets of Sodium Citrate B.P.

Size, 0.12 Gm. (2 gr.). Dissolve in water for use.

℃ Sodium citrate is often given orally to make the urine more alkaline for the treatment of cystitis. The tablets, however, are not for this purpose but to put in milk to prevent the formation of curds in the stomach, on the assumption that the digestibility of the milk may be improved.

Anticoagulant Injection of Sodium Citrate B.P. *Injectio Sodii Citratis Anticoagulans*

Sodium Citrate 25, Sodium Chloride 9, Water for Injection to make 1000.

Anticoagulant Sodium Citrate Solution U.S.P. *Liquor Sodii Citratis anticoagulans*

Sodium Citrate 25, Sodium Chloride 9, Water for Injection to make 1000 cc. Sterile and non-sterile solutions are also available.

Anticoagulant Acid Citrate Dextrose Solution U.S.P. *Liquor Acidi Citratis Dextrosi Anticoagulans*. (A.C.D. Solution)

Sodium Citrate 22, Citric Acid 8, Dextrose 24.5, Water for Injection to make 1000. A clear, colourless, odourless solution.

Injection of Sodium Citrate with Dextrose B.P.

A sterile solution containing in each 100 cc. Sodium Citrate 3.0 Gm., Dextrose 3.0 Gm.

℃ The preceding anticoagulant citrate solutions are used mostly to preserve blood for transfusion. One part of solution is added to 5 parts of blood. It is conceivable that the solutions might be used for purposes not requiring sterility, so that the U.S.P. permits three qualities to be supplied, (1) non-sterile, (2) sterile for external use, (3) sterile for injection (see Isotonic Solution of Sodium Chloride). Unless otherwise specified (3) will be supplied.

Sodium Hydroxide B.P. *Sodii Hydroxidi*. Caustic Soda

NaOH. Mol.wt. 40.01. S: 1 W; fs. A. White sticks, nearly white fused masses, small pellets or flakes; deliquescent, rapidly absorbing moisture and carbon dioxide when exposed to air.

℃ Caustic soda is seldom used as such for medicinal purposes.

Sodium Iodide. *Sodii Iodidum*.

DOSES: B.P. 0.3-2 Gm. (5-30 gr.); U.S.P. 0.3 (5 gr.). NaI.

Mol.wt. 149.92.   S: 0.6 W, 2 A, 1 G.   Odourless, colourless crystals or a white crystalline powder; taste saline and slightly bitter; deliquescent and may turn brownish when exposed to air.   See Potassium Iodide.

Sodium Lactate Injection U.S.P.   *Injectio Sodii Lactatis*

A sterile solution prepared for injection.   No strength specified.

℃ Sodium lactate is useful for increasing systemic and urinary alkalinity.   It is often given intravenously with Ringer's solution to correct the acid-base balance in severe systemic acidosis.   A 1.87% solution ($\frac{1}{6}$ Molar) is approximately isotonic with blood. Such a solution may be injected at rates up to 300 cc. per hour till the acidosis is corrected.   See also Lactated Ringer's Solution.

Sodium Lauryl Sulphate.   *Sodii et Laurylis Sulphas B.P.   Sodii Laurylis Sulfas U.S.P.*

S: 10 W, giving an opalescent solution; ss. A 90%.   Small white or yellow crystals having a slight characteristic odour.   A mixture of sodium alkyl sulfates consisting chiefly of $CH_3(CH_2)_{10}CH_2OSO_3Na$.

℃ Sodium lauryl sulphate is described as an anionic detergent. It lowers surface tension and is used as a soap substitute and also as an emulsifying agent in the manufacture of creams and hydrophilic ointments.   It has little antiseptic power, unlike the cationic detergents (see Benzalkonium Chloride).

Sodium Metabisulphite B.P.   *Sodii Metabisulphis*

$Na_2S_2O_5$.   Mol.wt. 190.1.   S: 2 W 15.5°; less sol. A.   Colourless prismatic crystals or a white powder which may become yellowish on keeping; odour sulphurous; taste acid and saline; slowly oxidizes to sulphate in moist air.

℃ Sodium metabisulphite may be used as a preservative in food, and in solutions of adrenaline, physostigmine, *et al.*, in concentrations of 0.1%.

Sodium Morrhuate Injection U.S.P.   *Injectio Sodii Morrhuatis*

An aqueous solution of sodium salts of the fatty acids of cod-liver oil with suitable preservative.   Strength, 5% solution in 2, 5 and 30 cc. containers.

℃ Sodium morrhuate injection is a sclerosing agent.   It is injected cautiously into varicose veins to produce local inflammation, thrombosis, and closure of the vein by fibrosis.

Sodium Nitrite. *Sodii Nitris*

DOSES: B.P. 0.03-0.12 Gm. ($\frac{1}{2}$-2 gr.); U.S.P. 60 mg. (1 gr.).
NaNO$_2$. Mol.wt. 69.01. S: 1.5 W; sps. A. Colourless or slightly
yellowish crystals; nearly white, opaque, fused masses; odourless;
taste saline; deliquescent.

Sodium Nitrite Tablets U.S.P.

Sizes, 30 and 60 mg. ($\frac{1}{2}$ and 1 gr.).

⊄ Nitrites are vasodilators by direct action on the smooth
muscle of blood vessels. The effects are some reddening of the skin
in the blush area, some decrease in blood pressure, and often
headache, which may be due to dilation of vessels within the cranium.
Flushing is seldom evident elsewhere in the skin, presumably because
vascular reflexes enforce some vasoconstriction, thus preventing a
serious fall in blood pressure.

Relief from angina pectoris may be obtained by the use of
nitrites. The action is by coronary dilatation and reduction of
venous return to the heart, thus reducing the work of the heart.

Sodium nitrite is slower and more persistent in action than amyl
nitrite or nitroglycerine. It may thus be used to abort repeated
attacks of angina. All the nitrites, if used too freely, will produce
methaemoglobinaemia. In chronic hypertension the nitrites are
of no value as they do not reduce the blood pressure without
producing headache or other undesirable effects.

Sodium Phosphate. *Sodii Phosphas.* (Disodium Hydrogen Phosphate, Disodium Orthophosphate, Dibasic Sodium Phosphate)

DOSES: B.P. 2-16 Gm. (30-240 gr.); U.S.P. 4 Gm. (1 dr.).
Na$_2$HPO$_4$.12H$_2$O (B.P.); Na$_2$HPO$_4$.7H$_2$O (U.S.P.). Mol.wt. 358.2
(B.P.); 268.09 (U.S.P.). S: sol. 4 W; ss. A. Colourless or white
crystals or a white granular salt; efflorescent; odourless; taste saline.

Effervescent Sodium Phosphate U.S.P. *Sodii Phosphas Effervescens*

DOSE: 10 Gm. (2$\frac{1}{2}$ dr.).

Exsiccated Sodium Phosphate 200, Sodium Bicarbonate 477,
Tartaric Acid 252, Citric Acid 162, to make about 1000 Gm.

⊄ The phosphate and tartrate ions are absorbed poorly from the
alimentary tract and thus act as saline purgatives or aperients.
This preparation is pleasant and popular.

Exsiccated Sodium Phosphate. *Sodii Phosphas Exsiccatus.* (Anhydrous Sodium Phosphate, Dried Sodium Phosphate)

DOSES: B.P. 0.6-5 Gm. (10-75 gr.); U.S.P. 2 Gm. (30 gr.). Na_2HPO_4. Mol.wt. 141.98. S: 8 W; ins. A. A white hygroscopic powder; odourless; taste saline.

℄ Sodium phosphate is a saline cathartic. The di-sodium salt is, to some extent, a systemic and urinary alkalizer.

Compound Effervescent Powder B.P. *Pulvis Effervescens Compositus.* (Seidlitz Powders)

Powder No. 1 *in Blue Paper*: Rochelle Salt (dry) 7.5, Sodium Bicarbonate (dry) 2.5. *Powder No.* 2 *in White Paper*: Tartaric Acid 2.5 Gm. Dissolve Powder No. 1 in half a glass of water, then add Powder No. 2. Drink while effervescing.

Sodium Salicylate. *Sodii Salicylas*

DOSES: B.P. 0.6-2 Gm. (10-30 gr.); U.S.P. 1 Gm. (15 gr.). $C_6H_4(OH)COONa$. Mol.wt. 160.11. S: 1 W, 10 A, 4 G; vs. W 100°, A 78°. A fine, white crystalline powder, scales, or an amorphous powder; usually odourless or may have a faint characteristic odour; taste sweet and saline; becomes slightly coloured in light.

Sodium Salicylate Injection U.S.P.

1 Gm. (15 gr.) in 5 cc.; 2 Gm. (30 gr.) in 10 or 20 cc.; for intravenous injection.

Sodium Salicylate Tablets U.S.P.

Sizes, 0.3 and 0.6 Gm. (5 and 10 gr.).

Tablets of Sodium Salicylate B.P.

Size, 0.3 Gm. (5 gr.). Dissolve in water before administration.

℄ Sodium Salicylate has analgesic and antipyretic actions. It is commonly given (with sodium bicarbonate) for the symptomatic treatment of rheumatic fever, and sometimes of rheumatoid arthritis. See also Acetylsalicylic Acid.

Sodium Stearate U.S.P. *Sodii Stearas*

S: slowly sol. in cold W and in A but readily in these solvents when hot. A fine white powder; soapy to the touch; odour tallow-like; it is affected by light. Contains varying porportions of sodium stearate and sodium palmitate.

℄ Sodium stearate may be used as an excipient for pills.

Sodium Sulphate. *Sodii Sulphas.* (Glauber's Salt)

DOSES: B.P. 2-16 Gm. (30-240 gr.); U.S.P. 15 Gm. (4 dr.). $Na_2SO_4.10H_2O$. Mol.wt. 322.21. S: 1.5 W; ins. A; sol. G. Large colourless, odourless, transparent crystals or a granular powder; effloresces rapidly in dry air; taste bitter and saline.

℄ Sodium sulphate is poorly absorbed from the gastrointestinal tract and hence acts as a saline cathartic. Most people prefer its taste to that of magnesium sulphate.

Exsiccated Sodium Sulphate B.P. *Sodii Sulphas Exsiccatus.*
(Anhydrous Sodium Sulphate, Exsiccated Glauber's Salt)
DOSES: 1-8 Gm. (15-120 gr.). Na_2SO_4. Mol.wt. 142.1. S: 8 W 15.5°. A white hygroscopic powder; odourless; taste bitter and saline.

Spearmint Oil U.S.P. *Oleum Menthae Viridis*
Sp.gr. 0.917-0.934. S: 1 A 80%. A colourless, yellow or greenish-yellow oil having the characteristic odour and taste of spearmint.

Spermaceti U.S.P. *Cetaceum*
M.p. 42-50°. S: ins. W; nearly ins. cold A; ss. cold petroleum benzin; sol. in A 78°, E, C, fixed and volatile oils. A waxy substance obtained from the head of the sperm whale.

℄ Cetaceum is used as a constituent of cold cream and other ointments. It consists chiefly of cetyl palmitate.

Absorbable Gelatin Sponge U.S.P. *Spongia Gelatini Absorbenda.*
(T.N. Gelfoam)
A sterile absorbable water-insoluble gelatin-base sponge. S: ins. W; absorbable by body tissue; completely digested in a solution of pepsin. Small pieces are applied to bleeding tissues to arrest haemorrhage.

Squill B.P. *Scilla*
The bulb of *Urginea scilla* or *Urginea maritima*, sliced and dried; taste bitter, mucilaginous and acrid; known in commerce as white squill.

Powdered Squill B.P. *Scillae Pulvis*
DOSES: 60-200 mg. (1-3 gr.). A white or yellowish-white powder.

Oxymel of Squill B.P. *Oxymel Scillae*

Doses: 2-4 cc. (30-60 min.). Squill 5, Acetic Acid 9, with Distilled Water and Purified Honey q.s. to make 100 cc. by maceration. Gm./cc. 1.26-1.27.

Syrup of Squill B.P. *Syrupus Scillae*

Doses: 2-4 cc. (30-60 min.). Vinegar of Squill 45, with Sucrose and Distilled Water to make 100 cc.

Tincture of Squill B.P. *Tinctura Scillae*

Doses: 0.3-2 cc. (5-30 min.). Squill 10, to make 100 cc. by maceration. Contains 52-57% v/v of C_2H_5OH.

Vinegar of Squill B.P. *Acetum Scillae*

Doses: 0.6-2 cc. (10-30 min.). Squill 10, Dilute Acetic Acid 100, by maceration. Gm./cc. 1.017-1.032.

⚌ Squill contains a number of glycosides with actions resembling those of digitalis. They are said to produce more coronary constriction than digitalis and for that reason are little used in the therapy of cardiac disease. The main use of preparations of squill is in cough mixtures, for an expectorant action. The cardioactive glycosides are destroyed in the acidic preparations. Squill is frequently used as a rat poison.

Starch. *Amylum*

S: ins. cold W and in A. Fine white powder or irregular angular masses; odourless. Obtained from rice, wheat, potatoes, or maize. (U.S.P. from maize only.)

⚌ Starch is an ingredient of mucilages, water-soluble lubricating jellies, ointments, and dusting powders. Ointments may be stiffened with starch to form pastes. In such, and in powders, starch helps to keep the skin dry by absorbing moisture.

Starch Glycerite U.S.P. *Glyceritum Amyli*

Starch 10, Benzoic Acid 0.2, Distilled Water 20, Glycerin 70 cc., to make about 100 Gm.

Glycerin of Starch B.P. *Glycerinum Amyli*

Wheat Starch 8.5, Distilled Water 17, Glycerin 74.5 Gm., to make about 100 Gm.

⚌ The starch glycerites are jelly-like preparations, used as lubricants and as vehicles for spermatocides.

Stibophen. *Stibophenum*

DOSES: B.P. intravenous, 0.1-0.3 Gm. (1½-5 gr.). U.S.P. intramuscular, 0.2 gm. (3 gr.). $C_{12}H_4O_{16}S_4Sb.Na_5.7H_2O$. Mol.wt. 895.3. S: sol. cold W; almost ins. dehydrated A, E, C, acetone and in light petroleum. A colourless, fine, crystalline powder; odourless.

Injection of Stibophen B.P.

DOSES: intravenous, 1.5-5 cc. (25-75 min.). Strength, Stibophen 6.4 Gm., Sodium Metabisulphite 0.1 Gm., Water for Injection to make 100 cc.

Stibophen Injection U.S.P.

225 mg. (3½ gr.) in 3.25 cc.; 325 mg. (5 gr.) in 5 cc.

℃ Stibophen is a systemic anti-infective agent. It is used principally to treat infections by the bilharzia parasites, and also to treat undulant fever, leishmaniasis, and granuloma inguinale. The drug is given by intravenous or intramuscular injection, usually once a day or every second day for several weeks. Toxic manifestations are nausea, epigastric pain, and occasionally liver damage. Bal is an effective antidote.

Powdered Stomach U.S.P. *Stomachus Pulveratus.* (Dried Stomach)

DOSE: one U.S.P. unit daily. The dried and powdered defatted wall of the stomach of the hog, containing anti-pernicious anaemia factors.

℃ Powdered Stomach contains the intrinsic factor which, acting on meat, produces anti-pernicious anaemia factor. For meaning of units, see Liver Extract. Powdered Stomach should not be given in hot fluids as its activity may be destroyed.

Prepared Storax B.P. *Styrax Praeparatus.* **Storax U.S.P.** *Styrax.* (Liquid Storax)

S: ins. W; almost completely sol. 1 A warm; sol. acetone, carbon disulfide and in E, some insoluble matter remaining. A brownish, viscous, sticky, opaque balsam obtained from the trunk of *Liquidamber orientalis* or *Liquidamber styraciflua* (U.S.P.); odour and taste characteristic. The B.P. requires purification by solution in alcohol, filtration, and evaporation of solvent.

℃ An ointment containing 25% of storax is sometimes used for scabies and other parasitic infections of the skin.

Stramonium B.P. *Stramonium.* (Jimson Weed, Jamestown Weed, Stramonium Leaves)

The dried leaves and flowering or fruiting tops of *Datura Stramonium* and of *Datura Tatula.* Yields not less than 0.25% of alkaloids calculated as hyoscyamine.

Powdered Stramonium B.P. *Stramonii Pulvis*

A green or light-brown powder; odour disagreeable; taste bitter.

Dry Extract of Stramonium B.P. *Extractum Stramonii Siccum*

DOSES: 15-60 mg. ($\frac{1}{4}$-1 gr.); or in post-encephalitic and similar conditions, 60-500 mg. (1-8 gr.). An alcoholic percolate of powdered stramonium, dried and adjusted to contain 0.9-1.1% of the alkaloids calculated as hyoscyamine. Contains in 60 mg., 0.6 mg. of alkaloid.

Liquid Extract of Stramonium B.P. *Extractum Stramonii Liquidum*

DOSES: 0.03-0.2 cc. ($\frac{1}{2}$-3 min.). An alcoholic extract adjusted to contain 0.225-0.275% w/v of alkaloids calculated as hyoscyamine. Contains 28-44% v/v of C_2H_5OH. Contains in 0.2 cc., 0.5 mg. of alkaloids.

Tincture of Stramonium B.P. *Tinctura Stramonii*

DOSES: 0.3-2 cc. (5-30 min.). Liquid Extract of Stramonium 10 cc., diluted to 100 cc. Contains 40-45% v/v of C_2H_5OH. and 0.0225-0.0275% of alkaloid.

❡ The alkaloids of stramonium consist mostly of hyoscyamine, the principal alkaloid of belladonna, but also include some hyoscine which contributes a sedative action, while the hyoscyamine has, if anything, a stimulating action on the central nervous system in addition to its paralysing action at the cholinergic endings of the automic nerves.

Stramonium preparations have come to be used principally for the tremor of Parkinsonian syndromes. They may also be used in the treatment of asthma. See Belladonna and Atropine.

Sucrose. *Sucrosum.* (Sugar, Refined Sugar, *Saccharum*)

$C_{12}H_{22}O_{11}$. Mol.wt. 342.30. S: 0.5 W, 170 A, about 0.2 W 100°; ins. C, E. White or colourless crystals or a white crystalline powder; odourless; taste sweet.

❡ A 50% solution of sucrose has been given intravenously to reduce intracranial pressure by osmotic action. There is reason, however, to think that sucrose given this way may produce kidney damage. Consequently, concentrated solutions of glucose are used more commonly for reducing cerebral oedema.

Sulphonal B.P. *Sulphonal*

DOSES: 0.3-1.2 Gm. (5-20 gr.). $(CH_3)_2.C(SO_2C_2H_5)_2$. Mol.wt. 228.3. S: 450 W, 80 A 90%, 90 E, 3 C, 15 W 100°. Colourless crystals or a white powder; odourless and nearly tasteless.

℃ Sulphonal is a hypnotic of rather slow and prolonged action. It should not be given repeatedly because it tends to accumulate, and to produce haematoporhpyrinuria.

SULPHONAMIDES

The sulphonamides may be described as internal antiseptics, or systemic anti-infectives. They check the growth and reproduction of micro-organisms at concentrations in the body fluids which are not too harmful to the patient. Micro-organisms vary greatly in their susceptibility to the sulphonamides and they can acquire resistance as a result of exposure to sublethal concentrations. The action of sulphonamides is thought to be a competitive inhibition of enzyme systems which use para-aminobenzoic acid in growth processes of the micro-organism. The chemical similarity of sulphonamides to PABA explains their combination with the specific enzymes. Excess PABA will displace the sulphonamide and thus antagonize its bacteriostatic action. Procaine and other para-amino compounds have a similar antagonistic effect. All sulphonamides except sulphamylon (Marfanil) and its congeners are thought to have the same mode of action but important quantitative differences exist which modify the apparent characteristics of the various compounds. These may depend on properties such as solubility, ionization, adsorbability on plasma proteins, and so on.

Most sulphonamides are absorbed rapidly from the small intestine. The notable exceptions are sulfathalidine, sulphaguanidine, and sulphasuxidine, which are absorbed so slowly that effective concentrations do not develop in the blood stream. For the others, excretion by the kidneys is somewhat slower than absorption so that fairly high concentrations of sulphonamides can be built up in the blood stream.

In the body the sulphonamides penetrate fairly freely into

various fluid compartments but the distribution is not uniform. Sulphathiazole concentrations, for example, are higher in the plasma than in other fluids, because as much as 75% of the sulphonamide in the plasma may be adsorbed to plasma protein. Only the remaining 25% is free to diffuse. The adsorbed fraction of sulphanilamide is much smaller (20%). It is evident that caution must be observed in reasoning about the effectiveness of concentrations in blood or plasma of different sulphonamides. Desirable or undesirable concentrations in the blood must be established empirically for each drug.

Sulphonamides are excreted for the most part by the kidney after a part has been conjugated with an acetyl radical. Many of the acetylated compounds are not readily soluble and may precipitate in the urinary passages causing various renal symptoms, and even death by anuria. Acetylsulphanilamide is an exception in being fairly soluble, which probably explains why death by renal damage with sulphanilamide was extremely uncommon during the years that this drug was in general use.

Toxic symptoms from full doses of sulphonamides are not uncommon. In order of increasing seriousness these are—mental depression, dizziness, nausea, vomiting, fever, skin rashes, haematuria, agranulocytosis, anuria. The fever and skin rashes resemble allergic reactions and often represent acquired sensitivities.

In giving sulphonamides, the object is to build up quickly a concentration of drug in the body fluids which will check the growth of micro-organisms and to maintain an adequate concentration till the infection is eradicated. The plan usually adopted is to give a large initial dose (4 Gm.) followed by 1 Gm. every 4 hours, night and day. Dosage should be altered if determinations of sulphonamide in the blood show that the concentrations are too high or too low. In general, blood levels should be kept between 5 and 15 mg. per 100 cc. A urinary volume of at least 1500 cc. daily should be maintained by forcing fluids if necessary. This is to assure enough urine to dissolve the less soluble sulphonamides and prevent precipitation of crystals within the kidney or ureters. Alkali in the form of sodium bicarbonate is often given to make the urine alkaline and thus increase the solubility of the sulphonamides. To make a real difference, large amounts of alkali must be given; enough to make the urine alkaline (pH 7.2-7.5).

More recently another procedure, known as "sulpha combination," has been introduced to diminish the hazards of supersaturation and precipitation in the urinary tract. It is based on the fact that the less soluble sulphonamides dissolve independently, i.e. they are each as soluble in the presence of the others as they are alone. On the other hand their antibacterial actions are additive. Consequently, if the total intake of sulphonamide is made up of three different sulphonamides, each in one-third of the usual dose, the therapeutic effect will be unimpaired but the danger of precipitation in the urinary tract will be greatly reduced.

Succinylsulphathiazole. *Succinylsulphathiazolum.* (T.N. Sulfasuxidine)

DOSES: B.P. 3-6 Gm. (45-90 gr.); U.S.P. 2 Gm. (30 gr.). $C_{13}H_{13}O_5N_3S_2.H_2O$. Mol.wt. 373.39. M.p. 188-195° with decomposition. S: 4800 W; sps. A, acetone; ins. C; sol. in solutions of alkali hydroxides and in solutions of sodium bicarbonate with effervescence. White or yellowish-white crystalline powder; odourless; slowly darkens on exposure to light.

Succinylsulfathiazole Tablets U.S.P. Tablets of Succinylsulphathiazole B.P.

Usual size, 0.5 Gm. (7½ gr.).

℡ Succinylsulphathiazole is poorly absorbed from the alimentary tract. It is useless for treating systemic infections but effective in bacillary dysenteries. Very large doses are given, for example, an average-sized adult may be given an initial dose of 12 Gm. and 2 Gm. every 4 hours thereafter.

Sulphacetamide B.P. *Sulphacetamidum.* (T.N. Albucid, Sulamyd)

$C_8H_{10}O_3N_2S$. Mol.wt. 214.2. M.p. 181-184°. S: at 20°, 150 W, 15 A, 7 acetone 15.5°, ins. E; sol. in mineral acids and solutions of alkali carbonates. White or yellowish-white crystalline powder; odourless; taste acid and slightly saline.

Sulphacetamide Sodium B.P. *Sulphacetamidum Sodium.* (Soluble Sulphacetamide)

$C_8H_9O_3N_2SNa.H_2O$. Mol.wt. 254.2. S: at 15.5° 1.5 W; sps. A and in acetone. A white or yellowish-white crystalline powder; odourless; taste slightly bitter.

℡ Sulphacetamide is not the same as the acetylated sulphanilamide produced in the body. In the former the acetyl radical is at the sulphone end of the molecule, in the latter at the opposite end (N position). Sulphacetamide is not acetylated further in the body but split into sulphanilamide. The latter is partly acetylated at the N position before excretion. Since N-acetyl sulphanilamide is fairly soluble, the danger of renal complications is minimal with sulphacetamide. One important feature of soluble sulphacetamide is that solutions of it are close to neutrality instead of strongly alkaline like other sodium salts of sulphonamides and consequently may be used in the eye. Its use is also advocated for urinary infections in doses of 2-4 Gm. daily.

Sulphadiazine. *Sulphadiazina B.P. Sulfadiazinum U.S.P.*
DOSES: B.P. initial, 2 Gm. (30 gr.); subsequent doses, 1 Gm. (15 gr.) every 4 hours; U.S.P. 2 Gm. (30 gr.). $C_{10}H_{10}N_4O_2S$. Mol.wt. 250.27. M.p. 252-256°. S: 13,000 W; sps. A and acetone; 620 human serum at 37°; fs. in dilute mineral acids and in solutions of sodium and potassium hydroxides and in ammonia. A white or slightly yellow powder; odourless or nearly so; slowly darkens when exposed to light.

⟪ Sulphadiazine is currently the most favoured sulphonamide for the treatment of systemic infections. Toxic side effects are said to be fewer with it than with other sulphonamides, but do occur. Its excretion is slower than that of others and a dosage interval of 6 hours will maintain adequate blood levels.

Sulphadiazine Sodium B.P. *Sulphadiazina Sodium.* **Sulfadiazine Sodium U.S.P.** *Sulfadiazinum Sodicum.* (Soluble Sulfadiazine)
DOSES: B.P., initial, 2 Gm. (30 gr.); subsequent doses 1 Gm. (15 gr.) every 4 hours; U.S.P. 2 Gm. (30 gr.). $C_{10}H_9N_4O_2SNa$. Mol.wt. 272.26. S: 2 W; ss. A. A white powder; on long exposure to humid air it will dissolve carbon dioxide and liberate sulfadiazine; odourless; almost tasteless. A $2\frac{1}{2}\%$ solution of soluble sulphadiazine, with some Triethanolamine, is known as Pickrell's Solution and is recommended for use as nose drops to abort colds.

Injection of Sulphadiazine Sodium B.P.
DOSE: intravenous, 0.5-2 Gm. (8-30 gr.). May be given as 5% solution.

Sulfadiazine Sodium Injection U.S.P.
2.5 Gm. ($37\frac{1}{2}$ gr.) in 50 cc. or in 10 cc.

Sterile Sulfadiazine Sodium U.S.P.
DOSE: 2 Gm. (30 gr.) intravenously.

Sulfadiazine Tablets U.S.P.
Sizes, 300 and 500 mg. (5 and 7½ gr.).

Tablets of Sulphadiazine B.P.
Usual size, 0.5 Gm. (7½ gr.).

Sulphadimidine B.P.C. (T.N. Sulphamezathine, Sulfamethazine)
DOSES: initial, oral, 4 Gm. (60 gr.) followed by 2 Gm. (30 gr.)
every six hours. 2(Sulphanilamido), 4:6, dimethylpyrimidine).
$C_{12}H_{14}O_2N_4S$. Mol.wt. 278.3. M.p. 196-199°. S: vss. W; sps.
A, E, C; sol. acids and alkalis. A white crystalline powder. Available in tablets, each containing 0.5 Gm. (7½ gr.).

℄ Sulphadimidine is one of the more soluble of the sulphonamides
and for that reason unlikely to cause renal damage by reason of
supersaturation in the urine, and precipitation of crystals in the
urinary tract. For the treatment of lobar pneumonia and other
infections susceptible to sulphonamides, sulphadimidine is considered to be about as effective as sulphathiazole of sulphadiazine.
One firm sells this sulfonamide under the name Sulphamezathine
for human use, and another firm sells it as Sulfamethazine for the
treatment of coccidiosis in chickens. It is also a common ingredient
of sulphonamide mixtures, and tablets containing two or more
sulphonamides.

Sulphaguanidine. *Sulphaguanidina B.P. Sulfaguanidinum U.S.P.*
DOSES: B.P. 2-4 Gm. (30-60 gr.); U.S.P. 2 Gm. (30 gr.).
$C_7H_{10}N_4O_2S.H_2O$. Mol.wt. 232.26. M.p. 190-193°. S: 1000 W,
10 W 100°; sps. A, acetone; fs. in dilute mineral acids; ins. in
solutions of alkali hydroxides at room temperature. White, needle-
like, crystalline powder; tasteless; odourless or nearly so; darkens on
exposure to light.

Sulfaguanidine Tablets U.S.P.
Sizes, 300 and 500 mg. (5 and 7½ gr.).

Tablets of Sulphaguanidine B.P.
Usual size, 0.5 Gm. (7½ gr.).

℄ Sulphaguanidine is poorly absorbed and hence used mainly for bacillary dysenteries or for prophylaxis (to reduce intestinal flora) preceding colonic operations.

Sulfamerazine U.S.P. *Sulfamerazinum*
Dose: 2 Gm. (30 gr.). $C_{11}H_{12}N_4O_2S$. Mol.wt. 264.30. M.p. 234-238°. S: 6250 W 20°, 3300 W 37°; readily sol. in solutions of dilute mineral acids and in sodium, potassium and ammonium hydroxides; sps. in acetone, A; ss. E, C. White or faintly yellowish crystals or powder; taste slightly bitter; almost odourless; darkens on exposure to light.

℄ The acetylated form of sulfamerazine is more soluble than most others and hence less likely to cause renal damage. It may be given in smaller quantities than sulfadiazine and adequate blood levels will still be maintained, e.g. 1 Gm. every 8 hours.

Sulfamerazine Tablets U.S.P.
Size, 0.5 Gm. (7½ gr.).

Sulfamerazine Sodium U.S.P. *Sulfamerazinum Sodicum.* (Soluble Sulfamerazine)
$C_{11}H_{11}N_4O_2SNa$. Mol.wt. 286.29. S: 3 W; ss. A; ins. E, C. White or faintly yellow crystalline powder; odourless or nearly so; taste bitter; slowly darkens on exposure to light; absorbs carbon dioxide from the air.

Sterile Sulfamerazine Sodium U.S.P.
Dose: 2 Gm. (30 gr.) intravenously.

Sulfamerazine Sodium Injection U.S.P.
2.5 Gm. (37½ gr.) in 10 cc.; 3 Gm. (45 gr.) in 50 cc.

Sulphanilamide. *Sulphanilamidum*
Doses: B.P. initial, 2 Gm. (30 gr.); subsequent doses, 1 Gm. (15 gr.) every 4 hours; U.S.P. 2 Gm. (30 gr.). $C_6H_8N_2O_2S$. Mol.wt. 172.20. M.p. 164.5-166.5°. S: 125 W, 37 A, 5 acetone; vs. W 100°; sol. G, hydrochloric acid and in solutions of potassium and sodium hydroxides; ins. C, E, B. White crystals, granules, or powder; odourless; affected by light; taste slightly bitter with a sweet after taste.

Sulfanilamide Tablets U.S.P.
Sizes, 300 and 500 mg. (5 and 7½ gr.).

Tablets of Sulphanilamide B.P.
Usual size, 0.5 Gm. (7½ gr.).

℃ Sulphanilamide is less effective against streptococcus, pneumococcus, and staphylococcus than the newer sulphonamides. It also has some toxic effects more or less peculiar to itself, such as producing methaemoglobinaemia and acidosis. On the other hand, anuria is exceedingly rare.

Sulfapyrazine N.N.R.   (2-Sulfanilamidopyrazine)
DOSES: initial, oral, 2-4 Gm. (30-60 gr.), followed by 1 Gm. (15 gr.) every 4-6 hours. $C_{10}H_{10}N_4O_2S$. Mol.wt. 250.27. M.p. 250-254°. S: 20,000 W at 25° and 37°; sol. alkalis and acids; ins. E, C; vss. A; ss. acetone. A white or yellowish white powder which may darken on exposure to light; odourless and tasteless. Available in tablets each containing 0.5 Gm. (7½ gr.).

℃ Sulfapyrazine is one of the more potent sulfonamides. It is about as effective as sulphadiazine for the treatment of pneumococcal, streptococcal, and *E. coli* infections. It is rather slowly absorbed and excreted. Considerable quantities reach the cerebrospinal fluid so that a concentration of ½ to 2/3 of that in the blood may be reached after 12 hours. A relatively small fraction of this sulfonamide is excreted in the acetylated form. Kidney damage has been reported with this drug, as with other sulfonamides of low solubility. It is a suitable ingredient for preparations of two or more sulfonamides in combination.

Sulphathiazole.   *Sulphathiazolum*
DOSES: B.P. initial, 2 Gm. (30 gr.); subsequent doses, 1 Gm. (15 gr.) every 4 hours; U.S.P. 2 Gm. (30 gr.). $C_9H_9N_3O_2S_2$. Mol.wt. 255.31. M.p. 200-204°. S: 1700 W, 200 A; sol. in acetone, in dilute mineral acids and in solutions of sodium, potassium, and ammonium hydroxides. White or faintly yellowish crystals, granules, or powder; odourless; almost tasteless; slowly darkens on exposure to light.

Sulfathiazole Tablets U.S.P.
Sizes, 300 and 500 mg. (5 and 7½ gr.).

Tablets of Sulphathiazole B.P.
Usual size, 0.5 Gm. (7½ gr.).

Sulphathiazole Sodium B.P. *Sulphathiazolum Sodium.* **Sulfa-thiazole Sodium U.S.P.** *Sulfathiazolum Sodicum*

DOSES: B.P. initial, 2 Gm. (30 gr.); subsequent doses, 1 Gm. (15 gr.) every 4 hours; U.S.P. 2 Gm. (30 gr.). $C_9H_8N_3O_2S_2Na.1\frac{1}{2}H_2O$ (U.S.P.), $C_9H_8N_3O_2S_2Na.5H_2O$ (B.P.). Mol.wt. 304.32 (U.S.P.), 367.4 (B.P.). S: 2.5 W, 15 A. A white or yellowish-white crystalline powder; odourless; almost tasteless; absorbs carbon dioxide from the air.

⊄ Sulphathiazole is one of the most effective of the sulphonamides against a wide range of infections. Dosage intervals must be shorter than with sulphadiazine or sulfamerazine, and various toxic effects are said to be more frequent.

Injection of Sulphathiazole Sodium B.P.

DOSE: intravenous, 0.5-2 Gm. (8-30 gr.).

Sulfathiazole Sodium Injection U.S.P.

2.5 Gm. (37$\frac{1}{2}$ gr.) in 10 cc.

Sterile Sulfathiazole Sodium U.S.P.

DOSE: 2 Gm. (30 gr.) intravenously.

Sulfisoxazole N. (T.N. Gantrisin)

DOSES: initial, oral, 4-6 Gm.; maintenance, 1 Gm. every 4 hours. 5-sulfanilamido-3, 4-dimethyl-isoxazole. S: 300 W at pH 6.0. Available in tablets of 0.5 Gm.

⊄ Sulfisoxazole is one of the more potent of the sulfonamides with the particular advantage of relatively good solubility at urinary pH's. This permits large doses with minimal danger of damage in the urinary tract due to supersaturation and precipitation of crystals. It is claimed to be particularly effective against urinary infections by *E. coli*, *B. proteus*, and *B. Pyocyaneus*.

Phthalylsulfathiazole U.S.P. (T.N. Sulfathalidine)

DOSE: 2 Gm. (30 gr.). $C_{17}H_{13}O_5N_3S_2$. Mol.wt. 403.42. M.p. 272-277° with decomposition. S: ins. W, C; ss. A; sol. 10% ammonia, KOH and conc. HCl. White or faintly yellow crystalline powder; odourless; taste slightly bitter.

❡ Sulfathalidine is almost insoluble and is poorly absorbed from the alimentary tract. It is, however, effective against infections in the digestive tract. About 5% of the amount given by mouth may appear in the urine, mostly in conjugated form. The latter is quite soluble in acid urine and thus causes no harm. Sulfathalidine may be used to treat various intestinal infections or to reduce bacterial content of the intestine prior to operations. Usual adult dosage is 4-6 Gm. daily, divided.

Phthalylsulfathiazole Tablets U.S.P.
Size 0.5 Gm. ($7\frac{1}{2}$ gr.).

Sulfobromophthalein Sodium U.S.P. *Sulfobromophthaleinum Sodicum.* (T.N. Bromsulphalein Sodium)
$C_{20}H_8Br_4O_{10}S_2Na_2$. Mol.wt. 838.04. S: sol. W; ins. A, acetone. A white crystalline powder; odourless; taste bitter; hygroscopic.

Sulfobromophthalein Sodium Injection U.S.P.
DOSE: 5 mg. ($\frac{1}{12}$ gr.) intravenously per kg. body weight. Strength, 150 mg. ($2\frac{1}{2}$ gr.) in 3 cc.

❡ The rate of disappearance of bromsulphalein from the blood after intravenous injection is used as a test of liver function.

Precipitated Sulphur. *Sulphur Praecipitatum.* (Milk of Sulphur)
DOSES: B.P. 1-4 Gm. (15-60 gr.); U.S.P. 4 Gm. (60 gr.). At.wt. 32.06. M.p. about 115°. S: ins. W; ss. A; incompletely in 2 of CS_2, 100 olive oil. A very fine, pale-yellow, amorphous or microcrystalline powder without taste or odour.

❡ Precipitated sulphur is softer and less gritty than sublimed sulphur. Either form taken internally is partly converted to sulphides which produce mild laxation. Sulphur ointment was formerly the standard treatment for scabies. It is still used for acne, often in lotions with wetting agents to favour its penetration.

Sublimed Sulphur B.P. *Sulphur Sublimatum.* (Flowers of Sulphur)
DOSES: B.P. 1-4 Gm. (15-60 gr.). At.wt. 32.06. M.p. 115°. S. ins. W; almost ins. A; incompletely in 2 of CS_2, 100 olive oil. A yellow, crystalline, slightly gritty powder with a faint odour and taste.

Sulphur Ointment. *Unguentum Sulphuris*
U.S.P.—Precipitated Sulfur 10, Liquid Petrolatum 10, White Ointment 80.

B.P.—Sublimed Sulphur 10, Simple Ointment (prepared with Soft White Paraffin) 90.

Sulfuric Acid U.S.P. XII. *Acidum Sulfuricum.* (Oil of Vitriol)

H_2SO_4. Mol.wt. 98.08. Sp.gr. 1.84. A colourless, corrosive, oily liquid; becomes very warm when diluted with water; contains about 95% H_2SO_4 by weight.

℟ Sulphuric acid may be used in 30% solution in dentistry to enlarge root canals and as a "pickle" to remove oxidized surface from gold after soldering or casting.

Diluted Sulfuric Acid U.S.P. XII. *Acidum Sulfuricum Dilutum*

A colourless liquid containing 10% by weight H_2SO_4.

℟ As a caustic, sulphuric acid is difficult to control and painful in its action.

Suramin B.P. *Suraminum.* **Suramin Sodium U.S.P.** *Suraminum Sodicum.* (T.N. Naphuride, Bayer 205, Antrypol, Germanin, Fourneau 309)

DOSES: B.P. intravenous, 1-2 Gm. (15-30 gr.); U.S.P. intravenous, 1 Gm. (15 gr.). $C_{51}H_{34}N_6O_{23}S_6Na_6$. Mol.wt. 1429.17. S: sol. W; ss. A; ins. E, C, B. A white or slightly pink powder; odourless; taste slightly bitter; very hygroscopic; affected by light.

Injection of Suramin B.P.

DOSES: intravenous, 1-2 Gm. (15-30 gr.). Supplied dry in sealed containers. Fresh solutions in Water for Injection are made immediately before use.

Sterile Suramin Sodium U.S.P.

DOSE: intravenous, 1 Gm. (15 gr.).

℟ Suramin is used to treat African sleeping sickness. It is particularly effective against infection by T. *gambiense.* The most important manifestation of toxicity is kidney damage.

Syrup. *Syrupus.* (Sirup, Simple Syrup)

U.S.P.—Sucrose 85, Distilled Water to make 100 cc. Sp.gr. about 1.313. B.P.—Sucrose 667, Water to produce 1000 Gm. Gm./cc. 1.315-1.327. The two syrups are of almost equal strength.

Talc U.S.P. *Talcum.* (Purified Talc)

Native hydrous magnesium silicate sometimes containing a small proportion of aluminium silicate.   A fine white or greyish-white crystalline powder; unctuous and free from grittiness.

℄ The smooth texture of talc makes it useful as a dusting powder. It is also used as a lubricant in tablet making.

Tannic Acid B.P. *Acidum Tannicum.* (Tannin, Gallotannic Acid)
S: vs. W, A, acetone; almost ins. B, C, E, petroleum benzin; 1 G warm.   Yellowish-white or brownish glistening scales; light masses or an impalpable powder; odour characteristic; taste strongly astringent; not a pure chemical; obtained from the galls of various species of oak (*Quercus*).

℄ Tannic Acid in 5-10% solution precipitates proteins and is used to produce a coagulum on the surface of burns, particularly extensive burns of the trunk.   Solutions should be freshly made, though a 10% solution with 0.1% salicylic acid is said to keep indefinitely.   Tannic acid is not used on burns of the face or flexor folds because it tends to kill epithelial cells which might otherwise survive.   Indeed, its use on burns of all kinds has declined.   If large areas of burn are tanned, there is some danger of damage to the liver by the absorption of tannic acid.

The suppository or ointment of tannic acid is useful for the symptomatic treatment of haemorrhoids.   The astringent and haemostatic properties of tannic acid have been applied in many ways, e.g. in styptic solutions to stop bleeding from tooth sockets. The solutions of tannic acid in glycerin serve as stock solutions which may be diluted for local application.

Tannic acid or one of its less soluble derivatives (Acetyltannic Acid) is sometimes effective in checking diarrhoea.

Glycerin of Tannic Acid B.P. *Glycerinum Acidi Tannici*
Tannic Acid 15, Glycerin to make 100 Gm.   Gm./cc. 1.288-1.298.

Lozenges of Tannic Acid B.P. *Trochisci Acidi Tannici*
Each lozenge contains 30 mg. ($\frac{1}{2}$ gr.) of Tannic Acid.   See Lozenges of Krameria and Cocaine.

Suppositories of Tannic Acid B.P. *Suppositoria Acidi Tannici*
Tannic Acid 0.2 Gm. (3 gr.) in each suppository.

Tar B.P. *Pix Liquida*
S: misc. A, E, C, glacial acetic acid, fixed and volatile oils; ss. W.
A bituminous liquid prepared from the wood of various species of
Pinus by destructive distillation, known in commerce as Stockholm
tar. A dark-brown or nearly black semi-liquid; heavier than water;
odour and taste characteristic and empyreumatic.

℃ Pine tar has actions like those of coal tar but is used in higher
concentrations (30-70%) in ointments. It is also given in cough
syrups for an expectorant action.

Coal Tar U.S.P. *Pix Carbonis*
S: ss. W; partly sol. A, acetone, methyl alcohol, petroleum benzin,
carbon disulfide, C, E. A by-product during the destructive distillation of bituminous coal; a nearly black, thick liquid; heavier
than water, with a characteristic naphthalene-like odour and a
sharp burning taste.

Prepared Coal Tar B.P. *Pix Carbonis Praeparata*
S: almost ins. W; partly sol. A, E; almost entirely sol. C, B. A
nearly black, viscous liquid, brown in very thin layers, with a
disagreeable empyreumatic odour; prepared by heating commercial
coal tar at 50° in a shallow vessel for 1 hour, stirring frequently.

Coal Tar Ointment U.S.P. *Unguentum Picis Carbonis*
Coal Tar 5, Zinc Oxide Paste 95.

Solution of Coal Tar B.P. *Liquor Picis Carbonis.* (*Liquor Picis
Detergens*)
Prepared Coal Tar 20, with Quillaia and Alcohol to make 100.
Contains 75-85% v/v of C_2H_5OH.

℃ Coal tars contain a great variety of aromatic organic compounds including phenols and cresols. They are accordingly antiseptic and antipruritic. They are also slightly irritant and promote
a mild inflammation with desquamation and proliferation of
epithelium. Coal Tar is used to treat eczema but is contraindicated
when the skin is inflamed. It is applied in lotions or ointments in
concentrations of 2-10%.

Tartaric Acid. *Acidum Tartaricum*
Doses: B.P. 0.3-2 Gm. (5-30 gr.). $(OH)_2.C_2H_2.(COOH)_2$. Mol.wt.

150.09. S: 0.8 W, 3 A, 0.5 W 100°. Colourless crystals or a white powder; odourless; taste strongly acid.

℀ Tartaric acid is used in effervescent powders (Seidlitz Powders). See Effervescent Potassium Citrate.

Tartrazine Can. Supp. *Tartrazina.* (F. D. & C. Yellow No. 5)
$C_{16}H_9N_4O_9S_2Na_3$. Mol.wt. 534.2. S: sol. W, giving a golden-yellow solution; incompletely sol. A. An orange-yellow powder.

℀ Tartrazine is a food dye, stable in acid and alkaline solutions. A concentration of 1:50,000 imparts a bright yellow colour.

Terramycin Hydrochloride N.
DOSES : 2-3 Gm. daily in divided doses at intervals of 4-6 hours. An antibiotic product of *Streptomyces rimosus.* A yellow crystalline powder. Available in capsules containing 50, 100, or 250 mg.; and also for intravenous administration in 10 cc. vials containing 250 mg. in buffered solution.

℀ Terramycin is effective against a wide spectrum of gram positive and gram negative organisms, rickettsial infections, and certain virus-like infections such as atypical pneumonia. It is not effective against measles, mumps, or smallpox; or against infections by *salmonella, B. proteus,* or *B. pyocyaneus.*

After oral administration, peak concentrations in the blood are attained in about 2 hours. At doses of 4 Gm. daily given at six hour intervals, blood levels range from 2-10 mcg. per cc. which are considered adequate for most infections. Nausea and diarrhoea are sometimes observed with large doses. These may be minimized by giving the drug with milk of other food. Serious toxic effects are rare.

Terpineol B.P. *Terpineol*
$C_{10}H_{18}O$. Mol.wt. 154.2. Gm./cc. 0.931-0.935. S: ss. W; sol. A, E. A colourless, viscous liquid which has a pleasant odour and a characteristic bitter and slightly pungent taste.

℀ Terpineol is an antiseptic and is used in the Solution of Chloroxylenol, and also in soaps.

Tetrachloroethylene. *Tetrachloroaethylenum.* (Perchloroethylene)
DOSES: B.P. 1-3 cc. (15-45 min.); U.S.P. 3 cc. (45 min.). C_2Cl_4. Mol.wt. 165.85. B.p. 118-122°. Gm./cc. 1.622-1.630. Sp.gr. 1.603-1.615. S: ins. W; sol. A; misc. E and with oils. A clear,

colourless, mobile liquid having a characteristic ethereal odour; non-inflammable.

Tetrachloroethylene Capsules U.S.P.

Sizes, 0.2, 1, 2.5 cc. (3, 15, 40 min.).

℆ Tetrachloroethylene is less toxic than carbon tetrachloride and is favoured in the treatment of hookworm. Three doses of 1 cc. of tetrachloroethylene are recommended at hourly intervals, followed in 3 hours by a saline purge. Alcohol and fats are witheld for 2-3 days before the treatment and the patient is kept in bed on a diet of skim milk during the treatment. Tetrachloroethylene is not recommended for roundworm infection because it may stimulate the worms so that they curl into a bolus and cause obstruction.

Oil of Theobroma B.P.   Theobroma Oil U.S.P.   *Oleum Theobromatis.* (Cacao Butter, Cocoa Butter)

M.p. 29-34°; Sp.gr. 0.858-0.864. S: ss. A; sol. in boiling dehydrated A; fs. E, C. A yellowish-white solid having a faint, agreeable odour; may have a bland, chocolate-like taste; brittle at temperatures below 25°.

℆ Cocoa butter is a useful base for suppositories.

Theobromine Calcium Salicylate U.S.P.   *Theobrominae Calcii Salicylas*

DOSE: 0.5 Gm. (7½ gr.). S: ss. W; ins. A. A double salt of theobromine calcium, $C_{14}H_{14}CaN_8O_4$ and calcium salicylate, $C_{14}H_{10}CaO_6$; contains not more than 50% of theobromine. A white powder; odourless; taste saline.

Theobromine Calcium Salicylate Tablets U.S.P.

Size, 500 mg. (7½ gr.).

Theobromine and Sodium Acetate U.S.P.   *Theobromina et Sodii Acetas*

DOSE: 0.5 Gm. (7½ gr.). S: 1.5 W; ss. A. A white crystalline powder; almost odourless; taste bitter; hygroscopic.

Theobromine and Sodium Acetate Capsules U.S.P.

Sizes, 100 and 200 mg. (1½ and 3 gr.).

Theobromine and Sodium Acetate Tablets U.S.P.

Sizes, 250, 500, and 750 mg. (4, 7½, and 12 gr.)

Theobromine and Sodium Salicylate B.P. *Theobromina et Sodii Salicylas*
DOSES: 0.6-1.2 Gm. (10-20 gr.). S: 1 W 15.5°; ins. A 90%, E, C. A white amorphous powder; odourless; taste sweetish and alkaline. Contains at least 46% of theobromine and 41% of sodium salicylate.

℄Theobromine, or 3-7 dimethylxanthine, is almost insoluble in water but its solubility is greatly increased by sodium acetate or sodium salicylate, which otherwise do not appreciably modify its action. Theobromine is related to caffeine but has less effect on the central nervous system, i.e. it is less likely to induce wakefulness. It is the principal alkaloid present in cocoa and chocolate. Like caffeine and theophylline, theobromine is a diuretic, but it is considered to be less effective than theophylline.

Theophylline. *Theophyllina.* (1-3 dimethylxanthine)
DOSES: B.P. 60-200 mg. (1-3 gr.); U.S.P. 0.2 Gm. (3 gr.). $C_7H_8N_4O_2.H_2O$. Mol.wt. 198.18. M.p. (B.P.) 269-272°; (U.S.P.) 270-274°. S: 120 W, 80 A, more sol. W 100°; sparingly sol. E; C; fs. solutions of sodium and potassium hydroxides and ammonia. A white crystalline powder; odourless; taste bitter.

Injection of Theophylline with Ethylenediamine B.P.
. See Aminophylline and Mersalyl.

Theophylline and Sodium Acetate B.P. *Theophyllina et Sodii Acetas.* (Theophylline with Sodium Acetate)
DOSES: B.P. 0.12-0.3 Gm. (2-5 gr.) S: 25 W; ins. A, E. C. A white crystalline powder; odourless; taste bitter and salty; gradually absorbs carbon dioxide from the air. Contains 55-65% of anhydrous theophylline.

Theophylline-Sodium Glycinate N.N.R. (T.N. Theoglycinate)
DOSES: 0.3-1.0 Gm. (5-15 gr.) orally, in tablets, powders or syrups. One mole of theophylline sodium with slightly more than 2 moles of glycine, contains 49-52% of theophylline. S: fs. W. Incompatible with acids. A white odourless powder with a bitter taste. Available in tablets containing 0.33 Gm.; suppositories containing 0.78 Gm. and in various proprietary syrups and elixirs.

℄ Theophylline-sodium glycinate has the same actions and uses as aminophylline and its most important use is in the treatment of asthma. The effects are thought to be due entirely to the theo-

phylline. Therefore it is important to realize that whereas aminophylline contains about 78% theophylline, the glycinate contains
only about 50% theophylline. In other words, 0.78 Gm. of theophylline-sodium glycinate is equivalent to about 0.5 Gm. of aminophylline.

Theophylline-sodium glycinate is claimed to be less irritant than
aminophylline when given orally. While aminophylline is often
given intravenously, the glycinate is recommended chiefly for oral
or rectal administration. It may, however, be given by inhalation
as an aerosol. For this purpose a 5-10% aqueous solution is nebulized with oxygen. About 2 cc. of this solution are given every
four hours.

Thiouracil B.P. *Thiouracilum*
DOSES: 0.1-0.2 Gm. (1½-3 gr.). $C_4H_4ON_2S$. Mol.wt. 128.2.
S: ss. W, A 90%, E and in acids; readily sol. in dil. solutions of
sodium hydroxide in water. A white or pale-cream powder; odourless; taste bitter.

Tablets of Thiouracil
Size, 0.1 Gm. (1½ gr.).

℄ Thiouracil and its various derivatives act on the thyroid gland,
preventing the production of thyroxine, perhaps by inhibiting a
peroxidase system. The lack of circulating thyroxin evokes a
secretion of thyrotropic hormone from the anterior pituitary, causing
hypertrophy and hyperplasia of the thyroid gland. Thus we have the
paradox that thiouracil is a goitrogenic agent but may be used to
treat hyperthyroidism. The metabolic rate is lowered but exophthalmos, if present, may be exaggerated because it is somehow
connected with excessive thyrotropic activity. Thiouracil and its
derivatives may be used to prepare patients for thyroid surgery or
they may be used for prolonged medical treatment of hyperthyroidism. Toxic effects are not uncommon. The most important
of these is agranulocytosis. If exophthalmos tends to increase
during treatment with thiouracil, dried thyroid may be given to
suppress thyrotropic activity.

Methylthiouracil B.P. *Methylthiouracilum.* (6-methylthiouracil)
DOSES: 0.05-0.2 Gm. (¾-3 gr.). $C_5H_6ON_2S$. Mol.wt. 142.2. S:
ss. W, A, and dilute mineral acids; readily sol. in dilute sodium
hydroxide solution. A white or pale-cream powder; odourless;
taste bitter.

Tablets of Methylthiouracil B.P.
Size, 0.1 Gm. (1½ gr.).

Propylthiouracil U.S.P. *Propylthiouracilum*
DOSE: 50 mg. (¾ gr.); 50-150 mg. daily. $C_7H_{10}N_2OS$. Mol.wt. 170.23. M.p. 218-221°. S: vss. W; ss. C, E; sparingly sol. A. A white powdery crystalline substance resembling starch in appearance; taste bitter.

Propylthiouracil Tablets U.S.P.
Sizes, 25 and 50 mg. (⅜ and ¾ gr.).

ℭ The occurrence of fever, rash, and other undesirable effects such as agranulocytosis, has been substantially less with propylthiouracil than with thiouracil, and in consequence it has become the drug of choice for treating hyperthyroidism. It is not clear yet whether it is any better than methylthiouracil.

Thrombin U.S.P. *Thrombinum*
A sterile protein substance prepared from prothrombin of animal (usually human or bovine) origin; for topical application to promote blood clotting.

Thymol B.P., N.F. *Thymol*
DOSES: B.P. 30-120 mg. (½-2 gr.); anthelmintic, 1-2 Gm. (15-30 gr.); N.F. anthelmintic, 2 Gm. (30 gr.) divided into 3 doses. $C_{10}H_{14}O$. Mol. wt. 150.21. M.p. 48-51°. S: 1000 W, 1 A, 1 C, 1.5 E, 2 olive oil; sol. glacial acetic acid and in fixed or volatile oils. Colourless crystals, often large, or a white crystalline powder; odour pungent, aromatic, and thyme-like. Prepared synthetically or from *Thymus vulgaris* or *Trachyspermum Ammi* or *Monarda punctata.*

ℭ Thymol in saturated aqueous solution is bacteriostatic and fungicidal and may be used as a preservative. It is used in mouth washes and gargles and leaves a pleasant sensation in the mouth and throat. In such concentration it has little or no germicidal effect. Thymol has been given by mouth for hookworm but is now superseded by tetrachloroethylene. It is a useful ingredient of dusting powders for the prophylaxis of fungal infections.

Thyroid. *Thyroideum.* (Dry Thyroid, Thyroid Extract, Thyroid Gland)
DOSES: B.P. 30-120 mg. (½-2 gr.); U.S.P. 60 mg. (1 gr.). *N.B.:*

Thyroid Extract differs in strength in Canada, U.S.A., and Great Britain. The cleaned, dried, and powdered thyroid glands, free from fat and connective tissue, are obtained from domesticated animals used for food by man. A yellowish to buff-coloured amorphous powder, having a slight characteristic meat-like odour and a saline taste. Contains: B.P. 0.09-0.11% of iodine in combination as thyroxine; U.S.P. 0.17-0.23% of iodine in thyroid combination and must be free from iodine in inorganic or any form of combination other than that peculiar to the thyroid gland; Can. Gaz. 0.27-0.33% of iodine and shall contain no added iodine in either organic or inorganic form.

Thyroid Tablets U.S.P.
Sizes, 15, 30, 60 and 120 mg. ($\frac{1}{4}$, $\frac{1}{2}$, 1 and 2 gr.).

Tablets of Thyroid B.P.
Size, 30 mg. ($\frac{1}{2}$ gr.).

❦ Dried thyroid is indicated in hypothyroid states but is used in many other conditions, sometimes as an adjunct to a reducing diet. Overdosage leads to nervousness, tachycardia, and sometimes diarrhoea.

Balsam of Tolu B.P. Tolu Balsam U.S.P. *Balsamum Tolutanum.* (Tolu)
S: nearly ins. W, petroleum benzin; sol. A, C, E. A brown or yellowish-brown plastic solid; brittle when old, dried, or exposed to cold; odour, vanilla-like; taste mild, aromatic; obtained from *Myroxylon Balsamum.*

Syrup of Tolu B.P. *Syrupus Tolutanus.* (Syrup of Balsam of Tolu)
DOSES: 2-8 cc. (30-120 min.). Balsam of Tolu 2.5, Sucrose 66, Distilled Water to make 100 Gm.

Tolu Balsam Syrup U.S.P. *Syrupus Balsami Tolutani.* (Syrup of Tolu)
Tolu Balsam Tincture 5, Magnesium Carbonate 1, Sucrose 82, Distilled Water to make 100 cc.

❦ The syrup is used as a flavour for cough mixtures. It is said to have expectorant properties but they must be feeble.

Tincture of Tolu B.P.   *Tinctura Tolutana.*   (Tincture of Balsam of Tolu)

DOSES: 2-4 cc. (30-60 min.).   Balsam of Tolu 10 Gm. to make 100 cc.   Contains 80-84% v/v of C_2H_5OH.

Tolu Balsam Tincture U.S.P.   *Tinctura Balsami Tolutani.*   (Tolu Tincture)

DOSE: 2 cc. (30 min.).   Tolu Balsam 20, Alcohol to make 100, by maceration.   Contains 77-83% v/v of C_2H_5OH.

℄ The tinctures of tolu are sometimes given by mouth as expectorants.   If given in mixtures with water, acacia is added to prevent settling out of the resin.

Totaquine B.P.   *Totaquina*

DOSES: B.P. 0.3-0.6 Gm. (5-10 gr.).   S: almost ins. W; most of it dissolves in warm A and in C; it is partly sol. in E.   A white to greyish-white or yellowish-white powder; odourless; taste bitter; contains not less than 14% of quinine and between 70-80% of the total anhydrous crystallizable cinchona alkaloids.

℄ Being less expensive than quinine, totaquine has a definite place in public health and institutional practice for suppressive or active treatment of malaria.

Tragacanth.   *Tragacantha.*   (Gum Tragacanth)

The dried gummy exudation from *Astragalus gummifer* and other species of *Astragalus*; odourless; taste insipid, mucilaginous.

Powdered Tragacanth B.P.   *Tragacanthae Pulvis*

A white powder.

℄ Tragacanth swells in water to form a thick gel which is useful for suspending insoluble material.   It is less useful than acacia as an emulsifying agent.

Mucilage of Tragacanth B.P.   *Mucilago Tragacanthae*

Powdered Tragacanth 12.5 Gm. with Alcohol and Chloroform Water to make 1000 cc.

Compound Powder of Tragacanth B.P.   *Pulvis Tragacanthae Compositus*

DOSES: 0.6-4 Gm. (10-60 gr.).   Tragacanth 15, Acacia 20, with Starch and Sucrose to make 100 Gm.

℟ The compound powder and mucilages of tragacanth are used to suspend insoluble materials in liquids.

Trichloracetic Acid. B.P. *Acidum Trichloraceticum.* **Trichloroacetic Acid U.S.P.** *Acidum Trichloroaceticum.*
$CCl_3.COOH$. Mol.wt. 163.4. M.p. 55-57°. S: 0.1 W; sol. A, E. Colourless, very deliquescent crystals; odour pungent and characteristic.

℟ Trichloracetic acid precipitates proteins. The acid may be applied undiluted to warts or callouses. It was at one time used to a considerable extent as a styptic and caustic in dentistry.

Trichloroethylene. *Trichloroaethylenum.* (T.N. Trilene)
DOSE: U.S.P. by inhalation, 1 cc. (15 min.). C_2HCl_3. Mol.wt. 131.40. B.p. 86-88°. Gm./cc. 1.462-1.468. Sp.gr. 1.456-1.462. S: ins. W; misc. A, E, C; dissolves most fixed and volatile oils. A clear, colourless, mobile liquid having an odour resembling that of chloroform; non-inflammable.

℟ Trichloroethylene may be used as a general anaesthetic but the boiling point is high and a special vaporizer is required. One cc. inhaled from a piece of gauze will induce analgesia and has been recommended for the treatment of trigeminal neuralgia. The patient should be lying down during the treatment, which may be repeated 4 or 5 times a day for several weeks. It has also been recommended as an obstetrical analgesic. *It should never be used in apparatus containing Soda Lime.*

Triethanolamine U.S.P. *Triethanolamina*
Sp.gr. 1.1204-1.1284. S: misc. W, A; sol. C. A mixture of alkanolamines consisting largely of triethanolamine with various amounts of di- and mono-ethanolamine. A colourless to pale-yellow, viscous, hygroscopic liquid having a slight ammoniacal odour.

℟ Triethanolamine is a base which reacts with fatty acids to form emulsifying soaps with excellent qualities. It is used in making vanishing creams and cold creams. It is also used in Pickrell's solution. See Sulphadiazine.

Trimethadione U.S.P. *Trimethadionum.* (T.N. Tridione)
USUAL DAILY DOSE: 1 Gm. (15 gr.). $C_6H_9NO_3$. 3, 5, 5-trimethyl-oxazolidine-2, 4-dione. Mol.wt. 143.14. M.p. 45-57°. S: sol. W; fs. A, E, C. White crystalline granules; odour resembling camphor.

Trimethadione Capsules U.S.P.
Size, 0.3 Gm. (5 gr.)

Trimethadione Tablets U.S.P.
Size, 0.15 Gm. (2½ gr.).

℮ Trimethadione is an anticonvulsant with some analgesic action.
It is particularly useful for the treatment of epilepsy of the *petit mal*
type but has little value for the control of *grand mal* epilepsy. It
may be given with phenytoin sodium (Dilantin) to control psycho-
motor epilepsy.

Toxic reactions are fairly common and include rashes and a
peculiar sensation of brightness or glare in the eyes. Agranulocytosis and aplastic anaemia occur occasionally.

Oil of Turpentine B.P. *Oleum Terebinthinae.* (Rectified Oil of
Turpentine)
DOSES: 0.2-0.6cc. (3-10 min.). Gm./cc. 0.855-0.865. S: 7 vols.
A 90% 15.5°; misc. A, E, C, and glacial acetic acid. The oil distilled
from the oleo-resin, turpentine, obtained from various species of
Pinus. A colourless, limpid liquid; odour characteristic; taste
pungent and somewhat bitter.

Liniment of Turpentine B.P. *Linimentum Terebinthinae*
Oil of Turpentine 65 cc., Camphor 5 Gm., with Soft Soap 7.5 Gm.,
and Distilled Water to make 100 cc.

℮ Turpentine is an old-fashioned remedy for coughs, colds, and
"kidney trouble." It has an expectorant action when taken
internally, and rubefacient and antiseptic actions when applied
externally. It may be irritant to the urinary tract when taken
orally or absorbed from large areas of skin.

Tyrothricin U.S.P. *Tyrothricinum*
An antibacterial substance produced by the growth of *Bacillus
brevis* (Dubos), consisting principally of gramicidin and tyrocidine.

Tyrothricin Spray U.S.P. *Nebula Tyrothricini*
A spray prepared by dissolving tyrothricin in water by the aid of
suitable, harmless, solubilizing and wetting agents.

Tyrothricin Troches U.S.P.
Sizes, 1 and 2 mg. (1/60 and 1/30 gr.).

❪ Tyrothricin is not effective when given orally, and too toxic for parenteral administration. Its use is limited to nasal sprays and local applications. Local allergic sensitization to tyrothricin may occur.

Urea. *Urea.* (Carbamide)
DOSES: B.P. 5-15 Gm. (75-225 gr.); U.S.P. 8 Gm. (2 dr.). CH_4N_2O. Mol.wt. 60.06. M.p. 131-133°. S: 1.5 W, 10 A, 1 A 78°; almost ins. C, E. White prismatic crystals or a white crystalline powder; odourless; cooling, saline taste.

❪ Urea is rapidly eliminated by the kidneys and hence may be used as a diuretic. Strong solutions of urea are useful for dissolving coagulated protein. Saturated solutions have been applied to foul ulcers and sloughing cancers. They do not delay the healing of healthy tissue.

Urethane. *Urethanum.* (Ethyl Carbamate)
DOSES: B.P. 1-2 Gm. (15-30 gr.). $C_3H_7O_2N$. Mol.wt. 89.09. M.p. 48-50°. S: 0.5 W, 1 A, 3 G, 1 C, 2 E, 35 olive oil. Colourless crystals or a white granular powder; odourless; taste cooling, saline and slightly bitter.

❪ Large doses of urethane are used for basal anaesthesia; it has been used as a hypnotic in medical practice but is regarded as too weak and unreliable. Urethane inhibits intracellular respiratory enzymes and has recently been reported to be beneficial in lymphatic leukaemia.

Valerian B.P. *Valeriana.* (Valerian Rhizome)
The rhizome and roots of *Valeriana officinalis* collected in the autumn and dried.

Powdered Valerian B.P. *Valerianae Pulvis*
A light brown powder.

Ammoniated Tincture of Valerian B.P. *Tinctura Valerianae Ammoniata*
DOSES: 2-4 cc. (30-60 min.). Valerian 20 Gm., with Oil of Nutmeg, Oil of Lemon, Dilute Solution of Ammonia, and Alcohol to make about 100 cc., by maceration. Contains 50-54% v/v of C_2H_5OH.

℄ Valerian has been used as a sedative in hysterical states. It is thought now to be effective mainly on account of its impressive and persistent odour, but it is still used to treat acute alcoholism.

Vanilla U.S.P. *Vanilla.* (Vanilla Bean)
The cured, full-grown, unripe fruit of *Vanilla planifolia* or of *Vanilla tahitensis.*

Vanilla Tincture U.S.P. *Tinctura Vanillae*
Vanilla 100, Sucrose 200, Alcohol and Water to make 1000 cc. by maceration and percolation. Contains 38%-42% C_2H_5OH.

Vanillin. *Vanillinum*
$C_8H_8O_3$. Mol.wt. 152.14. M.p. 81-83°. S: 100 W, 20 G, 20 W 80°; fs. A, C, E, and in solutions of fixed alkali hydroxides. Fine white to yellowish crystals, usually needle-like; odour and taste characteristic of vanilla.

℄ Vanillin is used only as a flavour.

Vasopressin Injection
See Pituitary.

Vinyl Ether. *Aether Vinylicus.* (Divinyl Oxide, Divinyl Ether)
C_4H_6O. Mol.wt. 70.09. Gm./cc. 0.770-0.778. B.p. 28-31°. S: ss. W; misc. A, acetone, C, E. A clear, colourless, volatile liquid having a characteristic odour. *Inflammable.* Contains about 4% of C_2H_5OH to reduce its volatility, and a suitable stabilizer.

℄ Inhalation of the vapour of vinyl ether produces anaesthesia with great rapidity (less than 2 minutes) so that great care is necessary in its administration. Recovery is rapid and vomiting uncommon. It is mostly used for induction of anaesthesia, or for short minor operations, and sometimes for obstetrical analgesia. Anaesthetic concentration in the blood is 15-30 mg. %, in air about 4% by volume. It is sometimes used in dentistry. Disadvantages are inflammability and danger of damage to the liver in long operations.

Vitamins are presented in the following order: A, B complex, C, D, K, A and D, multi-vitamin combinations.

VITAMIN A

Concentrated Solution of Vitamin A B.P. *Liquor Vitamini A Concentratus.* **Oleovitamin A U.S.P.** *Oleovitamina A.* (Natural Vitamin A in Oil)

DOSES: B.P. 0.06-0.6 cc. (1-10 min.) (2500-25,000 units) daily; U.S.P. as prescribed. S: ss. A; misc. E, C, light petroleum.

An oily solution of Vitamin A, containing a small amount of Vitamin D. U.S.P.—Vitamin A, 50,000-65,000 units per Gm., with not more than 1000 units of Vitamin D. B.P.—50,000 units of Vitamin A per Gm., with not more than 500 units of Vitamin D. U.S.P. and B.P. procedures for bioassay in units are not identical but probably give equivalent results. The international unit of Vitamin A is 0.6 microgram of beta-carotene.

Oleovitamin A Capsules U.S.P.

DOSE: daily prophylactic, 5000 U.S.P. units. Sizes, 5000 and 25,000 U.S.P. units of Vitamin A.

❡ Vitamin A is sometimes called the anti-infective vitamin but this description is misleading. Prolonged deficiency of this vitamin causes xerophthalmia and secondary infection of the conjunctivae. It also causes night blindness (nutritional nyctalopia or hemeralopia).

B VITAMINS

Aneurine Hydrochloride B P. *Aneurinae Hydrochloridum.* **Thiamine Hydrochloride U.S.P., Can. Supp.** *Thiaminae Hydrochloridum.* (Thiamin Chloride, Vitamin B_1 Hydrochloride, Vitamin B_1)

DOSES: B.P. daily prophylactic, 2-5 mg. ($\frac{1}{30}$-$\frac{1}{12}$ gr.) daily therapeutic, 20-50 mg.($\frac{1}{3}$-$\frac{3}{4}$ gr.); U.S.P. as prescribed. $C_{12}H_{17}Cl\ N_4OSHCl$ (U.S.P.); + $1H_2O$ (B.P.). Mol.wt. 337.27 (U.S.P.); 355.3 (B.P.). S: 1 W, 100 A; sol. G; ins. E, B. Small white crystals or a crystalline powder having a slight characteristic odour; taste bitter.

❡ Thiamine is specific for beri-beri. It has been used hopefully in a great variety of nervous diseases, sometimes with apparently beneficial effects. Alcoholic neuritis responds well to large doses. Prophylactic administration may be advisable during arsenical therapy to prevent arsenical encephalopathy and other toxic reactions to arsenic.

Injection of Aneurine Hydrochloride B.P.

DOSES: subcutaneous or intramuscular, 10-30 mg. ($\frac{1}{6}$-$\frac{1}{2}$ gr.). Strength, 25 mg. per cc. ($\frac{2}{5}$ gr. in 15 min.).

Thiamine Hydrochloride Tablets U.S.P.

Sizes, 3, 5, 10 mg. ($\frac{1}{20}$, $\frac{1}{12}$, $\frac{1}{6}$ gr.).

Tablets of Aneurine Hydrochloride B.P. (Tablets of Vitamin B₁)

Thiamine Hydrochloride Tablets
Size, 1 mg. ($\frac{1}{60}$ gr.).

Thiamine Hydrochloride Injection U.S.P.

Sizes, 10 mg. ($\frac{1}{6}$ gr.) in 1 cc.; 0.25 Gm. (4 gr.) in 10 cc.; 0.1, 0.5, 1.0 Gm. in 10 cc.; 3 Gm. in 30 cc.

Extract of Malt B.P. *Extractum Malti*

DOSES: 4-30 cc. (60 min.-1 fl.oz.) daily. S: misc. W, giving a translucent solution. An amber or yellowish-brown viscous liquid; odour agreeable and characteristic; taste sweet; may be prepared from malted barley or a mixture of barley and not more than 33% wheat.

❡ Malt extract contains easily digestible sugars and is a rich source of B vitamins. It is thus an agreeable and nutritive vehicle for tonics and other medications.

Nicotinamide. *Nicotinamidum.* (Nicotinic Acid Amide, Niacinamide)

DOSES: B.P. prophylactic, 15-30 mg. ($\frac{1}{4}$-$\frac{1}{2}$ gr.) daily; therapeutic, 50-250 mg. ($\frac{3}{4}$-4 gr.) daily; U.S.P. 25 mg. ($\frac{3}{8}$ gr.). $C_6H_6ON_2$. Mol.wt. 122.1. M.p. 128-131°. S: sol. 1 W, 1.5 A, 10 G. A white crystalline powder; almost odourless; taste bitter.

Nicotinamide Capsules U.S.P.

Size, 25 mg. ($\frac{3}{8}$ gr.).

Nicotinamide Injection U.S.P.

DOSE: 100 mg. ($1\frac{1}{2}$ gr.). Sizes, 100 mg. in 1 cc.; 100 mg. in 2 cc.

Nicotinamide Tablets U.S.P.

Sizes, 25 and 50 mg. ($\frac{3}{8}$ and $\frac{3}{4}$ gr.).

Tablets of Nicotinamide B.P. (Tablets of Nicotinic Acid Amide)

Size, 50 mg. ($\frac{3}{4}$ gr.)

Nicotinic Acid. *Acidum Nicotinicum.* (Niacin)

DOSES: 15-30 mg. ($\frac{1}{4}$-$\frac{1}{2}$ gr.) daily; therapeutic, 50-250 mg. ($\frac{3}{4}$-4 gr.) daily; U.S.P. 25 mg. ($\frac{3}{8}$ gr.). $C_5H_4N.COOH$. Mol.wt. 123.1. M.p. 234-237°. S: 60 W; ins. E; vs. W 100°; vs. A 78° and alkali hydroxides. White crystals; odourless; taste feebly acid.

Nicotinic Acid Capsules U.S.P.

Sizes, 25, 50 and 100 mg. ($\frac{3}{8}$, $\frac{3}{4}$ and 1$\frac{1}{2}$ gr.).

Nicotinic Acid Tablets U.S.P.

Sizes, 25, 50, 100 mg. ($\frac{3}{8}$, $\frac{3}{4}$, 1$\frac{1}{2}$ gr.).

Tablets of Nicotinic Acid B.P.

Size, 50 mg. $\frac{3}{4}$ gr.

⟨ Nicotinic acid and nicotinamide, once known as PP factor, form part of the vitamin B complex. They relieve most of the symptoms of pellagra. Doses of 50-100 mg. produce flushing and dizziness.

Riboflavine B.P. *Riboflavina.* **Riboflavin U.S.P.** *Riboflavinum.* (Lactoflavin, Vitamin B$_2$, Vitamin G)

DOSES: B.P. 1-4 mg. ($\frac{1}{60}$-$\frac{1}{16}$ gr.) daily; therapeutic, 5-10 mg. ($\frac{1}{12}$-$\frac{1}{6}$ gr.) daily; U.S.P. to be determined by the physician. $C_{17}H_{20}N_4O_6$. Mol.wt. 376.36. M.p. about 280°. S: 10,000 W; more sol. in isotonic sodium chloride solution; less sol. A; ins. E, C; vs. dilute alkalies. A yellow to orange-yellow crystalline powder; slight odour; taste slightly bitter; solutions, especially if alkaline, deteriorate rapidly in light.

Riboflavin Injection U.S.P.

Sizes, 0.2 mg. ($\frac{1}{300}$ gr.) in 1 cc.; 1 mg. ($\frac{1}{60}$ gr.) in 2 cc.; 5 mg. ($\frac{1}{12}$ gr.) in 1 cc.

Riboflavin Tablets U.S.P.

Sizes, 1 and 5 mg. ($\frac{1}{60}$ and $\frac{1}{12}$ gr.).

⟨ Riboflavine is a constituent of the intracellular respiratory enzyme system, sometimes known as yellow enzyme. A rich source of dietary intake is milk. Mild deficiency shows as soreness and reddening of the eyes, with some vascular invasion of the edges of the cornea. Typical lesions of more severe deficiency are glossitis and sores at the corners of the mouth.

Rice Polishings U.S.P. *Perpolitiones Oryzae.* (Rice Bran, Tikitiki)
Fine, flaky, yellowish or pale-orange powder; taste sweetish; odour characteristic and non-rancid.

Rice Polishings Extract U.S.P. *Extractum Perpolitionum Oryzae.* (Tikitiki Extract, Rice Bran Extract, Extracto de Salvado)
DOSE: 8 cc. (2 fl.dr.). A dark-brown, viscous liquid having the odour of burnt sugar and a sweetish taste. Each cc. contains not less than 0.06 mg. of vitamin B_1.

⚌ Although standardized only as to content of vitamin B_1, rice polishings are a rich source of other members of the B complex, and are favoured as a form of administering B complex when a multiple deficiency is suspected, for example in chronic infantile diarrhoea.

Triasyn B Capsules U.S.P. and Triasyn B Tablets U.S.P.
DOSE: to be determined by the physician. Each capsule or tablet contains 2 mg. Thiamine Hydrochloride, 3 mg. of Riboflavine, 20 mg. of Nicotinamide.

Dried Yeast U.S.P. *Saccharomyces Siccum.* (Dry Yeast)
DOSE: to be determined by the physician. The dried cells of any suitable strain of *Saccharomyces cerevisiae*; yellowish-white to yellowish-orange flakes, granules, or powder, having an odour and taste characteristic of the strain. Each Gm. contains not less than 0.12 mg. of Thiamine Hydrochloride, 0.04 mg. of Riboflavine, 0.25 mg. of Nicotinic Acid.

Dried Yeast Tablets U.S.P. *Tabellae Saccharomycitis Sicci*
DOSE: to be determined by the physician. Size, 0.5 Gm. (7½ gr.).

⚌ Dried yeast is a rich source of the various members of the vitamin B complex.

Vitamin B_{12} U.S.P. *Vitamina B_{12}.* (T.N. Cobione, Anacobin, Rubramine)
DOSES: 15-30 microgm. by injection once or twice weekly for macrocytic anaemias. M.p. above 300°. S: 80 W. A red crystalline powder; odourless and tasteless; decomposed by strong acids, alkalis, reducing or oxidizing agents, phenol, and by light.

⚌ Vitamin B_{12} is the most potent material yet found for the treatment of pernicious anaemia. It may well prove to be the long sought active principle of liver extract. It not only causes a prompt reticulocyte response in untreated cases of pernicious anaemia but it also causes improvement in the symptoms of subacute combined degeneration of the spinal cord. To produce effects when given orally to patients with macrocytic anaemia, the dose has had to be increased to about 30 microgm. or more daily. However, the addition of extracts of normal stomach or gastric juice greatly increased the potency of orally administered B_{12} so that 5-10 microgm. daily have given excellent responses. The addition of folic acid also increases the oral activity of B_{12}. Oral administration may, before long, replace therapy by injection.

Vitamin B_{12} is available in concentrates as well as in crystalline form. There is some reason to believe that some substance in the concentrate helps to stabilize B_{12}. In liver extract, or in concentrates, the B_{12} content has to be assayed by its action on humans with pernicious anaemia, or by a microbiological assay making use of its stimulating effect on growth of *L. lactis* or a certain species of algae. Three or four variants of B_{12} have been found. These are identified tentatively as B_{12a}, B_{12b}^{1}, and B_{12c}. B_{12} and B_{12b} are said to be equally active, while B_{12a} and B_{12c} are less active.

Vitamin B_{12} Injection U.S.P.
10 and 15 micrograms in 1 cc.

VITAMIN C

Ascorbic Acid. *Acidum Ascorbicum.* (Vitamin C, Cevitamic Acid)
DOSE: B.P. prophylactic, 25-75 mg. ($\frac{2}{5}$-1$\frac{1}{4}$ gr.) daily; therapeutic, 0.2-0.5 Gm. (3-8 gr.) daily; U.S.P. to be determined by the physician. $C_6H_8O_6$. Mol.wt. 176.12. M.p. 190-192°. S: 3 W, 30 A; ins. C, E, B. White or slightly yellowish crystals or powder; odourless; taste acid, resembling that of lemon juice; darkens on exposure to light; deteriorates in aqueous solution, especially if alkaline.

Ascorbic Acid Tablets U.S.P.
Sizes, 25, 50, 100 mg. ($\frac{3}{8}$, $\frac{3}{4}$, 1$\frac{1}{2}$ gr.).

℃ Ascorbic acid prevents and cures scurvy. In adults 15-25 mg. a day will prevent scurvy but there is much debate about the optimum daily intake, which is set as high as 50 mg. by some authorities. Very large doses, up to 10 Gm., have no demonstrable toxic effects.

Tablets of Ascorbic Acid B.P.   (Tablets of Vitamin C)
  Size, 50 mg.   ($\frac{3}{4}$ gr.)

Sodium Ascorbate Injection U.S.P.
  DOSE: 0.1 Gm. ($1\frac{1}{2}$ gr.).   Sizes, 0.1 Gm. ($1\frac{1}{2}$ gr.) in 2 cc.; 0.5 Gm.
($7\frac{1}{2}$ gr.) in 2 cc.; 0.5 Gm. ($7\frac{1}{2}$ gr.) in 5 cc.; 0.5 Gm. ($7\frac{1}{2}$ gr.) in 10 cc.;
1.0 Gm. (15 gr.) in 5 cc.

D VITAMINS

Calciferol.   *Calciferol.*   (Irradiated Ergosterol, Vitamin D_2, Vio-
    sterol)
  DOSES: for infants or adults, prophylactic, daily, 0.025-0.1 mg.
($\frac{1}{2400}$ - $\frac{1}{600}$ gr.) 1000-4000 units; therapeutic, daily, 0.05-0.5 mg.
($\frac{1}{1200}$ - $\frac{1}{120}$ gr.) 2000-20,000 units.   The minimum dose (0.025 mg.)
= 1000 International Units.   M.p. 115-118°.   S: ins. W; sol. 50-100
vegetable oils; sol. E, C, A, acetone.   Colourless, acicular needles;
odourless; tasteless.

Solution of Calciferol B.P.   *Liquor Calciferolis* .   (Viosterol in Oil)
  DOSES: infants or adults, prophylactic, daily, 0.3-1.2 cc. (5-20
min.) (1000-4000 units); therapeutic, 0.6-6 cc. (10-100 min.) 2000-
20,000 units daily.   Six cc. contain 20,000 units.   Calciferol dissolved in a suitable oil.   A pale yellow, oily liquid; odour slight but
not rancid; taste bland.   Contains 3000 units of antirachitic activity
per Gm.

Synthetic Oleovitamin D U.S.P.   *Oleovitamina D Synthetica.*
    (Vitamin D_2 or D_3 in oil)
  DOSE: as prescribed.   S: ss. A; misc. E, C.   Activated ergosterol
or activated 7-dehydrocholesterol in an edible vegetable oil; each
Gm. contains not less than 10,000 U.S.P. Units of Vitamin D.

Activated 7-Dehydrocholesterol U.S.P.   *7-Dehydrocholesterol Acti-
    vatum.*   (Vitamin D_3)
  $C_{27}H_{44}O$.   Mol.wt. 384.62   M.p. 82.-86°.   S: ins. W; sol. A, C
and in fatty oils.   White odourless crystals, affected by air and light.

Concentrated Solution of Vitamin D B.P.   *Liquor Vitamini D
    Concentratus*
  DOSES: prophylactic, daily, 0.1-0.4 cc. ($1\frac{1}{2}$-6 min.) 1000-4000
units; therapeutic, daily, 0.2-2 cc. (3-30 min.) 2000-20,000 units.

S: ss. A; misc. E, C, and light petroleum. A solution of vitamin D containing in 1 Gm. 10,000 units of vitamin D. It may consist of a suitable fish-liver oil or blend of fish-liver oils, or have been formed by dissolving a suitable source of vitamin D, including calciferol, in a suitable vegetable oil. A pale-yellow or yellow oily liquid having a faint but not rancid fishy odour and taste; contains not more than 5000 units of vitamin A per Gm.

⟪ In addition to the prevention or cure of rickets and osteomalacia, mobilization of calcium into the blood stream can be accomplished by rather large doses of calciferol. Hypoparathyroid tetany may be treated by large doses. Very large doses, used sometimes for the treatment of arthritis, are dangerous. Calcium deposits may be formed in the kidney, resulting in hypertension or urolithiasis. There is some evidence that synthetic vitamin D may not be as effective in preventing or curing rickets in humans as vitamin D from natural sources.

K VITAMINS

Acetomenaphthone B.P. *Acetomenaphthonum.*
DOSES: 2-10 mg. ($\frac{1}{30}$ - $\frac{1}{6}$ gr.). 1 : 4-diacetoxy-2-methylnaphthalene. $C_{15}H_{14}O_4$. Mol.wt. 258.3. M.p. 112-114°. S: almost ins. W; ss. cold A, 3.3 A 78°. A white crystalline powder; odourless or with a slight odour of acetic acid.

⟪ Acetomenaphthone and Menadione have the actions of vitamin K. They are given to restore plasma prothrombin when this is depleted, as in obstructive jaundice or in conditions of faulty absorption of fat. They are also given to infants with haemorrhagic disease. Acetomenaphthone is said to be less irritant than Menadione and better absorbed when taken by mouth.

Tablets of Acetomenaphthone B.P.
Size, 5 mg. ($\frac{1}{12}$ gr.)

Menadione U.S.P. *Menadionum.* **Menaphthone B.P.** *Menaphthonum.* (2-methyl-naphthoquinone, menaphthene)
DOSES: B.P. 1-5 mg. ($\frac{1}{60}$ - $\frac{1}{12}$ gr.) intramuscular, daily; U.S.P. 1 mg. ($\frac{1}{60}$ gr.). $C_{11}H_8O_2$. Mol.wt. 172.17. M.p. 105-107°. S: ins. W; sol. 60 A, 10 B; sol. C, CCl$_4$; sol. vegetable oils. A bright-yellow crystalline powder; odourless; irritating to respiratory tract and skin; an alcoholic solution is vesicant.

Menadione Capsules U.S.P.
Sizes, 1 and 2 mg. (1/60 and 1/30 gr.).

Menadione Injection U.S.P.
Sizes, 1 and 2 mg. (1/60 and 1/30 gr.) in 1 cc. of vegetable oil.

Menadione Tablets U.S.P.
Sizes, 1 and 2 mg. ($\frac{1}{60}$ and $\frac{1}{30}$ gr.).

Menadione Sodium Bisulfite U.S.P. *Menadioni Sodii Bisulfis.*
(Menadione Bisulfite)
DOSE: intramuscular or intravenous, 2 mg. ($\frac{1}{30}$ gr.).
$C_{11}H_8O_2.NaHSO_3.3H_2O$. Mol.wt. 330.29. S: 2 W; ss. A; almost ins. E, B. A white, crystalline, odourless, hygroscopic powder.

Menadione Sodium Bisulfite Injection U.S.P.
Size, 2 mg. in 1 cc.

Injection of Menaphthone B.P.
Strength, 5 mg. per cc. ($\frac{1}{12}$ gr. in 15 min.).

COMBINED A AND D VITAMINS

Cod Liver Oil. *Oleum Morrhuae*
DOSES: B.P. 4-12 cc. (60-180 min.) daily in divided doses; U.S.P. 8 cc. (2 fl.dr.) for infants or adults, daily. Gm./cc. 0.917-0.924. S: ss. A; fs. E, C, ethyl acetate, CS_2. A pale-yellow oil having a slightly fishy but not rancid odour and taste; obtained from the fresh liver of the cod (*Gadus morrhua* and other species of *Gadus*); partially destearinated by cooling and filtering; 1 Gm. contains not less than 600 units of Vitamin A (B.P.) or 850 units (U.S.P.); and not less than 85 units of antirachitic activity (B.P. and U.S.P.).

Non-Destearinated Cod Liver Oil U.S.P. *Oleum Morrhuae Non-Destearinatum*
Entire cod-liver oil containing not more than 0.5% v/v of water and some liver tissue. Potency as above. Deposits stearin on chilling.

Concentrated Solution of Vitamins A and D B.P. *Liquor Vitaminorum A et D Concentratus*

Doses: 0.06-0.6 cc. (1-10 min.) daily (Vitamin A 2500-25,000 units; vitamin D 250-2500 units). S: ss. A; misc. E, C, light petroleum. A solution in oil of Vitamins A and D containing in 1 Gm. 50,000 units of Vitamin A activity and 5000 units of vitamin D activity.

Oleovitamin A and D U.S.P. *Oleovitamina A et D*
Average Daily Dose: infants or adults, 8 cc. (2 fl.dr.). Prepared in a manner similar to Oleovitamin A, but Vitamin D may be synthetic Oleovitamin D; each Gm. contains between 850 and 1100 U.S.P. units of Vitamin A and between 85 and 110 U.S.P. units of Vitamin D.

Concentrated Oleovitamin A and D U.S.P. *Oleovitamina A et D Concentrata*
Dose: as prescribed. Prepared in a manner similar to Oleovitamin A and D; each Gm. contains 50,000-65,000 U.S.P. units of Vitamin A and 10,000-13,000 U.S.P. units of Vitamin D.

Concentrated Oleovitamin A and D Capsules. (Concentrated Vitamin A and D Capsules)
Average Daily Dose: 1 capsule. Size, 5000 U.S.P. units of Vitamin A, with 1000 U.S.P. units of Vitamin D.

Emulsion of Cod-liver Oil B.P. *Emulsio Olei Morrhuae*
Doses: 8-24 cc. (120-360 min.) daily, in divided doses; 10 cc. contain about 2750 units of A and 390 units of D. Cod-liver Oil 50 cc., with Acacia, Tragacanth, Purified Volatile Oil of Bitter Almond, Saccharin Sodium, Chloroform, and Distilled Water to make 100 cc.

Extract of Malt with Cod-liver Oil B.P. *Extractum Malti cum Oleo Morrhuae*
Doses: 4-30 cc. (60 min.-1 fl.oz.) daily. Extract of Malt 90 Gm., Cod-liver Oil 10 Gm. Contains in 30 cc. about 2450 units of Vitamin A and about 350 units of Vitamin D.

₡ Extract of malt with cod-liver oil is an old and popular tonic for undernourished children. It combines vitamins A, B, and D in a vehicle of high caloric value.

Halibut Liver Oil. *Oleum Hippoglossi*
Doses: B.P. 0.06-0.5 cc. (1-8 min.) daily; U.S.P. 0.1 cc. (1½

min.) daily, prophylactic. Sp.gr. 0.920-0.930. S: ins. W; ss. A; fs. E, C, carbon disulfide, and in ethyl acetate. The fixed oil from the fresh or suitably preserved livers of *Hippoglossus hippoglossus*. Each Gm. contains not less than 30,000 units of Vitamin A activity (B.P.); not less than 60,000 international units of Vitamin A activity (Can. Supp.); not less than 60,000 U.S.P. units of Vitamin A and not less than 600 U.S.P. units of Vitamin D (U.S.P.). A yellow to brownish-yellow liquid having a characteristic fishy but not rancid odour or taste.

Halibut Liver Oil Capsules U.S.P.
Sizes, 5000 and 25,000 U.S.P. units of Vitamin A per capsule.

Hexavitamin Capsules U.S.P.
DOSE: as prescribed. Strength, each capsule contains not less than 5000 U.S.P. units of Vitamin A from natural sources and 400 U.S.P. units of Vitamin D from natural sources or as activated ergosterol or activated 7-dehydrocholesterol, 75 mg. of Ascorbic acid, 2 mg. of Thiamine hydrochloride, 3 mg. of Riboflavin and 20 mg. of Nicotinamide.

Hexavitamin Tablets U.S.P.
Strength, vitamin content as for Hexavitamin Capsules.

Water U.S.P. *Aqua*
H_2O. Mol.wt. 18.02.

Distilled Water. *Aqua Destillata*
H_2O. Mol.wt. 18.02. Water purified by distillation.

Sterile Distilled Water U.S.P. *Aqua Destillata Sterilis*
Sterile Distilled Water and Distilled Water are not to be used for parenteral administration or in preparations to be used par-enterally.

Water for Injection. *Aqua pro Injectione*
Water for parenteral use which meets the requirements of B.P. or U.S.P. tests for sterility, clarity, and freedom from pyrogens.

Wild Cherry Bark B.P. *Prunus Serotina*. Wild Cherry U.S.P. *Prunus Virginiana*. (Wild Black Cherry Bark)
The stem bark of *Prunus serotina* collected in the autumn and dried.

Powdered Wild Cherry Bark B.P. *Pruni Serotinae Pulvis*
A light-brown powder.

Syrup of Wild Cherry B.P. *Syrupus Pruni Serotinae.* **Wild Cherry Syrup U.S.P.** *Syrupus Pruni Virginianae.* (Syrup of Virginian Prune)
DOSES: B.P. 2-8 cc. (30-120 min.). An extract of Wild Cherry Bark 15 Gm., with Sucrose, Glycerin, and Water to make 100 cc.

℃ Syrup of Wild Cherry is a popular ingredient of cough syrups. It is said to have a mild depressant effect on cough, due perhaps to the presence of minute amounts of HCN. The amount is, however, probably too small to have any noticeable action.

White Beeswax B.P. **White Wax U.S.P.** *Cera Alba.* (Bleached Beeswax)
M.p. 62-64°. S: ins. W; ss. cold A. A yellowish-white solid; odour faint and characteristic; made by bleaching Yellow Beeswax.

℃ White wax is used in cold cream, in other creams and ointments, and in certain injections of penicillin to delay absorption.

Yellow Beeswax B.P. **Yellow Wax U.S.P.** *Cera Flava*
M.p. 62-65°. S: ins. W; sps. cold A; sol. warm E, C. A yellow to greyish-brown solid; odour honey-like; obtained from the honey comb.

℃ Used in ointments and to make bone wax (Horsley's Wax).

Ointment of Zinc Oleate B.P. *Unguentum Zinci Oleatis.* (Zinc Oleate Ointment)

Contains Zinc Sulphate, Hard Soap, Distilled Water, and White Soft Paraffin. The content of zinc is equivalent to 5.2% w/w of zinc oxide.

Zinc Oxide. *Zinci Oxidum*
ZnO. Mol.wt. 81.38. S: ins. W, A; dissolves in dilute acids and in solutions of sodium hydroxide. A very fine, odourless, amorphous, white or yellowish-white powder, free from gritty particles.

℃ The actions of zinc oxide are mainly protective, soothing and absorbent. It is credited with a drying action on moist lesions of the skin. In the presence of acids, soluble zinc salts may be formed with the liberation of sufficient zinc ion to be astringent.

Compound Paste of Zinc Oxide B.P. *Pasta Zinci Oxidi Composita.*
Zinc Oxide Paste U.S.P. *Pasta Zinci Oxidi.* (Lassar's Plain
Zinc Oxide Paste, Zinc Paste)
Zinc Oxide 250, Starch 250, White Petrolatum to make 1000 Gm.

Hydrous Ointment of Zinc Oxide B.P. *Unguentum Zinci Oxidi
Aquosum*
Zinc Oxide 15, Hydrous Ointment 85.

Zinc Oxide Ointment. *Unguentum Zinci Oxidi.* (Zinc Ointment)
U.S.P.—Zinc Oxide 20%, with Wool Fat and White Ointment.
B.P.—Zinc Oxide 15%, with Simple Ointment.

Zinc Peroxide B.P. *Zinci Peroxidum.* **Medicinal Zinc Peroxide
U.S.P.** *Zinci Peroxidum Medicinale*
S: almost ins. W and organic solvents; sol. in dil. mineral acids.
A mixture of zinc peroxide, zinc carbonate, and zinc hydroxide.
Contains not less than 45% ZnO_2. A fine white or only faintly
yellow, odourless powder.

⟪ Zinc peroxide on exposure to water gradually liberates nascent
oxygen and thus acts as an oxidizing antiseptic and deodorant.
It is applied to foul wounds in the form of a cream or suspension.

Zinc Stearate. *Zinci Stearas*
S: ins. W, A, E. A fine, white, bulky powder, free from grittiness;
odour faint and characteristic.

⟪ The smooth, slippery feel of zinc stearate makes it popular
for application as a dusting powder to chafed surfaces. The zinc
content is equivalent to 13-15.5% of ZnO.

Zinc Sulphate. *Zinci Sulphas*
Doses: B.P. 0.6-2 Gm. (10-30 gr.) emetic. $ZnSO_4.7H_2O$. Mol.wt.
287.55. S: 0.6 W, 2.5 G; ins. A. Odourless transparent needles or
a granular crystalline powder; taste astringent and metallic;
efflorescent in dry air.

⟪ Solutions of zinc sulphate are antiseptic, irritant, and astringent.
A dose of 2 Gm. by mouth is emetic by local irritation. A 0.2-0.3%
solution may be used as an eye wash for conjunctivitis.

Index

Lightning Source UK Ltd.
Milton Keynes UK
UKHW010005210722
406167UK00001B/106